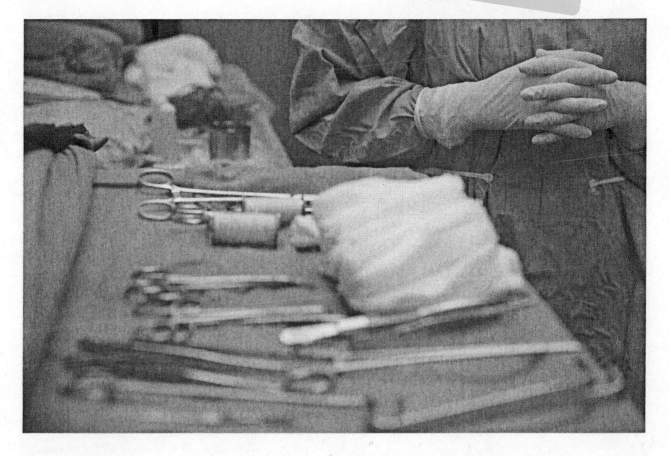

Succeeding in the MRCS Part B Exam

Nikhil Pawa & Efthymios Ypsilantis

BPP
LEARNING MEDIA

First edition April 2013

ISBN 9781 4453 8227 2
e-ISBN 9781 4453 8580 8

British Library Cataloguing-in-Publication Data
A catalogue record for this book is available from the British Library

Published by

BPP Learning Media Ltd
BPP House, Aldine Place
142–144 Uxbridge Road
London W12 8AA

www.bpp.com/health

Printed in the United Kingdom by

Ricoh
Ricoh House
Ullswater Crescent
Coulsdon
CR5 2HR

Your learning materials, published by BPP Learning Media Ltd, are printed on paper obtained from traceable sustainable sources.

BPP
LEARNING MEDIA

Contents

BPP
LEARNING MEDIA

Contents

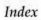

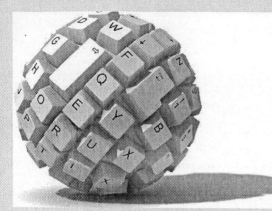

Free Companion Material

Readers can access free additional material including example examination questions. Please visit:
www.bpp.com/freehealthresources

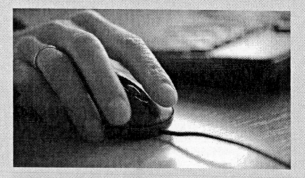

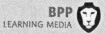

About the Publisher

BPP Learning Media is dedicated to supporting aspiring professionals with top quality learning material. BPP Learning Media's commitment to success is shown by our record of quality, innovation and market leadership in paper-based and e-learning materials. BPP Learning Media's study materials are written by professionally-qualified specialists who know from personal experience the importance of top quality materials for success.

Every effort has been made to ensure the accuracy of the material contained within this guide. However it must be noted that medical treatments, drug dosages/formulations, equipment, procedures and best practice are currently evolving within the field of medicine.

Readers are therefore advised always to check the most up-to-date information relating to:

- The applicable drug manufacturer's product information and data sheets relating to recommended dose/formulation, administration and contraindications.
- The latest applicable local and national guidelines.
- The latest applicable local and national codes of conduct and safety protocols.

It is the responsibility of the practitioner, based on their own knowledge and expertise, to diagnose, treat and ensure the safety and best interests of the patient are maintained.

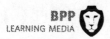

Preface

The MRCS Part B examination is a crucial landmark during a surgical career, associated with high levels of anxiety. The recent changes in the exam format and the ongoing updates of the syllabus according to newly generated evidence render effective preparation a challenging process. Considering that revision is usually undertaken beyond the working hours of a busy surgical job (sometimes in a means of transportation during commuting!), with limited available study leave (or none at all!), a stand-alone revision aid that would consolidate the knowledge and methodology you need to master in order to succeed, would be a valuable guide for your preparation.

Having been through the same stressful process ourselves not so long ago, we prepared this book having in mind your needs and aimed to:

- Incorporate an overview of the topics that need to be covered during preparation;
- Arrange the order of chapters to follow the following examined key areas: anatomy and surgical pathology, applied surgical science and critical care, communication skills in giving and receiving information, history taking and clinical and procedural skills;
- Classify pieces of information in tables easy to access and refer to;
- Offer additional sources of information for further study, recommending dynamic resources (web-based and videos), to ensure that your preparation is kept up-to-date with changing evidence;
- Present the topics by simulating exam questions and conditions, when possible;
- Offer tips for a successful performance, beyond the sterile reproduction of knowledge, focusing on aspects of communication and examination skills.

We hope that, by achieving the above, this book will guide you through a strong preparation and will help you face the examination confidently reaching a high performance. You have our warmest wishes for your efforts in succeeding in the MRCS Part B.

Nikhil Pawa and Efthymios Ypsilantis

About the Authors

Nikhil Pawa is a General Surgery Specialist Registrar in the London Deanery. Following on from obtaining his primary medical qualification he completed an LLM in Medical Law (Kent) and an MSc in Surgical Technology (London). He has been a member of the Royal College of Surgeons of England since 2008.

Efthymios Ypsilantis is a General Surgery Specialist Registrar in the London Deanery. He qualified from the Medical School of Athens and has been a member of the Royal College of Surgeons of England since 2006. He is also qualified with an MPhil in Surgery (Cambridge), an MSc in Advanced Surgical Practice (Cardiff) and the USMLEs.

Acknowledgements

We would like to thank Matt Green and BPP for giving us the opportunity to write this book and for all their support and flexibility during this effort. In particular we would like to thank our Development Editor, Jennifer Brookbanks, who has been a constant source of help and encouragement. We are indebted to Matthew Tutton who kindly reviewed the work and contributed with valuable suggestions. Finally, and most importantly, we would both like to thank our families and wives Jasmin and Tina for their support and patience during this period of commitment to researching and writing.

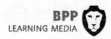

Foreword

Part B of the MRCS examination enables a thorough investigation of candidates' knowledge and understanding in all areas of the core surgical curriculum. At times there seems to be a never ending amount of information that can be examined and this can be a daunting challenge, especially while working an intensive clinical job.

This excellent new book will help to manage this stress. It takes the candidate through the MRCS syllabus, focusing on information not only needed to pass the examination but also to be a safe and competent surgeon.

The approach throughout each chapter is clear and logical. Relevant topics, examination questions and cases are taken and discussion placed in a simple list format to aid quick and concise revision; with summary tables providing focal points as aide memoires. Candidates are also directed to up-to-date national guidance by NICE, Cochrane reviews and national institutes to ensure best current practice. Links to relevant multimedia web based videos allow candidates to fully appreciate the procedures and operations being discussed.

Armed with the knowledge within this book, the MRCS examination becomes a more manageable challenge, and it also ensures a rounded knowledge base for individuals completing core surgical training.

Mr Matthew G. Tutton BSc MS FRCS (Gen. Surg.)
Consultant General and Laparoscopic Surgeon
Colchester Hospital University NHS Foundation Trust

The exam and preparation for succeeding

The aim of the MRCS exam is to assure the knowledge, skills and attributes that you need in order to proceed to the various pathways of higher specialty training. As the conditions in undergraduate and postgraduate medical training are subject to ongoing dynamic changes, the MRCS exam has inevitably evolved over the years. Since 2008 the MRCS Part B has been set up to be the last checkpoint before acquisition of the Membership Diploma, and has been formatted as an Objective Structured Clinical Examination (OSCE). You are no longer requested to strictly reproduce knowledge only; instead, you are expected to demonstrate additional aptitudes relevant to a successful surgical career, such as strong communication skills, effective hand-over strategies, empathetic bedside manners and the ability to make safe decisions under pressure.

The current exam format

All these skills are examined in eighteen stations, each of nine minutes' duration, where you will be assessed in five main subject areas; anatomy and surgical pathology; applied surgical science and critical care; communication skills in giving and receiving information and history taking; and clinical and procedural skills. The majority of stations test generic knowledge and are compulsory for all candidates and, to allow for differences in training, there are also speciality stations that are to be selected at the time of application. In each of the main subject areas, six domains are tested (clinical knowledge, clinical skill, technical skill, communication, decision making and problem solving and organisation and planning), against which you will be marked according to a predefined marking scheme. There is an overall pass mark set for Part B, but also minimum score has to be achieved in each of the domains.

The stations

The stations can be manned, i.e. examiners will be present, or unmanned. The anatomy and surgical pathology can be manned, where there is questioning of applied anatomy, and unmanned with prosections, images and photographs. In the surgical skills and patient safety stations (manned) examiners will assess skills such as knot tying and suturing, hand-washing, patient positioning and use of tourniquets. The communication skills station can be manned, where you may be assessed during referring a patient to a colleague or talking to relatives, or unmanned, where you may be asked to prepare a transfer letter or a discharge summary. In the applied surgical science and critical care stations, examiners will evaluate your knowledge on the application of pathophysiological processes (manned) or you may be asked to interpret images and results (unmanned). The clinical skills stations are manned and you are tested in taking history from or examining a patient or actor. In these stations you will be examined in your preferred specialty-specific stations as well.

Forthcoming changes

With effect from February 2013 some changes are planned to the format of the Intercollegiate MRCS Part B OSCE examination. The exam stations are reconfigured, with the specialty-choice station being removed from the examination, and the specialty-specific stations becoming generic stations.

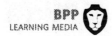

The addition of a surgical pathology/medical microbiology station is planned at the expense of one history-taking station. The examination is now divided in two components that are renamed as Broad Content Areas (BCAs): one BCA evaluating knowledge and its application ('applied knowledge'), which is dealt with in Chapters 1 to 4 of this book; and a BCA assessing communication, clinical and procedural skills ('skills'), which is covered by Chapters 5 to 8. Candidates must pass both BCAs and there will be no overall pass mark. A failure in one BCA only will mean that a candidate must repeat the whole examination.

Additionally, the number of examiners is reduced from two to one in one surgical science and critical care station. The history-taking stations will be examined by a clinician and a lay examiner. Finally, generic physical examination stations will be developed, with specific questioning of candidates, dependent on the actual case under consideration.

(For further updates on the exact dates and definitive format of the planned changes, please refer to the official Intercollegiate MRCS website www.intercollegiatemrcs.org.uk/new/announcements_html.)

Preparation

It is easily understood from the above that a successful outcome in the MRCS Part B depends on a combination of wide background knowledge and strong clinical, technical and communication skills, all of which have to be effectively demonstrated on the day of the exam, under stressful conditions! In order to achieve this, it is wise to decide that a specific time for preparation is devoted to the task, the length of which varies individually, depending on your confidence of your established knowledge, skills and performance in previous similar exams (e.g. medical school finals).

During this period, it is important to organise a balanced revision schedule that would ideally include:

- Bookwork, including use of all available resources such as atlases or videos for surgical techniques, usually out of hours.
- Practising history taking and clinical examinations during your working time on the wards/emergency rooms/outpatient clinics, trying to simulate the exam, without cutting corners (as it is tempting to do when busy).
- Organising teaching by seniors on relevant topics, possibly with mock exams (preferably not only during the last week before the exam, as this will maximise stress and will have doubtful benefit - plan it in advance).
- Organising groups of candidates sitting the same exam; you can benefit from other colleagues critique.

All these will require a well organised preparation plan, making good use of the working time, out-of-hours revision and study leave time, if available! You must not neglect, however, your need for rest and recreation, all necessary to maximise your performance.

Timing of sitting the exam

Although you could be using this book as a reference source for the MRCS Part A as well, it is likely that you have already passed this step and you are about to sit the Part B; therefore the timing of sitting the exam has already been decided! The Royal Colleges of Surgeons have set no restrictions regarding when to sit the exam, but recommend against doing so too soon. In our opinion it is wise to take advantage of as many training opportunities offered in a surgical job as possible; on the other hand do not allow too much time between Part A and Part B, because revised knowledge can fade after a few months!

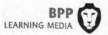

Further reading

- Surgical Royal Colleges of Great Britain (2011). *Regulations for the Intercollegiate Membership Examination of the Surgical Royal Colleges of Great Britain*. Available at: www.intercollegiatemrcs.org.uk/new/pdf/regulations.html
- Surgical-tutor-org.uk. *Surgical-tutor.org.uk. A free online resource*. Available at: www.surgical-tutor.org.uk (2011) default-home.htm?amazon/mrcs.htm~right

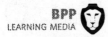

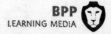

Chapter 1
Anatomy

Anatomy

Overview

The study of surgical anatomy can be labour intensive because of the need to learn complex terms and understand topographic relations between structures in a three-dimensional level from descriptive text. The purpose of exam preparation – and also the aim of this chapter – is to not to exhaust you with endless memorisation of tables, but to focus on the understanding of important aspects of anatomy with emphasis on their clinical significance. Although a compilation of lists of anatomical structures and their features is unavoidable, for reference purposes, this chapter emphasises their surgical and pathological importance. This chapter is also best used in combination with an anatomical atlas or model that is likely to be presented in the exam situation. For this purpose a non-exhaustive list of further reading is provided at the end of each chapter where appropriate. Finally, you are advised to practise drawing anatomical graphs and schemes, to help reproduce your understanding of the subjects, which also seems to be increasingly requested on the exam day!

Head
Base of skull

The base of skull is the floor of the cranial cavity and separates the brain from the facial structures. It is made by seven bones: the ethmoid, sphenoid, occipital, paired frontal, and paired parietal bones. It is subdivided into three regions, the anterior, middle, and posterior cranial fossae.

Anterior cranial fossa (Figure 1.1)

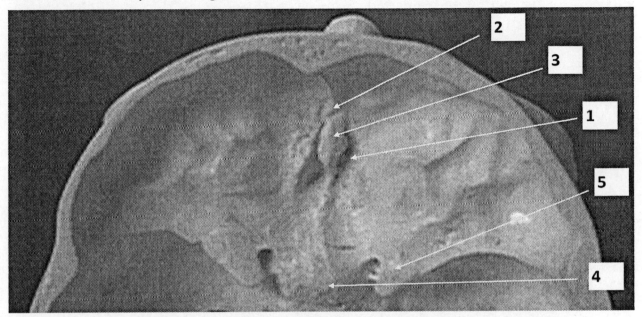

Figure 1.1. The anterior cranial fossa. The numbered structures refer to the text below.

Boundaries

It is bounded anteriorly by the posterior wall of the frontal sinus, posteriorly by the anterior clinoid processes and root of the sphenoid sinus, laterally by the frontal bone, and inferiorly (floor) by the orbital portion of the frontal bone and the ethmoid bone.

Features

The anterior skull base features:

- The cribriform plate through which the olfactory tracts run (1).
- The foramen caecum (2), between the frontal crest and the prominent crista galli, (a site of communication between the draining veins of the nasal cavity and the superior sagittal sinus).
- The crista galli (3), which projects up centrally between the cerebral hemispheres, providing site of attachment for the falx cerebri.
- The chiasmatic sulcus (4) for the optic chiasm.
- The anterior clinoid process (5), formed by the lesser wing of the sphenoid, an important landmark for the optic nerve and supracavernous internal carotid artery (ICA).

Relations

The anterior skull base lies in relation to, inferiorly,

- The paranasal sinuses and
- Each orbit, the posterior aspect of which includes:
  - The optic canal, transmitting the optic nerve (CN II) and the ophthalmic artery.

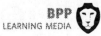

- The superior orbital fissure, conveying the oculomotor, trochlear, abducens, and ophthalmic nerves (CN III, IV, VI, and V_1, respectively), and the ophthalmic veins.
- The inferior orbital fissure (IOF), conveying the maxillary nerve (CN V_2) and infraorbital vessels.

Contents

The anterior skull base contains:

- The dura matter attaches anteriorly at the frontal crest and crista galli to form the falx cerebri, which transmits the superior and inferior sagittal sinuses.
- The foramen caecum, anterior to the crista galli, which usually ends blindly.
- The frontal cerebral lobes which occupy the anterior fossa.

Middle cranial fossa (Figure 1.2)

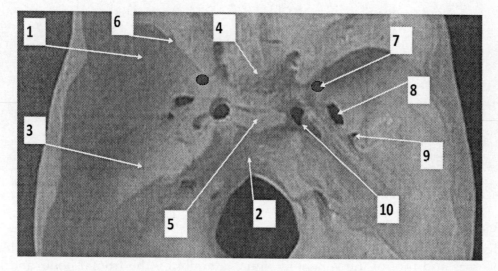

Figure 1.2. Middle cranial fossa. The numbered structures refer to the text on pages 4 and 5.

Boundaries

The medial cranial fossa is bounded by: anteriorly, the greater wings of the sphenoid (1); posteriorly the clivus (2); posteromedially the petrous portion of the temporal bone (3); laterally the greater wings of the sphenoid; and inferiorly (floor) by the greater wings of the sphenoid bone and the petrous temporal bone. The body of the sphenoid makes up the central portion of the middle fossa and houses the sella turcica, bounded by the anterior (4) and posterior clinoid processes (5).

Clinically important: The middle meningeal artery (MMA) courses anterolaterally from the foramen spinosum and divides into frontal and parietal branches. The anterior branch ascends across to the **pterion**, an H-shaped suture (found 3cm behind the zygomaticofrontal suture and 4cm above the zygomatic arch), where the frontal bone, the greater wing of the sphenoid bone, the squamous temporal bone and the parietal bone meet. The pterion is made up of thin bone that can be easily fractured, resulting in injury to the MMA and epidural haematoma.

Features and foramina of the middle skull base

- The superior orbital fissure (SOF) (6).
- The foramen rotundum (7), (posteroinferior to the base of SOF), transmitting the maxillary division (CN V$_2$) of the trigeminal nerve into the pterygopalatine fossa.
- The foramen ovale (8), posterolaterally, transmitting the mandibular division (CN V$_3$) of the trigeminal nerve, along with the accessory meningeal artery, the lesser superficial petrosal nerve (LSPN), and emissary veins to the pterygoid plexus into the infratemporal fossa.
- The foramen spinosum (9), further posterolaterally, transmitting the middle meningeal artery and the meningeal branch of the facial nerve (CN VII).
- The carotid canal which continues into the foramen lacerum (10) on the undersurface of the skull base.

Contents of the middle cranial fossa

The middle skull base contains the temporal lobe, the pituitary gland, the trigeminal or gasserian ganglion, the greater superficial petrosal nerve (GSPN), the intracranial portion of the internal carotid artery (ICA), and the cavernous sinus.

The cavernous sinus is a complex plexus of veins in the dura, lateral to the sphenoid sinus, extending from the SOF to the petrous temporal bone. Along its lateral wall run the ICA, the oculomotor nerve (CN III), the trochlear nerve (CN IV), the ophthalmic nerve (CN V$_1$), and the maxillary nerve (CN V$_2$). Basilar skull fracture can result to a carotid-cavernous fistula, manifesting with proptosis, chemosis, and pulsating exophthalmos.

Posterior cranial fossa (Figure 1.3)

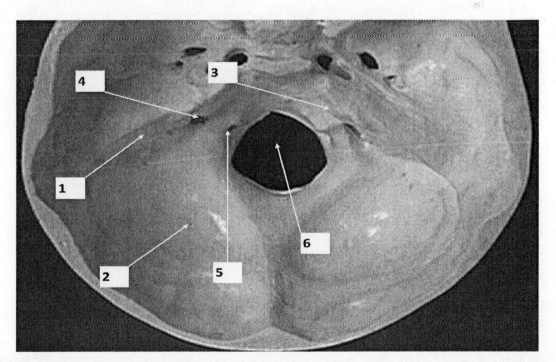

Figure 1.3. The posterior cranial fossa. The numbered structures refer to the text on the next page.

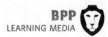

Boundaries

It is bounded by: anteriorly, the basal portion of the occipital bone (the basiocciput) and the basisphenoid, which combine to form the midline clivus; laterally, the posterior surface of the petrous temporal bones (1) and the lateral aspect of the occipital bone (2); inferiorly (floor) the occipital bone; and superiorly, the overlying tentorium cerebelli, that separates the cerebellum from the cerebral hemispheres.

Features and foramina of the posterior skull base

- The porus acousticus (3), which is the opening of the internal auditory canal (IAC) and transmits; the CNs VII and VIII, the nervus intermedius, and the labyrinthine vessels (branches of the anterior inferior cerebellar artery en route to the inner ear).
- The jugular foramen (4), extending laterally from the posterior aspect of the occipital condyle; it receives the sigmoid sinus and the jugular bulb and transmits the IX, X, and XI cranial nerves.
- The hypoglossal foramen (5), transmitting the hypoglossal nerve (CN XII), a meningeal branch of the ascending pharyngeal artery, and the hypoglossal venous plexus.
- The foramen magnum (6) that transmits the medulla oblongata, the spinal accessory nerve, the vertebral and posterior spinal arteries, and the apical ligament of the dens and membrane tectoria.

Contents

The posterior skull base includes the midbrain, the pons, the medulla, and the cerebral and cerebellar hemispheres. Dura and the tentorium cerebelli enclose the occipital sinus, the superior sagittal sinus and the paired transverse sinuses.

Neck

Knowledge of the anatomy of the neck is paramount for the surgical trainee, because of its important implications in the management of airway, the assessment of abdominal disease, neck surgical oncology, trauma cases, the assessment of central nervous system perfusion and in central vascular access.

Surface landmarks

The neck extends from the base of the skull to the thoracic inlet. You should familiarise yourself with the following important surface landmarks and structures:

- Superiorly, the inferior margin of mandible, the mastoid process, and the external occipital protuberance.
- Posteriorly, the spinous process of axis (C2) and vertebral prominence (C7).
- Laterally, the transverse process of atlas (C1), between the angle of mandible and mastoid process.
- Anteriorly, the hyoid bone, at the level of C3 vertebra; the laryngeal prominence (formed by the thyroid cartilage at C4–5 vertebral level); the cricoid cartilage (C6 level); the suprasternal or jugular notch (above the manubrium sterni) and the supraclavicular fossa (above the middle part of clavicle).
- Platysma muscle: It is a broad thin subcutaneous sheet of muscle, superficial to the external jugular vein (EJV) and the main cutaneous nerves of the neck. It is attached, superiorly, to the inferior border of mandible and the tissues of lower face and, inferiorly, to the fascia covering the pectoralis major and deltoid muscles. Its nerve supply derives from the cervical branch of facial nerve. Its main action is to tense the skin and depress the mandible.

Fasciae of the neck

The neck fasciae determine the division of tissues in separate compartments and help contain neck infections within defined planes; understanding of these planes allows easy and bloodless dissection in neck operations.

Superficial fascia: It is a thin layer of subcutaneous tissue that contains cutaneous nerves, blood vessels and lymphatics, superficial lymph nodes and fat and the platysma muscle.

Deep fascia: It surrounds viscera and vessels, limits the spread of infections and provides slippery surface for movement of neck viscera, e.g. during swallowing. It consists of four layers:

- Investing layer
  It surrounds the entire neck deep to the superficial fascia and splits to envelope two muscles (sternocleidomastoid and trapezius) and two salivary glands (submandibular and parotid). It splits above the manubrium sterni to form the suprasternal space (that contains the inferior end of anterior jugular veins, the jugular venous arch, lymphnodes and fat) and above the middle third of clavicle, below which it continues as *clavi-pectoral fascia*.
- Pretracheal layer
  It lies anterior to the trachea and consists of two parts: a thin muscular layer enclosing the infrahyoid muscles and a visceral layer enclosing the thyroid gland, trachea and oesophagus.
- Prevertebral layer
  It is a tubular layer around the vertebral column and muscles, containing the sympathetic trunks.
- Carotid sheath
  It is a tubular sheath containing the common and internal carotid arteries, the internal jugular vein (IJV), the vagus nerve, the carotid sinus nerve (a branch from glossopharyngeal nerve), the carotid sympathetic plexus and deep cervical lymphnodes.

Compartments of the neck

They are enclosed by the investing layer of deep cervical fascia and are classified into:

- Visceral (anteriorly): includes air and food passages covered by the pretracheal fascia.
- Vertebral (posteriorly): includes vertebrae and muscles covered by the prevertebral fascia.
- Vasculo-neural (laterally): includes the great neck vessels and vagus nerve covered by carotid sheath.

Triangles of the neck

For descriptive purposes, the surface anatomy of neck structures is classified into triangles bounded by neck muscles, as presented in Figure 1.4.

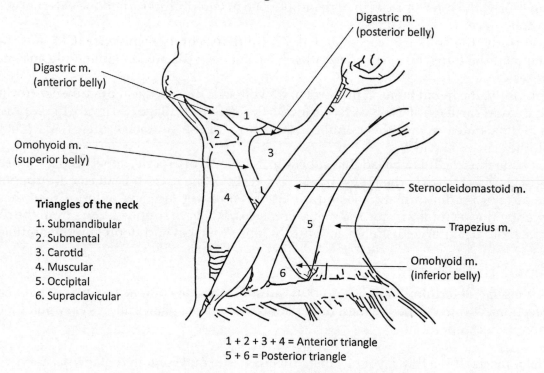

Triangles of the neck

1. Submandibular
2. Submental
3. Carotid
4. Muscular
5. Occipital
6. Supraclavicular

1 + 2 + 3 + 4 = Anterior triangle
5 + 6 = Posterior triangle

Figure 1.4. The triangles of the neck
Based on Gray H (1918) Anatomy of the Human Body. 20th edition, Lea & Febiger, Philadelphia.
(*This image is in the public domain because its copyright has expired. This applies worldwide.*)

There are two major triangles, containing multiple smaller triangles:

Anterior triangle: It is bounded by the anterior border of the sternocleidomastoid (SCM), the midline of the neck, and the mandible and is further subdivided into:

- Muscular triangle, formed by the midline, superior belly of the omohyoid, and SCM (contains the infrahyoid muscles, the thyroid and parathyroid glands).
- Carotid triangle, formed by the superior belly of the omohyoid, SCM, and posterior belly of the digastric (contains the common carotid artery, the internal jugular vein and the vagus nerve CN X).
- Submental triangle, formed by the anterior belly of the digastric, the hyoid bone, and the midline (contains the submental lymph nodes).
- Submandibular triangle, formed by the mandible, posterior belly of the digastric and anterior belly of the digastric (contains the submandibular gland, lymph nodes and the hypoglossal cranial nerve XII).

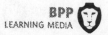

Posterior triangle: It is bounded by the posterior border of the SCM, trapezius, and clavicle, and is further divided into:

- Supraclavicular triangle, formed by the inferior belly of the omohyoid, clavicle, and SCM (contains the superior, middle and lower trunks of the brachial plexus, the third part of the subclavian artery and the external jugular vein).
- Occipital triangle, formed by the inferior belly of the omohyoid, trapezius, and SCM (contains the spinal accessory nerve XI, the great auricular nerve, part of the occipital and parts of the transverse cervical and suprascapular arteries).

The thyroid gland

Location and morphology: The thyroid gland is enclosed in the pretracheal fascia, anterior to the larynx and trachea, covered by the strap muscles and overlapped by the sternocleidomastoids. It consists of the *isthmus* (over the second and third rings of the trachea), the *lateral lobes*, (each extending from the thyroid cartilage downwards to the sixth tracheal ring) and an inconstant *pyramidal lobe*, which can project upwards from the isthmus (embryological residual). The anterior jugular veins course over the isthmus and the carotid sheaths run on either side of the gland.

Important nerve relations: The recurrent laryngeal nerve lies in the tracheoesophageal groove and the external branch of the superior laryngeal nerve lies deep to the upper pole.

Arterial supply: By the superior thyroid artery (from the external carotid), the inferior thyroid artery (from the thyrocervical trunk of the subclavian artery) and the inconstant thyroidea ima artery (from the aortic arch).

Venous drainage: Through the superior and middle thyroid veins to the internal jugular vein and through the inferior thyroid veins to the brachiocephalic veins.

Embryology: The first of the body's endocrine glands to develop. It arises from the floor of the pharynx between the first and second pharyngeal pouches (foramen caecum of the tongue). It descends to the neck initially remaining connected to the tongue via the thyroglossal duct which obliterates later (tenth gestational week). Abnormalities in the embryological descend or failure of obliteration of the thyroglossal duct can result in ectopic (lingual) thyroid, pyramidal lobe, a patent thyroglossal duct or cyst and a retrosternal thyroid.

The larynx

Location: Between the laryngeal part of the pharynx and the trachea (C3–C6 vertebrae).

Functions: They are achieved by its skeletal components and the muscles that act on them and include the control of airflow during breathing, protection of the inlet of air passages and voice production.

Morphology: The larynx consists of the laryngeal folds, cavity, cartilages, membranes, ligaments and muscles. These are described below and need to be studied along with a detailed atlas or anatomical model.

Laryngeal folds

- Aryepiglottic folds (upper rim of the larynx): fibrous membrane that connects the lateral walls of the epiglottis to the arytenoid cartilage complex. The epiglottis cartilage folds posteriorly and inferiorly over the laryngeal vestibule, separating the pharynx from the larynx.
- Ventricular folds (not normally active during phonation): they help increase intrathoracic pressure by blocking the outflow of air from the lungs and compress tightly during coughing, sneezing or vomiting.
- True vocal folds: they provide a vibrating source for phonation, close tightly for coughing, throat clearing, and help protect the trachea and lungs from foods and liquids during swallowing actions.

Laryngeal cavity

It is covered by mucous membrane with ciliated columnar epithelium, extends from the laryngeal inlet to the lower border of the cricoid cartilage and is divided into:

- Upper part or vestibule (from the inlet to the vestibular folds).
- Middle part (from the vestibular folds to the vocal folds).
- Lower part (from the vocal folds to the lower border of the cricoid cartilage).

Laryngeal cartilages

- Thyroid cartilage (two laminae of hyaline cartilage meeting in the midline in the prominent V angle of the Adam's apple) providing surface for attachment of the sternothyroid, thyrohyoid, inferior constrictor muscles, the anterior end of vocal ligaments and the cricothyroid muscle.
- Cricoid cartilage (a complete ring of hyaline cartilage). It articulates with the inferior cornu of the thyroid cartilage and the base of the arytenoid cartilages. It provides surface for the origin of the cricothyroid, the lateral and posterior cricoarytenoid muscles.
- Arytenoid cartilages (pair): They are attached by the vocal folds and are attached to the cricoid cartilages through the cricoarytenoid joint.
- Corniculate cartilages (pair): They provide attachment to the aryepiglottic folds.
- Cuneiform cartilages (pair): They support the aryepiglottic folds.

Laryngeal membranes and ligaments

These include the thyrohyoid membrane, cricothyroid ligament, vocal ligaments (the gap between them is the glottis), vestibular ligament and the cricotracheal ligament.

Muscles of the larynx

- The extrinsic muscles consist of two opposing groups:
  - Elevators of the larynx: digastric, stylohyoid, mylohyoid and geniohyoid. (The stylopharyngeus, the salpingopharyngeus and the palatopharyngeus, which are inserted into the thyroid cartilage, also elevate the larynx.)
  - Depressors of the larynx: sternothyroid, sternohyoid and omohyoid.
- The intrinsic muscles can be divided into two groups:
  - Muscles that move the vocal folds (Table 1.1)
  - Muscles that control the laryngeal inlet: Transverse and oblique interarytenoid muscles (adductors), supplied by the recurrent laryngeal nerve.

Muscle	Action	Nerve supply
Cricothyroid	Tensor	External laryngeal nerve
Thyroarytenoid	Relaxor	Recurrent laryngeal nerve
Lateral cricoarytenoid	Adductor	
Posterior cricoarytenoid	Abductor	

Table 1.1. The intrinsic muscles that move the vocal cords

Nerve supply of the larynx

- Sensory: Above the vocal folds, from the internal laryngeal branch of the superior laryngeal branch of the vagus nerve and below the level of the vocal folds, by the recurrent laryngeal nerve.
- Motor: Intrinsic muscles – recurrent laryngeal nerve, except for the cricothyroid muscle, which is supplied by the external laryngeal branch of the superior laryngeal branch of the vagus.

Blood supply and lymph drainage

The upper half of the larynx is supplied by the superior laryngeal branch of the superior thyroid artery and the lower half by the inferior laryngeal branch of the inferior thyroid artery. The venous return is transmitted through the jugular vein.

Arteries of head and neck

It is important that you know the course, branches and basic relations of the arteries that supply the head and neck and be familiar with the surface points for auscultation and palpation of the carotid arteries.

Common carotid artery

The right common carotid arises from the brachiocephalic artery and the left one from the aortic arch. It is embedded in the carotid sheath with the internal jugular vein and the vagus nerve. It divides at the upper border of thyroid cartilage into internal and external carotid arteries. Just proximal to the bifurcation is the carotid sinus that receives nerve endings from the glossopharyngeal nerve and functions as baroreceptor. Posterior to the bifurcation is the carotid body, also innervated by glossopharyngeal nerve that functions as chemoreceptor.

External carotid artery

The external carotid artery begins at the level of upper border of thyroid cartilage after bifurcation of the common carotid artery and terminates in the substance of the parotid gland. It gives off the following branches (see also Figure 1.5).

- Superficial temporal artery (terminal)
- Maxillary artery (terminal)
- Superior thyroid artery
- Ascending pharyngeal artery
- Lingual artery
- Facial artery
- Occipital artery
- Posterior auricular artery

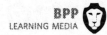

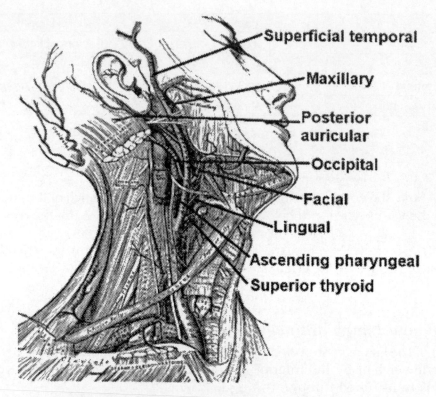

Figure 1.5. Branches of the external carotid artery
Based on Gray H (1918) Anatomy of the Human Body, 20th edition, Lea & Febiger, Philadelphia.
(This image is in the public domain because its copyright has expired. This applies worldwide.)

Internal carotid artery

It begins at the level of the upper border of thyroid cartilage and has no branches in the neck.

The internal carotid artery is divided into four parts:

- Cervical: It passes near the C3 and C4 vertebrae and enters the petrous bone through the carotid foramen to run cranially into the foramen lacerum.
- Intratemporal: It courses medial to the eustachian tube and anterolateral and inferior to the cochlea (tinnitus in carotid artery stenosis).
- Cavernous: It runs medial to the anterior clinoid process.
- Supracavernous: It courses under the optic nerve, branches to the terminal anterior and middle cerebral arteries that join the Circle of Willis (Figure 1.6).

Vertebral artery

The vertebral artery originates from the subclavian artery and has four parts, the cervical, foraminal, atlantic and subarachnoid part. On entering the posterior fossa through the foramen magnum it branches to the *posterior inferior cerebellar artery* and subsequently joins the opposite at the midline to form the *basilar artery* at the base of the pons. The basilar artery then branches into the *anterior inferior cerebellar arteries*, the *labyrinthine artery*, the *pontine arteries*, and, finally, the *superior cerebellar arteries*, which make up the posterior portion of the Circle of Willis (Figure 1.6).

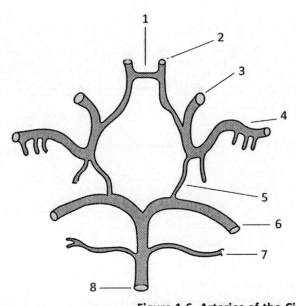

1. Anterior communicating
2. Anterior cerebral
3. Internal carotid
4. Middle cerebral
5. Posterior communicating
6. Posterior cerebral
7. Superior cerebellar
8. Basilar

Figure 1.6. Arteries of the Circle of Willis
Based on Gray H (1918) Anatomy of the Human Body, 20th edition, Lea & Fibeger, Philadelphia.
(*This image is in the public domain because its copyright has expired. This applies worldwide.*)

Upper extremity

In this section emphasis is given on the presentation of the main joints and their components, the neurovascular supply of the upper extremity and the relevant clinical implications.

The brachial plexus

The brachial plexus is a somatic nerve plexus formed by intercommunications among the ventral rami of the lower four cervical nerves (C5 – C8) and the first thoracic nerve (T1), although it can occasionally receive fibres from C4 or T2. It supplies the muscles of the upper limb, except from the trapezius and levator scapulae. It provides the cutaneous innervation of the upper limb except from the axilla (which is supplied by the intercostobrachial nerve), an area above the shoulder (by the supraclavicular nerves) and the dorsal scapular area (cutaneous branches of dorsal rami). It communicates with the sympathetic trunk by gray rami communicates that join all the roots of the plexus and are derived from the middle and inferior cervical sympathetic ganglia and the first thoracic sympathetic ganglion. Topographically it is divided into:

- Roots: the ventral rami of spinal nerves C5 to T1
- Trunks:
    - The ventral rami of C5 and C6 unite to form the Upper Trunk.
    - The ventral ramus of C7 continues as the Middle Trunk.
    - The ventral rami of C8 and T1 unite to form the Lower Trunk.
- Divisions: Each trunk splits into an anterior division and a posterior division. (The anterior divisions usually supply flexor muscles and the posterior divisions usually supply extensor muscles.)
- Cords (named according to their position relative to the axillary artery).
    - The anterior divisions of the upper and middle trunks unite to form the lateral cord.
    - The anterior division of the lower trunk forms the medial cord.
    - All three posterior divisions from each of the three cords all unite to form the posterior cord.
- Branches (see Figure 1.7 and Table 1.2).

You are expected to be able to draw the figure and name the numbered parts and divisions, which are detailed below in Table 1.2.

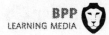

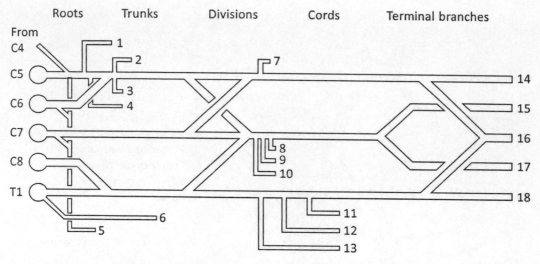

Figure 1.7 Schematic representation of the brachial plexus

Origin	Nerve (number in Figure 1.7)	Root value	Muscles	Cutaneous
Roots	Dorsal scapular (1)	C5	Rhomboid and levator scapulae	–
	Long thoracic (5)	C5, C6, C7	Serratus anterior	–
Upper trunk	N. to subclavius m.(3)	C5, C6	Subclavius	–
	Suprascapular (2)	C5, C6	Supraspinatus and infraspinatus	–
Lateral cord	Lateral pectoral (7)	C5, C6, C7	Pectoralis major and minor (by communicating with medial pectoral nerve)	–
	Musculocutaneous (14)	C5, C6, C7	Coracobrachialis, brachialis and biceps brachii	Lateral forearm (Lateral cutaneous n. of forearm)
	Lateral root of median n.	C5, C6, C7		–
Posterior cord	Upper subscapular (8)	C5, C6	Subscapularis (upper part)	–
	Thoracodorsal (9)	C6, C7, C8	Latissimus dorsi	–
	Lower subscapular (10)	C5, C6	Subscapularis and teres major	–
	Axillary (15)	C5, C6	Deltoid, small area of overlying skin, teres minor	Lateral arm (Upper lateral cutaneous n. of arm)
	Radial (17)	C5, C6, C7, C8, T1	Triceps brachii, anconeus, the extensor muscles of the forearm, and brachioradialis	Posterior arm (Post. cutaneous n. of arm)
Medial cord	Medial pectoral (11)	C8, T1	Pectoralis major and minor	–
	Medial root of median n.	C8, T1		
	Medial cutaneous n. of the arm (12)	C8, T1	–	Anteromedial arm
	Medial cutaneous n. of the forearm (13)	C8, T1	–	Medial forearm
	Ulnar nerve (18)	C8, T1	Flexor carpi ulnaris, medial 2 bellies of flexor digitorum profundus, most of the small muscles of the hand	Palmar: medial side of hand and medial $1\frac{1}{2}$ fingers Dorsal: medial $2\frac{1}{2}$ fingers

The median nerve (16) is formed by the lateral and medial roots that originate from the lateral and medial cords. The phrenic nerve (4) (originates from C4 ramus, with contributions from C3 and C5 of the brachial plexus).

Table 1.2. Components and role of the brachial plexus

Brachial plexus injury

Aetiology and classification

It is usually caused by high-energy trauma to the upper extremity and neck by traction injuries, in which the head and neck are moved away violently from the ipsilateral shoulder (most common), compression between the clavicle and first rib, penetrating injuries, direct blows, and dystocia. It can be classified as *preganglionic*, proximal to the dorsal root ganglion, or *postganglionic*, distal to the dorsal root ganglion.

Clinical manifestations

- Local complications of trauma (open wound, shoulder girdle fractures/dislocations, oedema, and vascular compromise).
- Upper limb muscle weakness and sensory loss with or without severe pain.
- Horner syndrome: Ptosis (lid droop), enophthalmos (sinking of the eye into the orbit), anhydrosis (dry eye), and miosis (small pupil), because of damage of the sympathetic ganglion (in close proximity to T1).
- Erb's palsy (commonly birth-related): C5 and C6 root injury, affecting the axillary, musculocutaneous, and suprascapular nerve. The affected muscles (supraspinatus and infraspinatus and in more severe cases the deltoid, biceps, brachialis and subscapular) result in chronic internal rotation contracture, secondary osseous changes and shoulder subluxation. The arm hangs by the side and is rotated medially, the forearm is extended and pronated, the arm cannot be raised from the side.
- Klumpke palsy (also commonly birth-related): Lower plexus injury affecting C8 and T1, resulting in impairment of the long flexors of the fingers, short muscles of the hand, and sensory loss at the ulnar side of the hand and forearm; it is often associated with Horner syndrome.

Investigations

Plain neck and chest radiographs, MRI, CT-myelogram and neurophysiological studies (nerve conduction studies and electromyography) are used for diagnosis and to plan management.

Management

- Initial trauma management as per ATLS protocol.
- Priority to potential vascular injuries aiming to restore perfusion.
- Referral to specialist centre where individualised management applies: direct repair, nerve grafting, nerve transfer or decompression.

The shoulder joint

The shoulder complex consists of the following joints: the sternoclavicular joint (SCJ), acromioclavicular joint (ACJ), glenohumeral (GH) joint, and scapulothoracic (ST) joint (pseudoarticulation).

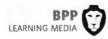

Bones (Figure 1.8)

The scapula (1), clavicle (2) and proximal humerus (3) take part in the shoulder joint.

Cartilage

The labrum is a fibrocartilagenous circle that provides area for attachment of glenohumeral ligaments, increases the surface area of contact for the humeral head and provides much of the socket function.

Ligaments (Figure 1.8)

- Coraco-acromial ligament (4)
- Coracohumeral ligament (5)
- Superior glenohumeral ligament (6)
- Middle glenohumeral ligament (7)
- Inferior glenohumeral ligament complex (8) (most important ligament in preventing anterior dislocation)
- Coracoclavicular ligaments: Trapezoid (9) and conoid (10)

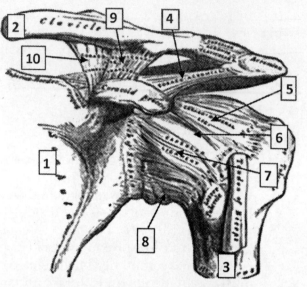

Figure 1.8. Ligaments of the shoulder
Based on Gray H (1918) Anatomy of the Human Body,
20th edition, Lea & Febiger, Philadelphia
(This image is in the public domain because its copyright has expired. This applies worldwide.)

Nerves

- Axillary nerve: A terminal branch of the posterior cord of the brachial plexus that passes into the quadrilateral space with the posterior circumflex humeral artery and vein and runs on the deep surface of the deltoid muscle, 5–6cm below the acromion.

The borders of the quadrilateral space (Figure 1.9) are: superiorly the lower margin of subscapularis, the axillary fold of the capsule and the lower border of teres minor (1); inferiorly the upper margins of tendons of latissimus dorsi and teres major (2); medially the long head of triceps (3) and laterally the humerus (4).

- Musculocutaneous nerve: A terminal branch of the lateral cord of brachial plexus. It is the most superficial nerve of brachial plexus. It enters the conjoint tendon 2cm distal to coracoid, supplying coracobrachialis and short head of biceps.
- Suprascapular: Nerve from upper trunk of brachial plexus. It travels with the suprascapular artery to the scapular notch, where the artery passes over the transverse ligament and the nerve below it. It gives two branches to supraspinatus and passes around the spine of scapula to supply infraspinatus.

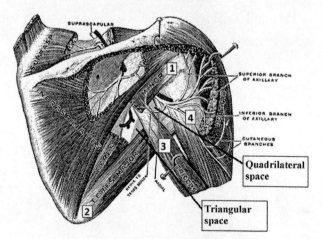

Figure 1.9. The quadrilateral space
Based on Gray H (1918) Anatomy of the Human Body,
20th edition, Lea & Febiger, Philadelphia
(This image is in the public domain because its copyright has expired. This applies worldwide.)

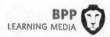

Muscle	Origin	Insertion	Action	Innervation
Subscapularis	Subscapular fossa	Lesser tubercle of humerus	Stabilisation, internal rotation of humerus	Subscapular
Supraspinatus	Supraspinous fossa	Greater tubercle of humerus	Stabilisation, abduction	Suprascapular
Infraspinatus	Infraspinous fossa	Greater tubercle of humerus	Stabilisation, external rotation of humerus	Suprascapular
Teres minor	Lateral border of scapula	Greater tubercle of humerus	Stabilisation, external rotation of humerus	Axillary
Pectoralis major	Medial clavicle, sternum and cartilage of ribs 2–6	Lateral lip of intertubercular groove	Horizontal adduction, internal rotation, flexion, extension, adduction	Medial and lateral pectoral
Biceps brachii	Coracoid process (short head), supraglenoid tubercle (long head)	Radial tuberosity	Shoulder flexion. Short head adducts and long head abducts. Horizontal adduction	Musculocutaneous
Coracobrachialis	Coracoid process of scapula	Medial shaft of humerus	Shoulder flexion, adduction, horizontal adduction	Musculocutaneous
Anterior deltoid	Lateral clavicle	Deltoid tuberosity of humerus	Shoulder flexion, abduction, medial rotation, horizontal adduction	Axillary
Latissimus dorsi	Spinous processes of lower thoracic and lumbar vertebra, ribs 8–12	Floor of intertubercular groove	Extension, adduction, medial rotation, horizontal abduction	Thoracodorsal
Teres major	Inferior angle of scapula	Medial lip of intertubercular groove	Extension adduction, medial rotation, horizontal abduction	Lower subscapular
Triceps brachii (long head)	Infraglenoid tubercle	Olecranon process	Shoulder extension, adduction, horizontal abduction	Radial
Posterior deltoid	Spine of scapula	Deltoid tuberosity of humerus	Extension, lateral rotation, abduction, horizontal abduction	Axillary
Middle deltoid	Acromion process	Deltoid tuberosity of humerus	Abduction	Axillary
Serratus anterior	Anterior shaft of ribs 1–9	Vertebral border of scapula	Scapular abduction, upward rotation	Long thoracic
Subclavius	Medial first rib	Lateral clavicle	Downward rotation, abduction of scapula	Subclavian
Pectoralis minor	Ventral surfaces of ribs 3–5	Coracoid process of scapula	Downward rotation, abduction, anterior tilt, depression	Medial pectoral
Rhomboid minor	Spinous processes of C7–T1	Vertebral border of scapula near spine	Adduction and downward rotation	Dorsal scapular
Rhomboid major	Spinous processes of upper thoracic vertebra	Vertebral border of scapula below spine	Adduction and downward rotation	Dorsal scapular
Levator scapulae	Transverse process of C1–C4	Superior angle of scapula	Elevates scapula, downward rotation	Cervical nerves C3–C4 and dorsal scapular

Table 1.3. Muscles of the shoulder joint

Blood supply of humeral head

- The anterolateral branch of anterior humeral circumflex artery, which passes laterally to the long head of biceps and forms the arcuate artery.
- The posterior circumflex artery that supplies only a small area in the posteroinferior aspect of the humeral head.

The elbow joint

The elbow is a *trochoginglymoid* joint, formed between three bones, the humerus of the arm and the paired radius and ulna of the forearm, with main function to position the hand in space. It consists of three different portions, enveloped by a common synovial membrane:

- Humeroulnar joint, between the trochlear notch of the ulna and the trochlea of humerus. Is a simple *hinge-joint*, allowing movements of flexion and extension only.
- Humeroradial joint, between the head of the radius and the capitulum of the humerus. It is an *arthrodial (gliding)* joint.
- Proximal radioulnar joint, between the head of the radius and the radial notch of the ulna, allowing rotation of the radius during pronation and supination.

The joint capsule is attached around the articular surfaces and its fibres are arranged in such a way as to provide stabilisation in flexion and in full extension.

The stability of the elbow joint is ensured (Figure 1.10):

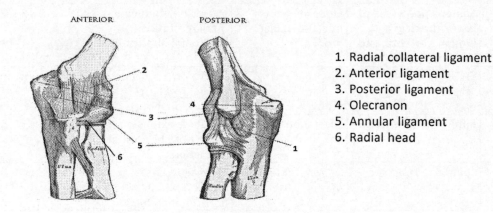

1. Radial collateral ligament
2. Anterior ligament
3. Posterior ligament
4. Olecranon
5. Annular ligament
6. Radial head

Figure 1.10. Ligaments of the elbow joint
Based on Gray H (1918) Anatomy of the Human Body, 20th edition, Lea & Febiger, Philadelphia
(*This image is in the public domain because its copyright has expired. This applies worldwide.*)

- Medially, by the medial collateral ligament: a strong and well-demarcated structure that consists of three bundles, the oblique anterior bundle, oblique posterior bundle and the oblique transverse ligament.
- Laterally, by five structures: the lateral (radial) collateral ligament, the annular ligament, the lateral ulnar collateral ligament, the accessory lateral collateral ligament and the anconeus muscle.

The movements of the elbow joint are affected by the muscles presented in Table 1.4.

The antecubital fossa

The antecubital fossa is an important anatomical area, allowing palpation and auscultation of the brachial artery (blood pressure measurement) and offering access for venipuncture (cubital vein).

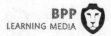

Movement	Muscle	Nerve supply	Nerve root
Elbow flexion	Brachialis	Musculocutaneous	C5 C6 (C7)
	Biceps brachii	Musculocutaneous	C5 C6
	Brachioradialis	Radial	C5 C6 (C7)
	Pronator teres	Median	C6 C7
	Flexor carpi ulnaris	Ulnar	C7 C8
Elbow extension	Triceps	Radial	C6 C7 C8
	Anconeus	Radial	C7 C8 (T1)
Forearm supination	Supinator	Posterior interosseous (radial)	C5 C6
	Biceps brachii	Musculocutaneous	C5 C6
Forearm pronation	Pronator quadratus	Anterior interosseous (median)	C8 T1
	Pronator teres	Median	C6 C7

Table 1.4. Movements and muscles moving the elbow joint

Boundaries

This is the triangular area on the anterior (flexor) aspect of the elbow, bounded by:

- Superiorly: A line connecting the medial and lateral epicondyles of the humerus.
- Medially: The lateral border of pronator teres muscle.
- Laterally: The medial border of brachioradialis muscle.
- An apex, formed by the meeting point of the lateral and medial boundaries.
- A superficial boundary (roof) that consists of skin and superficial fascia and contains the medial cubital vein, the lateral cutaneous nerve of the forearm and the medial cutaneous nerve of the forearm. The deep fascia is reinforced by the bicipital aponeurosis (a sheet of tendon-like material that arises from the tendon of the biceps).
- A deep boundary (floor) that consists of the brachialis and supinator muscles.

Contents (from lateral to medial)

- The biceps brachii tendon.
- The brachial artery, which usually bifurcates near the apex (inferior part) of the cubital fossa into the radial artery (superficial) and ulnar artery (deeper).
- The median nerve.

The radial nerve lies in the vicinity, between the brachioradialis and brachialis muscles.

Muscles of upper extremity

The muscles of the upper limb are presented below, classified in tables into muscles of the arm, forearm (anterior and posterior) and hand (Tables 1.5–1.8). In these tables, the origin, insertion, action and innervation of each muscle is summarised, to facilitate easy reference and revision.

Group	Muscle	Origin	Insertion	Action	Nerve
Arm, anterior deep	Brachialis	Middle 3rd humerus	Ulna coronoid process	Elbow: flexion	Musculocutaneous
	Coracobrachialis	Coracoid process of scapula	Middle 3rd humerus		
Arm, anterior superficial/ rotator cuff	Biceps brachii	Short head: coracoid process; Long head: supraglenoid tubercle	Tuberosity of radius	Elbow: flexion Forearm: forceful supination	
Arm, posterior	Triceps brachii	Long head: infraglenoid tubercle of scapula; lateral and medial heads: above and below radial groove of humerus	Olecranon of ulna	Elbow: extension	Radial

Table 1.5. Muscles of the arm

Group	Muscle	Origin	Insertion	Action	Nerve
Forearm, anterior deep	Flexor digitorum profundus	Common flexor tendon and radius	Distal phalanges of 2nd – 5th digits	Digits: flexion of fingers	Lateral half: anterior interosseus n. Medial half: ulnar n.
	Flexor pollicis longus	Volar radius, interosseus, ulnar coronoid	The 1st distal phalanx	Digits: flexion of thumb	Anterior interosseus n.
	Pronator quadratus	The distal ulna	The distal radius	Forearm: pronation with elbow extended	Anterior interosseus n.
Forearm, anterior middle	Flexor digitorum superficialis	Common flexor tendon	Middle phalanges of the 2nd through 5th digits	Digits: flexion of fingers	Median n.
Forearm, anterior superficial	Flexor carpi radialis	Common flexor tendon	Base of index finger metacarpal	Wrist: flexion, abduction (radial deviation)	Median n.
	Flexor carpi ulnaris	Common flexor tendon and proximal ulna	The pisiform bone	Wrist: flexion and adduction (ulnar deviation)	Ulnar n.
	Palmaris longus	Common flexor tendon	Superficial palmar fascia	Wrist: flexion	Median n.
	Pronator teres	Humeral head: medial epicondyle; ulnar head: proximal ulna	Distal third of radius	Forearm: pronation (radius over ulna)	Median n.

Table 1.6. Muscles of the anterior forearm

Group	Muscle	Origin	Insertion	Action	Nerve
Forearm, posterior deep	Abductor pollicis longus	Radius, ulna and interosseus membrane	1st metacarpal base	Digits: abduction of thumb	Radial
	Extensor indicis	Radius, ulna and interosseus membrane	Proximal phalanx of the 2nd digit	Digits: extension of index finger	
	Extensor pollicis brevis	Radius, ulna and interosseus membrane	Proximal phalanx of the 1st digit	Digits: extension of thumb	
	Extensor pollicis longus	Radius, ulna and interosseus membrane	Distal phalanx of the 1st digit	Digits: extension of thumb	
	Supinator	Proximal ulna and lateral epicondyle of humerus	Proximal radius	Forearm: supination	
Forearm, posterior superficial	Anconeus	Common extensor tendon	Lateral olecranon and posterior ulna	Elbow: extension, abduction of ulna during pronation	
	Brachioradialis	Common extensor tendon	Styloid process of the radius	Elbow: power flexion	
	Extensor carpi radialis brevis	Common extensor tendon	Base of the metacarpal bones	Wrist: extension and radial deviation (abduction)	
	Extensor carpi radialis longus	Common extensor tendon	Base of the metacarpal bones	Wrist: extension and radial deviation (abduction)	
	Extensor carpi ulnaris	Common extensor tendon	The base of the metacarpal bones	Wrist: extension and adduction (ulnar deviation)	
	Extensor digiti minimi	Common extensor tendon	The proximal phalanx of the 5th digit	Digits: extension of little finger	
	Extensor digitorum	Common extensor tendon	All phalanges of 2nd – 5th digits	Digits: extension of fingers	

Table 1.7. Muscles of posterior forearm

Arteries of the upper extremity

The upper limb is perfused by the subclavian artery and its continuations, axillary and brachial arteries, then by the terminal branches brachial and ulnar arteries and their branches (Figure 1.11).

Subclavian artery

The right subclavian artery arises from the *innominate* artery behind the right sternoclavicular articulation and the left from the arch of the aorta. Each subclavian artery is divided into three parts with reference to the relation of each part to the scalenus anterior muscle. The branches of the subclavian artery are the *vertebral* artery, the *internal mammary (thoracic)* artery, the *dorsal scapular* artery, and the *thyrocervical* and *costocervical* trunks.

Group	Muscle	Action	Innervation
Intrinsic Hand Hypothenar Eminence	Abductor Digiti Minimi	Digits: Abduction of little finger	Ulnar N.
	Flexor Digiti Minimi	Digits: Flexion of the little finger	
	Opponens Digiti Minimi	Digits: Opposition of little finger	
	Palmaris brevis	Tightens and corrugates the hypothenar skin, may deepen the concavity of the palm	
Intrinsic Hand Middle Hand	Dorsal Interossei	Digits: Abduction of fingers	Ulnar N.
	Lumbricals	Digits: Flexion of MCP joints; Extension of PIP and DIP joints	1st and 2nd: Median N., 3rd and 4th: Ulnar N.
	Palmar Interossei	Digits: Adduction of fingers	Ulnar N.
Intrinsic Hand Thenar Eminence	Abductor Pollicis Brevis	Digits: Abduction of thumb	Median N.
	Adductor Pollicis	Digits: Adduction of thumb	Ulnar N.
	Flexor Pollicis Brevis	Digits: Flexion of thumb	Median N.
	Opponens Pollicis	Digits: Opposition of thumb	Median N.
	1st dorsal interosseous	Index MCP joint: flexion, radial deviation and pronation; Thumb basal joint: adduction	Ulnar N.

Table 1.8. Intrinsic muscles of the hand (excluding thumb muscles)

Subclavian steal syndrome: a constellation of signs and symptoms that arise from retrograde flow of blood in the vertebral artery, due to a proximal stenosis (narrowing) and/or occlusion of the subclavian artery. Clinical manifestations include presyncope (sensation that one is about to faint) or syncope (fainting), neurologic deficits, blood pressure differential between the arms, distal upper limb vasculopathy. The diagnosis is confirmed by angiography and the treatment consists of surgical or endovascular treatment of the underlying cause of stenosis.

Axillary artery

The axillary artery is the continuation of the subclavian artery and extends from the lateral margin of the first rib to the lateral margin of the teres major muscle. It is divided into three segments based on its relation to the pectoralis minor muscle. It has six arterial branches that contribute to the rich collateral circulation around the shoulder girdle; the *superior thoracic, thoracoacromial, lateral thoracic, subscapular,* and the *anterior* and *posterior circumflex arteries*.

Brachial artery

The brachial artery is the continuation of the axillary artery and extends from the lateral margin of the teres major muscle to 1 inch below the elbow crease. It gives off the following branches: *profunda brachii,* the *superior* and *inferior ulnar collaterals* and the *terminal radial* and *ulnar arteries*.

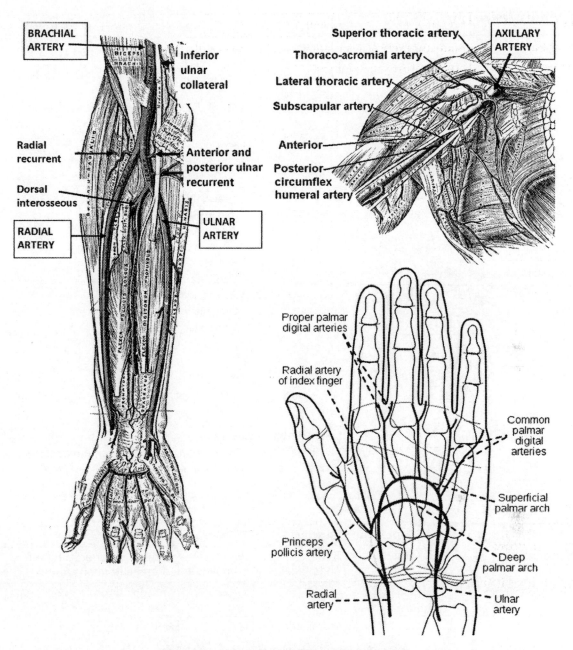

Figure 1.11. Arteries of the upper extremity
Based on Gray H (1918) Anatomy of the Human Body, 20th edition, Lea & Febiger, Philadelphia
(*These images are in the public domain because their copyright has expired. This applies worldwide.*)

Radial and ulnar arteries

Each artery terminates in the deep and superficial palmar arches, respectively.

Their main arterial branches are the *radial recurrent*, the *ulnar recurrent* and the *interosseous artery* (from the ulnar artery). The ulnar artery is the larger of the two and the major source of blood flow to the digits. The superficial arch is incomplete in approximately 20% of patients.

Lower extremity

The following sections present a summary of the nerves and muscles related to the lower limb along with the anatomy of the large joints.

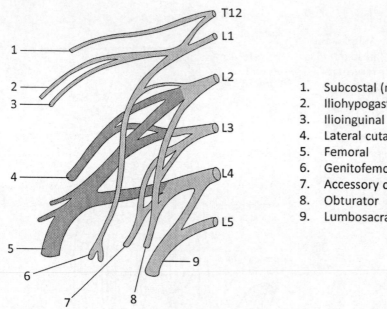

1.   Subcostal (not part of lumbar plexus)
2.   Iliohypogastric
3.   Ilioinguinal
4.   Lateral cutaneous of the thigh
5.   Femoral
6.   Genitofemoral
7.   Accessory obturator
8.   Obturator
9.   Lumbosacral trunk

Figure 1.12. Lumbar plexus nerves
Based on Gray H (1918) Anatomy of the Human Body, 20th edition, Lea & Febiger, Philadelphia
(*This image is in the public domain because its copyright has expired. This applies worldwide.*)

Nerve	Root value	Muscles	Cutaneous branches
Iliohypogastric	T12–L1	Transversus abdominis Abdominal internal oblique	Anterior cutaneous ramus Lateral cutaneous ramus
Ilioinguinal	L1		Anterior scrotal nerves (male) Anterior labial nerves (females)
Genitofemoral	L1, L2	Cremaster in males	Femoral ramus Genital ramus
Lateral cutaneous of the thigh	L2, L3		Lateral femoral cutaneous
Obturator	L2–L4	Obturator externus Adductor longus Gracilis Pectineus Adductor magnus	Cutaneous ramus
Femoral	L2–L4	Iliopsoas Pectineus Sartorius Quadriceps femoris	Anterior cutaneous branches Saphenous
Short, direct muscular branches	T12–L4	Psoas major Quadratus lumborum Iliacus Lumbar intertransverse	

Table 1.9. Nerves of the lumbar plexus

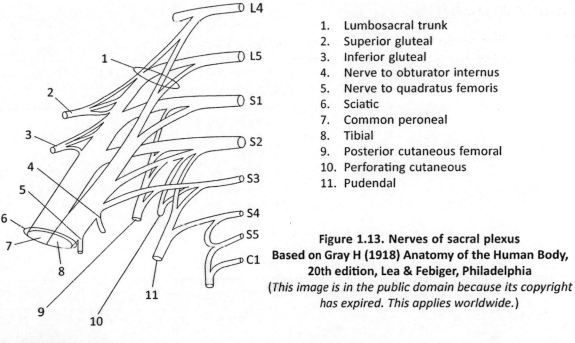

1. Lumbosacral trunk
2. Superior gluteal
3. Inferior gluteal
4. Nerve to obturator internus
5. Nerve to quadratus femoris
6. Sciatic
7. Common peroneal
8. Tibial
9. Posterior cutaneous femoral
10. Perforating cutaneous
11. Pudendal

Figure 1.13. Nerves of sacral plexus
Based on Gray H (1918) Anatomy of the Human Body,
20th edition, Lea & Febiger, Philadelphia
(*This image is in the public domain because its copyright
has expired. This applies worldwide.*)

The lumbar plexus

The lumbar plexus is formed from the ventral rami of nerves L1–L4 and some fibres from T12. It provides branches that pass in front of the hip joint and mainly support the anterior part of the thigh (Figure 1.12 and Table 1.9).

The sacral plexus

It is a nerve plexus that provides motor and sensory nerves for the posterior thigh, most of the lower leg, the entire foot, and part of the pelvis. It emerges from the sacral vertebrae (S2–S4) and is formed by the lumbosacral trunk, the anterior division of the first sacral nerve and portions of the anterior divisions of the second and third sacral nerves (Figure 1.13). A detailed presentation of the nerves of the sacral plexus, their route value and their function (motor and sensory) follows in Table 1.10.

Nerve	Segment	Innervated muscles	Cutaneous branches
Superior gluteal	L4–S1	Gluteus medius and minimus Tensor fascia latae	
Inferior gluteal	L5–S2	Gluteus maximus	
Posterior cutaneous femoral	S1–S3		• Inferior cluneal and perineal nerves
Direct branches from plexus			
Nerve to piriformis	L5, S2	Piriformis	
Nerve to obturator internus	L5, S1	Obturator internus	
Nerve to quadratus femoris	L4–S1	Quadratus femoris	
Sciatic	L4–S3	Semitendinosus (Tibial) Semimembranosus (Tibial) Biceps femoris • Long head (Tibial) • Short head (Fibular) Adductor magnus (medial part, Tibial)	

Table 1.10. Nerves of the sacral plexus

Nerve	Segment	Innervated muscles	Cutaneous branches
Common peroneal	L4–S2		Lateral sural cutaneous Communicating fibular
Superficial peroneal		Peroneus longus and Peroneus brevis	Medial and Intermediate dorsal cutaneous
Deep peroneal		Tibialis anterior Extensor digitorum longus and brevis Extensor hallucis longus and brevis Peroneus tertius	Lateral cutaneous nerve of big toe Intermediate dorsal cutaneous
Tibial nerve	L4–S3	Triceps surae, Plantaris, Popliteus, Tibialis posterior Flexor digitorum longus Flexor hallucis longus	Medial sural cutaneous Lateral calcaneal Medial calcaneal Lateral dorsal cutaneous
Medial plantar		Abductor hallucis Flexor digitorum brevis Flexor hallucis brevis (medial head) Lumbricals (first and second)	Proper digital plantar
Lateral plantar		Flexor hallucis brevis (lateral head) Quadratus plantae Abductor, Flexor and Opponens digiti minimi Lumbricals (third and fourth) Plantar interossei (first to third) Dorsal interossei (first to fifth) Adductor hallucis	Proper plantar digital

Pudendal (Pudendal plexus)	S1–S4	Muscles of the pelvic floor:
		  Levator ani
		  Superficial transverse perineal
		  Deep transverse perineal
		  Bulbospongiosus
		  Ischiocavernosus
		  Shpincter anus externus
		  Urethral sphincter
			Inferior rectal
			Perineal
			• Posterior scrotal/labial
			• Dorsal penis/clitoris

Coccygeal	S5–Co1	Coccygeus	Anococcygeal

Table 1.10 (continued). Nerves of the sacral plexus

The hip joint

The hip joint is a 'ball and socket' synovial joint, formed by the articulation of the rounded head of the femur and the cup-like acetabulum of the pelvis, with both articular surfaces covered by hyaline cartilage. The cup-like acetabulum forms at the union of three pelvic bones, the ilium, pubis, and ischium.

Capsule

It extends from outside the acetabular lip of the pelvis to the base of the femoral neck, leaving a wide extracapsular part of the neck.

Ligaments

There are four extracapsular ligaments (iliofemoral, ischiofemoral, pubofemoral and zona orbicularis) and one intracapsular (ligamentum teres); the latter contains a small artery to the head of the femur, important in femoral neck fractures, where it can become the only blood supply to the bone.

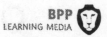

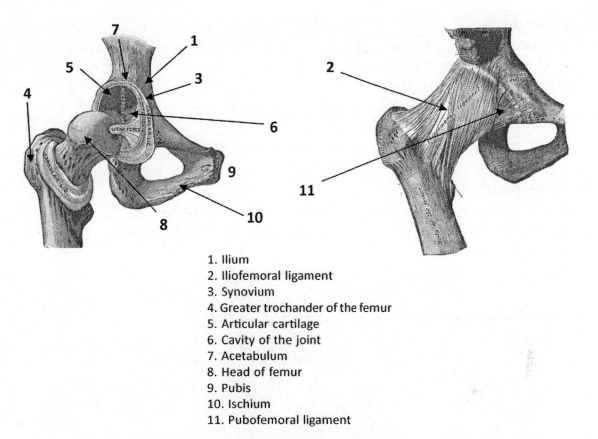

1. Ilium
2. Iliofemoral ligament
3. Synovium
4. Greater trochander of the femur
5. Articular cartilage
6. Cavity of the joint
7. Acetabulum
8. Head of femur
9. Pubis
10. Ischium
11. Pubofemoral ligament

Figure 1.14. The hip joint
Based on Gray H (1918) Anatomy of the Human Body, 20th edition, Lea & Febiger, Philadelphia
(*This image is in the public domain because its copyright has expired.This applies worldwide.*)

Movement	Range	Muscles
External rotation	30° (hip extended), 50° (hip flexed)	Gluteus maximus, quadratus femoris, obturator internus, gluteus medius and minimus (dorsal fibres), iliopsoas (including psoas major from the vertebral column), obturator externus, adductor magnus, longus, brevis, and minimus, piriformis and sartorius.
Internal rotation	40°	Anterior fibres of gluteus medius and minimus, tensor fasciae latae, adductor magnus and the pectineus.
Extension	20°	Gluteus maximus, dorsal fibres of gluteus medius and minimus, adductor magnus, piriformis and the hamstrings, semimembranosus, semitendinosus, and long head of biceps femoris.
Flexion	140°	Iliopsoas (with psoas major from vertebral column); tensor fasciae latae, pectineus, adductor longus, adductor brevis, gracilis and the thigh muscles rectus femoris and sartorius.
Abduction	50° (hip extended), 80°(hip flexed)	Gluteus medius, tensor fasciae latae, gluteus maximus, gluteus minimus, piriformis and obturator internus.
Adduction	30° (hip extended), 20° (hip flexed)	Adductors (magnus, minimus, longus, brevis), gluteus maximus, gracilis, pectineus, quadratus femoris, obturator externus and semitendinosus.

Table 1.11. Muscles moving the hip joint and range of movement

Blood supply

From the *medial circumflex femoral* and *lateral circumflex femoral arteries*, branches of the *profunda femoris*, with a small contribution from a *small artery in the ligament of the head of the femur* which is a branch of the *obturator* artery.

Muscles and movements

The range of movement of the hip joint and the relevant muscles are presented in Table 1.11.

The knee joint

The knee is the largest joint in the human body. It is a mobile, synovial, *trocho-ginglymus* joint (i.e. a pivotal hinge joint), permitting flexion, extension and a slight medial and lateral rotation.

Morphology (Figure 1.15)

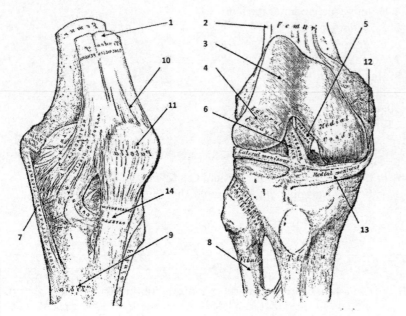

1. Quadriceps muscle
2. Femur
3. Articular cartilage
4. Lateral femoral condyle
5. Posterior cruciate ligament (PCL)
6. Anterior cruciate ligament (ACL)
7. Lateral collateral ligament
8. Fibula
9. Tibia
10. Quadriceps tendon
11. Patella
12. Medial collateral ligament
13. Medial meniscus
14. Patellar tendon (ligament)

Figure 1.15. Schematic anatomy of the knee joint
Based on Gray H (1918) Anatomy of the Human Body, 20th edition, Lea & Febiger, Philadelphia
(*This image is in the public domain because its copyright has expired. This applies worldwide.*)

Compartments

It consists of three functional compartments: the femoro-patellar articulation between the patella and the patellar groove of the femur, and the medial and lateral femoro-tibial articulations between the femur and the tibia. The joint is bathed in synovial fluid which is contained inside the synovial membrane (joint capsule). The articular surfaces are covered by cartilage of two types: hyaline and fibrous cartilage (the menisci).

Menisci

The medial and lateral meniscus consist of connective tissue with extensive collagen fibres containing cartilage-like cells; they serve to protect the ends of the bones from rubbing on each other and play a role in shock absorption.

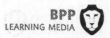

Ligaments of the knee

They can be divided into:

- Extracapsular ligaments: the patellar ligament, medial collateral ligament (MCL), lateral collateral ligament (LCL), oblique popliteal ligament, and arcuate popliteal ligament.
- Intra-articular ligaments: the anterior cruciate ligament (ACL), posterior cruciate ligament (PCL), and the posterior meniscofemoral ligament.

Bursae

Many bursae surround the knee with the medial group (anserine bursa and semimembranosus bursa) more clinically important, as they can become inflamed with excessive physical activity.

Blood supply

Arterial supply from the femoral artery, popliteal artery, and their branches:

1. Superior medial genicular artery
2. Superior lateral genicular artery
3. Inferior medial genicular artery
4. Inferior lateral genicular artery
5. Descending genicular artery
6. Recurrent branch of anterior tibial artery

Innervation

The sensory innervation of the knee derives from the sciatic nerve as well as from the obturator, femoral, and lateral femoral cutaneous nerves.

Movements of the knee joint (Table 1.12)

See also clinical examination of the knee joint.

Extension (5–10°)	Flexion (120–150°)
Quadriceps (with some assistance from the tensor fasciae latae)	Semimembranosus Semitendinosus Biceps femoris Gracilis Sartorius Popliteus Gastrocnemius
Internal rotation with knee flexed (10°)	External rotation with knee flexed (30–40°)
Semimembranosus Semitendinosus Gracilis Sartorius Popliteus	Biceps femoris

Table 1.12. Movements of the knee joint (range) and relevant muscles

Muscles of the lower extremity

The muscles of the gluteal region, thigh, leg and foot are presented below, classified in tables detailing their origin, insertion, action and innervation. The tables summarise the features of each muscle and are best used as reference sources along with an atlas.

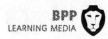

Muscle	Origin	Insertion	Action	Nerve
Gluteus maximus	Outer surface of ilium, sacrum, coccyx, sacrotuberous ligament	Iliotibial tract and gluteal tuberosity of femur	Extends and laterally rotates thigh; through iliotibial tract, it extends knee joint	Inferior gluteal nerve
Gluteus medius	Outer surface of ilium	Greater trochanter of femur	Abducts thigh. Tilts pelvis when walking	Superior gluteal nerve
Gluteus minimus	Outer surface of ilium	Greater trochanter of femur	Abducts thigh; anterior fibres medially rotate thigh	Superior gluteal nerve
Tensor fasciae latae	Iliac crest	Iliotibial tract	Assists gluteus major in locking the knee into full extension	Superior gluteal nerve
Piriformis	Anterior surface of sacrum			1st and 2nd sacral nerves
Superior gemellus	Spine of ischium	Greater trochanteric fossa of femur	Lateral rotators of thigh	Sacral plexus
Obturator internus	Inner surface of obturator membrane			Sacral plexus
Inferior gemellus	Ischial tuberosity			Sacral plexus
Obturator externus	Outer surface of obturator membrane			Obturator nerve

Table 1.13. Muscles of the gluteal region

Muscle	Origin	Insertion	Action	Nerve
Sartorius	Anterior superior iliac spine	Upper medial surface of tibia	Flexes, abducts, laterally rotates thigh; flexes and medially rotates leg	Femoral nerve
Iliacus	Iliac fossa	With psoas into the lesser trochanter of femur	Flexes thigh on trunk; if thigh is fixed, it flexes the trunk onto the thigh as in sitting up	Femoral nerve
Psoas	12th thoracic body; transverse processes, bodies and intervertebral discs of the 5 lumbar vertebrae	Lesser trochanter of femur along with iliacus	Flexes thigh on trunk; if thigh fixed, it flexes trunk onto thigh as in sitting up	Lumbar plexus
Pectineus	Superior ramus of pubis	Upper end shaft of femur	Flexes and adducts thigh	Femoral nerve
Quadriceps femoris, rectus femoris	Straight head from anterior inferior iliac spine; reflected head from ilium above acetabulum	Quadriceps tendon into patella; into tibial tuberosity by patellar tendon	Extension of leg	Femoral nerve
Quadriceps femoris, vastus lateralis	Upper end and shaft of femur	Quadriceps tendon into patella; into tibial tuberosity by patellar tendon	Extension of leg	Femoral nerve
Quadriceps femoris, vastus medialis	Upper end and shaft of femur	Quadriceps tendon into patella; into tibial tuberosity by patellar tendon	Extension of leg	Femoral nerve
Quadriceps femoris, vastus intermedius	Shaft of femur	Quadriceps tendon into patella; into tibial tuberosity by patellar tendon	Extension of leg	Femoral nerve

Table 1.14. Muscles of the thigh – anterior compartment

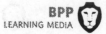

Muscle	Origin	Insertion	Action	Nerve
Gracilis	Inferior ramus of pubis; ramus of ischium	Upper part of shaft of tibia on medial surface	Adducts thigh and flexes leg	Obturator nerve
Adductor longus	Body of pubis	Posterior surface of shaft of femur	Adducts thigh; assists in lateral rotation	Obturator nerve
Adductor brevis	Inferior ramus of pubis	Posterior surface of shaft of femur	Adducts thigh; assists in lateral rotation	Obturator nerve
Adductor magnus	Inferior ramus of pubis; ramus of ischium, ischial tuberosity	Posterior surface of shaft of femur near linea aspera; adductor tubercle of femur	Adducts thigh and assists in lateral rotation; hamstring part extends thigh	Obturator nerve; tibial nerve to hamstring part

Table 1.15. Muscles of the thigh – medial compartment

Muscle	Origin	Insertion	Action	Nerve
Biceps femoris	Long head from ischial tuberosity; short head from shaft of femur	Head of fibula	Flexes and laterally rotates leg; long head extends thigh	Long head: tibial; short head: common peroneal
Semitendinosus	Ischial tuberosity	Upper part medial surface of shaft of tibia	Flexes and medially rotates leg; extends thigh	Tibial nerve
Semimembranosus	Ischial tuberosity	Medial condyle of tibia; forms oblique popliteal ligament	Flexes and medially rotates leg; extends thigh	Tibial nerve
Adductor magnus (hamstring part)	Ischial tuberosity	Adductor tubercle of femur	Extends thigh	Tibial nerve

Table 1.16. Muscles of the thigh – posterior compartment

Muscle	Origin	Insertion	Action	Nerve
Tibialis anterior	Shaft of tibia and interosseous membrane	Medial cuneiform and base of first metatarsal	Extends the foot; inverts foot at subtalar and transverse tarsal joints; supports medial longitudinal arch	
Extensor digitorum	Shaft of fibula and interosseous membrane	Extensor expansion of lateral four toes	Extends toes; dorsiflexes (extends) foot	
Peroneus tertius	Shaft of fibula and interosseous membrane	Base of 5th metatarsal bone	Dorsiflexes (extends) foot; everts foot at subtalar and transverse tarsal joints	Deep peroneal nerve
Extensor hallucis longus	Shaft of fibula and interosseous membrane	Base of distal phalanx of big toe	Extends big toe; dorsiflexes (extends) foot; inverts foot at subtalar and transverse tarsal joints	

Table 1.17. Muscles of the leg – anterior compartment

Muscle	Origin	Insertion	Action	Nerve
Peroneus longus	Shaft of fibula	Base of 1st metatarsal and medial cuneiform	Plantar flexes foot; everts foot at subtalar and transverse tarsal joints; supports lateral longitudinal arch	Superficial peroneal nerve
Peroneus brevis		Base of 5th metatarsal bone		

Table 1.18. Muscles of the leg – lateral compartment

Muscle	Origin	Insertion	Action	Nerve
Gastrocnemius	Medial and lateral condyles of femur	By way of Achilles tendon to calcaneum	Plantar flexes foot; flexes leg	Tibial nerve
Plantaris	Lateral supracondylar ridge of femur	Calcaneum	Plantar flexes foot; flexes leg	
Soleus	Shafts of tibia and fibula	By way of Achilles tendon into calcaneum	With gastrocnemius and plantaris is powerful plantar flexor of foot; provides main propulsive force in walking and running	
Popliteus	Lateral condyle of femur	Shaft of tibia	Flexes leg; unlocks full extension of knee by laterally rotating femur on tibia	
Flexor digitorum longus	Shaft of tibia	Distal phalanges of lateral four toes	Flexes distal phalanges of lateral four toes; plantar flexes foot; supports medial and lateral longitudinal arches of foot	
Flexor hallucis longus	Shaft of fibula	Base of distal phalanx of big toe	Flexes distal phalanx of big toe; plantar flexes foot; supports medial longitudinal arch	
Tibialis posterior	Shafts of tibia and fibula and interosseous membrane	Tuberosity of navicular bone	Plantar flexes foot; inverts foot at subtalar and transverse tarsal joints; supports medial longitudinal arch of foot	

Table 1.19. Muscles of the leg – posterior compartment

Muscle	Origin	Insertion	Action	Nerve
Dorsum of foot				
Extensor digitorum brevis	Calcaneum	By four tendons into the proximal phalanx of big toe and long extensor tendons to 2nd, 3rd and 4th toes	Extends toes	Deep peroneal
Sole of the foot (first layer)				
Abductor hallucis	Medial tubercle of calcaneum; flexor retinaculum	Medial side, base of proximal phalanx of big toe	Flexes, abducts big toe; supports medial arch	Medial plantar
Flexor digitorum brevis	Medial tubercle of calcaneum	Middle phalanx of four lateral toes	Flexes lateral four toes; supports medial and lateral longitudinal arches	Medial plantar
Abductor digiti minimi	Medial and lateral tubercles of calcaneum	Lateral side base of proximal phalanx of 5th toe	Flexes, abducts 5th toe; supports lateral longitudinal arch	Lateral plantar nerve
Sole of foot (second layer)				
Flexor accessorius (quadratus plantae)	Medial and lateral sides of calcaneum	Tendons flexor digitorum longus	Aids long flexor tendon to flex lateral four toes	Lateral plantar nerve

Table 1.20. Muscles of the foot

Muscle	Origin	Insertion	Action	Nerve
Flexor digitorum longus tendon	Shaft of tibia	Base of distal phalanx of lateral four toes	Flexes distal phalanges of lateral four toes; plantar flexes foot; supports longitudinal arch	Tibial nerve
Lumbricals	Tendons of flexor digitorum longus	Dorsal extensor expansion of lateral four toes	Extends toes at interphalangeal joints	1st lumbrical from medial plantar; remainder lumbricals from deep branch of lateral plantar nerve
Flexor hallucis longus	Shaft of fibula	Base of distal phalanx of big toe	Flexes distal phalanx of big toe; plantar flexes foot; supports medial longitudinal arch	Tibial nerve
Muscles of sole of foot (third layer)				
Flexor hallucis brevis	Cuboid, lateral cuneiform bones; tibialis posterior insertion	Medial and lateral sides of base of proximal phalanx of big toe	Flexes metatarsophalangeal joint of big toe; supports medial longitudinal arch	Medial plantar nerve
Adductor hallucis (oblique head)	Bases of 2nd, 3rd and 4th metatarsal bones	Lateral side base of proximal phalanx big toe	Flexes big toe, supports transverse arch	Deep branch of lateral plantar
Adductor hallucis (transverse head)	Plantar ligaments	Lateral side of base of proximal phalanx big toe	Flexes big toe; supports transverse arch	Deep branch of lateral plantar nerve
Flexor digiti minimi brevis	Base of 5th metatarsal bone	Lateral side of base of proximal phalanx of little toe	Flexes little toe	Superior branch of lateral plantar nerve
Muscles of sole of foot (fourth layer)				
Dorsal interossei (4)	Adjacent sides of metatarsal bones	Bases of phalanges and dorsal expansion of corresponding toes	Abduct toes with 2nd toe as the reference; flex metatarsophalangeal joints; extend interphalangeal joint	Lateral plantar nerve
Plantar interossei (3)	3rd, 4th, and 5th metatarsal bones	Bases of phalanges and dorsal expansion of corresponding toes	Adduct toes with 2nd toe as reference; flex metatarsophalangeal joints; extend interphalangeal joints	Lateral plantar nerve
Tendon of peroneus longus and tibialis posterior	See Tables 1.18 and 1.19			

Table 1.20 (continued). Muscles of the foot

The thorax

The thorax or chest refers to the region between the neck and the abdomen; it hosts the all important organs of the cardio-respiratory system and parts of the gastrointestinal and immune systems. Finally, the thorax provides support for the breasts.

The mediastinum

The mediastinum is the central compartment of the thoracic cavity, containing the heart, with its great vessels, the oesophagus, trachea, phrenic nerve, cardiac nerve, thoracic duct, thymus, and lymph nodes of the central chest, all surrounded by loose connective tissue.

Boundaries

The mediastinum is bounded by the:

- Thoracic inlet, superiorly
- Diaphragm, inferiorly
- Sternum, anteriorly
- Vertebral bodies, posteriorly
- Pleura, laterally on either side

As shown in Figure 1.16, the mediastinum is classified into a superior (S) and an inferior portion, divided by a plane extending from the sternal angle to the T4/5 vertebral disk. The inferior portion is further subdivided into anterior (A, in front of the pericardium), middle (M, containing the pericardium and its contents) and posterior mediastinum behind the pericardium. A detailed description of the mediastinal compartments and their contents follows in Table 1.21.

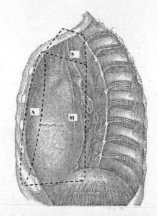

Figure 1.16. Schematic division of the mediastinum
Based on Gray H (1918) Anatomy of the Human Body,
20th edition, Lea & Febiger, Philadelphia
(*This image is in the public domain because its copyright has expired. This applies worldwide.*)

Mediastinal Compartment	Boundaries	Contents
Superior	Between the manubrium sterni anteriorly and the upper thoracic vertebrae posteriorly	The aortic arch, innominate artery, the thoracic portions of the left common carotid and left subclavian arteries, the innominate veins, the upper half of the superior vena cava, the left highest intercostal vein, the vagus, cardiac, phrenic, and left recurrent nerves, the trachea, oesophagus, thoracic duct, the remains of the thymus and some lymph glands
Anterior	The sternum anteriorly, pleurae laterally and pericardium posteriorly	Loose areolar tissue, some lymphatic vessels which ascend from the liver, lymph glands, and the small mediastinal branches of the internal mammary artery
Middle	Within the pericardium	The heart enclosed in the pericardium, the ascending aorta, the lower half of the superior vena cava with the azygous vein, the bifurcation of the trachea and the two bronchi, the pulmonary artery dividing into right and left, pulmonary veins, the phrenic nerves and some bronchial lymph glands
Posterior	The pericardium anteriorly, diaphragm inferiorly, vertebral column posteriorly, and mediastinal pleura on either side laterally	<ul><li>Thoracic part of the descending aorta</li><li>The azygous and the two hemiazygous veins</li><li>The vagus and splanchnic nerves</li><li>The oesophagus, the thoracic duct, and some lymph glands</li></ul>

Table 1.21. Mediastinal compartments, borders and contents

The heart

Location and morphology

The heart lies in the middle mediastinum within the pericardium. It has the shape of an irregular cone, with the base posteriorly (where it connects to the great vessels) and the apex pointing antero-inferiorly to the left.

It has three surfaces:

- Sterno-costal: Right atrium and ventricle and partly left ventricle and atrium.
- Diaphragmatic: Right and left ventricles.
- Base: Left (mainly) and right atrium.

It also bears three surface grooves:

- Atrioventricular groove: Separates the right and left atrium from the ventricles.
- Anterior and posterior interventricular grooves: Separate the ventricles and join each other.

The heart consists of four chambers that contain four valves. The heart possesses a 'fibrous skeleton' (composed of dense collagen) that provides anchorage for the myocardium of the cardiac chambers and for the cusps of the heart valves.

- The *right atrium* hosts the openings of the *superior* and *inferior vena cavae*, the opening of the *coronary sinus* and the *tricuspid* opening (guarded by the tricuspid valve) that leads to the *right ventricle*.
- The *left atrium* receives the *upper* and *lower pulmonary veins* and via the *mitral* opening (guarded by the mitral valve) continues to the *left ventricle*.
- The *right* and *left ventricle* walls show prominent muscular ridges on the interior, termed *trabeculae*; some of these form *papillary muscles*, which are connected to the cusps of the corresponding atrioventricular valve (tricuspid/mitral) by inelastic cords called *chordae tendinae*. The outflow tract of the right ventricle, the *infundibulum*, leads to the *pulmonary trunk* through the *pulmonary valve*. The outflow tract of the left ventricle leads to the *aortic root*, through the *aortic valve*. The left ventricular wall is three times as thick as the wall of the right ventricle.

Relations

- Laterally: Phrenic nerves, adjacent to the pericardium.
- Posteriorly: Oesophagus (behind the left atrium), descending thoracic aorta, azygous vein, thoracic duct.

Blood supply

Left coronary artery (LCA)

The LCA arises from the left aortic sinus, passes between the left atrial appendage and pulmonary trunk. It gives off the following branches:

1. *Sinoatrial nodal* artery (40% of individuals).
2. *Anterior interventricular* artery or *left anterior descending* artery: it continues in the anterior interventricular groove, anastomoses with the *posterior interventricular* branch of the RCA and gives the *diagonal* and *obtuse marginal* arteries.
3. *Circumflex artery*: It winds around the left heart border, passes in the atrioventricular groove, gives branches to left atrium and anastomoses with RCA.

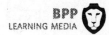

Right coronary artery (RCA)

The RCA arises from the anterior aortic sinus, continues between the right auricle and infundibulum of the right ventricle, then downwards in the atrioventricular groove on the anterior aspect of the heart. On reaching the inferior heart border, it turns backwards to continue in the atrioventricular groove on the inferior (diaphragmatic) surface of the heart and it ends by anastomosing with the *circumflex artery* of the LCA. It gives of the following branches:

1. *Sinoatrial* artery (60% of individuals).
2. Branches to the right atrium.
3. A branch to the infundibulum of the right ventricle (right conus branch).
4. *Right marginal* artery.
5. *Atrioventricular* nodal artery (in 90% of individuals).
6. Posterior interventricular artery (also known as posterior descending artery, which supplies the posterior one-third of the interventricular septum, the atrioventricular node, the inferior surface of the right ventricle and a portion of the inferior surface the left ventricle).

Venous drainage

- Coronary sinus: It is a continuation of the great cardiac vein, lies in the posterior part of the atrioventricular groove and drains into the right atrium. Receives the tributaries:
    1. Great cardiac vein.
    2. Middle cardiac vein.
    3. Small cardiac vein.
    4. Posterior vein of the left ventricle.
    5. Oblique vein of the left atrium.
- Anterior cardiac vein: Drains directly into the right atrium.
- Thebesian veins (Venae cordae minimae): They drain directly into the chambers of the heart.

Innervation of the heart

- Sympathetic, by the cervical and upper thoracic portions of the sympathetic chain through the *stellate* ganglion.
- Parasympathetic, by the vagus nerves.

Conducting system of the heart

It co-ordinates the contraction of the cardiac chambers and is made up of a continuum of highly specialised cardiac myocytes arranged along the following sequence of anatomical components:

- Sinoatrial node (normally the pacemaker of the heart).
- Atrioventricular node.
- Atrioventricular bundle of His.
- Right and left branches of the atrioventricular bundle.
- Subendocardial fibres of Purkinje.

The heart on chest radiograph

Four borders of the cardiac silhouette can be described on a chest radiograph (anteroposterior view). The right border is formed by the lateral edge of the right atrium; the left border, by the lateral edge of the left ventricle with the left atrial appendage; the superior (oblique) border, by the roots of the aorta and pulmonary trunk; and the inferior border, by the lower edge of right ventricle and part of the left ventricle.

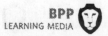

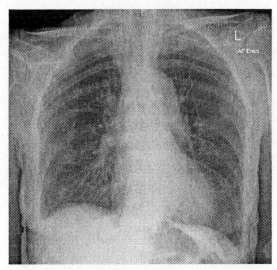
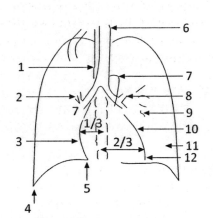

1. Superior vena cava
2. Right hilum and right main bronchus
3. Right atrium
4. Right costo-phrenic angle
5. Right cardio-phrenic angle
6. Trachea

7. Aortic arch
8. Left hilum
9. Branches of pulmonary artery
10. Left atrium
11. Lung peripheries
12. Left ventricle

Figure 1.17. A normal chest radiograph and the radiological features of thoracic structures. Reproduced with permission from Maidstone Hospital

The pericardium

The pericardium is a fibroserous sac enclosing the heart and roots of great vessels. It comprises two layers, the *fibrous* pericardium, (outer layer) and the *serous* pericardium that is double layered, with an inner visceral layer (epicardium) and an outer parietal layer. Between the parietal and visceral layers of the serous pericardium is the *pericardial cavity*, which contains a thin film of fluid that enables the pulsating heart to glide with no friction within the pericardium. Both layers are continuous around the great vessels and the pulmonary veins. There are two prominent recesses in the pericardial cavity, the pericardial sinuses (oblique sinus and transverse sinus).

The pleura

Morphology

The pleura is a serous membrane which folds back onto itself to form a two-layered membrane structure surrounding the lungs. Each pleura has two parts, the *parietal layer* that lines the thoracic wall and diaphragm and the *visceral layer* that covers the outer surface of lungs; the pleurae are continuous with each other at the root of lung. The two pleural layers are separated by the pleural cavity that contains a small amount of pleural fluid.

Innervation

The costal pleura is supplied by intercostal nerves, the mediastinal pleura by the phrenic nerves and the diaphragmatic pleura by both intercostal and phrenic nerves.

Surface anatomy

On the right side: the line of reflection of the pleura follows the following course: from the sternoclavicular articulation, downward and medially to the midpoint of the junction between

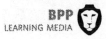

the manubrium and body of the sternum and along the midsternal line to the xiphoid process; then laterally and downward across the seventh sternocostal articulation, across the eighth costochondral junction in the mammary line, the tenth rib in the midaxillary line, and thence to the spinous process of the twelfth thoracic vertebra.

On the left side: from the sternoclavicular articulation, to the midpoint of the junction between the manubrium and body of the sternum, down the midsternal line in contact with that of the opposite side to the level of the fourth costal cartilage. From this point it diverges laterally and downwards lateral to the sternal border, as far as the sixth costal cartilage, then crosses the seventh costal cartilage, and from there onward it is similar to the line on the right side.

The trachea
Morphology

The trachea is a cartilaginous and membranous tube, extending from the lower part of the larynx, below the cricoid cartilage at level of C6 vertebra, to the upper border of the fourth–fifth thoracic vertebra at the level of sternal angle, where it divides into the two bronchi, one for each lung. It has a fibroelastic wall with 16–20 incomplete U-shaped hyaline cartilage rings. It is 10–11cm long, the upper half in the neck and the lower half in the superior mediastinum. The most distal ring has a triangular lower border forming an anteroposterior internal ridge, the *carina*.

Relations

The anterior relations of the trachea are particularly important (tracheostomy).

- Fascial layers: The investing lamina of the deep cervical fascia and the pretracheal lamina enclosing the thyroid isthmus.
- Veins: Tributaries of the anterior jugulars (jugular arch), inferior thyroids and the left brachiocephalic (in children).
- Arteries: The thyroidea ima (when present), branches of the superior thyroids; brachiocephalic (in children) and left common carotid at the root of the neck.
- The thyroid isthmus crosses rings 2–4.
- The thymus may extend into the neck in infants.
- The sternohyoid and sternothyroid muscles overlap the lateral borders.

Blood supply: from the inferior thyroid and bronchial arteries.
Venous drainage: to the inferior thyroid venous plexus.
Lymph drainage: to the pretracheal, paratracheal and posteroinferior deep cervical nodes.
Innervation: from vagus and recurrent laryngeal nerves and from the sympathetic trunk.

Tracheostomy
Indications

- To relieve upper airway obstruction (foreign body, trauma, facial fractures, burns, acute epiglottitis, diphtheria, glottic oedema, bilateral abductor paralysis of the vocal cords, tumours of the larynx, congenital web or atresia).
- To improve respiratory function (bronchopneumonia, chronic bronchitis and emphysema, chest injury, subcutaneous emphysema).
- Respiratory paralysis (unconscious head injury, bulbar poliomyelitis, tetanus).

- To provide a long-term route for mechanical ventilation in cases of respiratory failure.
- To provide pulmonary toilet when cough is inadequate due to chronic pain or weakness.
- To prevent aspiration and the ability to handle secretions.
- Prophylaxis (preparation for extensive head and neck procedures).
- Severe sleep apnoea not amenable to continuous positive airway pressure (CPAP) devices or other, less invasive surgery.

Surgical tracheostomy technique – steps

1. The patient is positioned supine with a sandbag between the scapulae.
2. A transverse skin incision is made 1cm above the sternal notch, extending to the sternocleidomastoid muscles.
3. Dissection through fascial planes is performed and the anterior jugular veins and strap muscles are retracted laterally.
4. The thyroid isthmus is divided and each cut end is oversewn to prevent bleeding.
5. The stoma is fashioned between third and fourth tracheal rings.
6. The anterior portion of tracheal ring is removed.
7. The endo-tracheal tube is withdrawn to sub-glottis and a tracheostomy tube is inserted using obturator.
8. When correct position is confirmed the endotracheal tube is removed and the tube is secured with tapes.

Complications of tracheostomy

Immediate

- Haemorrhage
- Surgical trauma – oesophagus, recurrent laryngeal nerve
- Pneumothorax

Intermediate

- Tracheal erosion
- Tube displacement or obstruction
- Subcutaneous emphysema
- Aspiration and lung abscess

Late

- Persistent tracheo-cutaneous fistula
- Laryngeal and tracheal stenosis
- Tracheomalacia
- Tracheo-oesophageal fistula

Percutaneous tracheostomy

It is usually performed at the bedside in an ITU by using a guide-wire and dilators. It bears reduced risk of bleeding and infection.

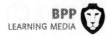

The bronchi

Morphology

The bronchial tree starts at the tracheal bifurcation that gives the two *main (primary) bronchi*. The right main bronchus is wider, shorter and more vertical than the left and divides at the hilum of right lung into three branches. The left main bronchus passes in front of the oesophagus and divides at the hilum of left lung into two branches. From these, a series of multiple divisions gives rise to the *lobar (secondary) bronchi* and the *segmental (tertiary) bronchi* that become *terminal bronchi*. These give the *lobular bronchioles*, the *terminal bronchioles* and finally the *respiratory bronchioles* that lead into the *alveolar ducts* and *sacs*.

Blood supply

The bronchi and their branches are perfused by the *bronchial arteries*, direct branches of the thoracic aorta. The bronchial veins drain into the *azygous* and *hemiazygous* veins.

The lungs

The lungs are located in the thoracic cavity and are the essential respiration organs. Their principal function is to transport oxygen from the atmosphere into the bloodstream, and release carbon dioxide from the bloodstream into the atmosphere (the lung functions are presented in Table 1.22).

Morphology

The lungs are conical in shape with a rounded convex apex, a concave diaphragmatic surface (base), a concave mediastinal surface and a convex costal surface. They are covered by visceral pleura. The apex extends into the base of the neck, surrounded by the first rib and costal cartilage, and extends about 2.5cm above the middle of the clavicle. The base of the lung overlies the dome of the diaphragm. Each lung root lies at T5–T7 level and consists of the *hilum* and the *pulmonary ligament*.

Each hilum contains: the bronchus posteriorly; the pulmonary vein anteriorly and inferiorly to the bronchus; the pulmonary artery superiorly; the bronchial vessels; autonomic nerve plexuses and lymph nodes.

The phrenic nerve and pericardiacophrenic vessels run anterior, and the vagus posterior, to each lung root. On the right there is a 'double section' of both the main bronchus and the pulmonary artery, as both structures bifurcate outside the lung. The left lung has two lobes – upper and lower, separated by the oblique fissure. The right lung has three lobes – upper, middle and

Metabolic	• Gas exchange • Acid-base
Endocrine	• Production of angiotensin-converting enzyme • Secretion of vasoactive peptides (part of amine precursor uptake and decarboxylation APUD system) • Removal of prostaglandins, bradykinin, 5- HT, amide, local anaesthetic agents
Synthesis	• Surfactant, mucopolysaccharides, collagen
Immune	• Production of alveolar IgA and alveolar macrophages
Other	• Removal of small blood clots and microbubbles • Reservoir for blood

Table 1.22. Functions of the lungs

 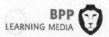

lower, separated by the oblique and horizontal fissures. The lobes of the lung are divided into bronchopulmonary segments (each receiving a segmental bronchus, artery and vein) that are further subdivided into lobules.

Blood supply

Arterial supply – bronchial arteries, venous drainage – bronchial veins.

Pulmonary circulation

The gaseous exchange is subserved by the pulmonary vessels:

- The pulmonary trunk divides into the two pulmonary arteries, right and left, with the branches of each artery following those of the bronchi.
- The pulmonary veins, two on each side, form intersegmental tributaries and empty separately into the left atrium.

The diaphragm

The diaphragm is a thin sheet of muscle that separates the thoracic cavity from the abdominal cavity and performs an important function in respiration.

Morphology

The muscle fibres converge from its periphery on to a central tendon. The peripheral attachments are lumbar (crura and the arcuate ligaments), costal and sternal.

Structures that pass through or behind the diaphragm cross three major openings and a number of minor ones:

- Aortic hiatus, between the vertebral column and the median arcuate ligament (T12): conveys the aorta, azygous vein and thoracic duct. The cisterna chyli lies behind the right crus.
- Oesophageal hiatus (T10): conveys the oesophagus, branches of the left gastric vessels, the two vagal trunks, and the phreno-oesophageal ligament.
- Vena caval hiatus (T8): in the central tendon and conveys the inferior vena cava and the right phrenic nerve.
- The crura are pierced by the greater and lesser splanchnic nerves and by the hemiazygous vein.
- The sympathetic trunks pass behind the medial and the subcostal nerves behind the lateral arcuate ligaments.
- The left phrenic nerve pierces the diaphragm just anterior to the central tendon.

Innervation

- Motor nerve supply: Exclusively from the phrenic nerves (C3, 4, 5).
- Sensory supply: The central part by the phrenic nerves, the peripheral part by the lower six intercostal nerves.

Blood supply

Blood supply is from the intercostal, superior and inferior phrenic branches of the aorta, and from branches of the internal thoracic artery.

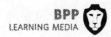

The abdomen

The abdomen is the largest cavity in the body. It is mainly bounded by muscles and fasciae, which accounts for its variation in capacity and shape, depending on age, sex and the condition of the contained viscera.

Boundaries

- Superior – diaphragm
- Inferior – pelvic inlet
- Anterior – anterior abdominal wall
- Posterior – lumbar vertebrae, upper bony pelvis, psoas and quadratus lumborum.

Anterior abdominal wall

Knowledge of the anatomy and layers of the abdominal wall is of paramount importance, because it is relevant to the operative surgery of the abdomen and pelvis (abdominal incisions) and to the pathology of herniae.

From superficial to deep the following layers/structures are encountered:

1. Skin
    - Nerve supply: by the anterior rami of the T7–L1 (T7 innervates the epigastrium, T10 the umbilicus, L1 the inguinal ligament).
    - Arterial supply: by branches of the superior and inferior epigastric arteries (which anastomose within the rectus sheath), intercostal and lumbar arteries.
    - Venous drainage: into the axillary and femoral veins, with few small paraumbilical veins draining into the portal vein.
    - Lymphatic drainage: into axillary and superficial inguinal nodes.
2. Superficial fascia, divided into a superficial fatty layer (Camper's fascia) and a deep membranous layer (Scarpa's fascia).
3. Muscles and their fasciae (and rectus sheath)
    - External oblique
    - Internal oblique
    - Transversus abdominis
    - Rectus abdominis
    - Pyramidalis
4. Preperitoneal fat.
5. Parietal peritoneum.

The rectus sheath

Each rectus sheath is formed by the aponeuroses of three lateral abdominal muscles (external oblique, internal oblique and transversus abdominis) on either side and the two sheaths are separated by the linea alba. The rectus sheath has different configuration above and below the level of the anterior superior iliac spine.

Between the costal margin and the anterior superior iliac spine

The external oblique aponeurosis passes anterior (superficial) to the rectus muscle. Under the external oblique lies the internal oblique muscle, whose aponeurosis splits in two layers, one that passes anterior and one posterior to the rectus, enclosing the muscle. Further deep is the

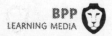

aponeurosis of the transversus abdominis (posterior to the rectus), the transversalis fascia, some pre-peritoneal fat and the parietal peritoneum.

Between the anterior superior iliac spine and pubis

The anterior wall of rectus sheath is formed by the aponeurosis of all three muscles and behind the rectus muscle lies only the transversalis fascia, fat and peritoneum. This curved line marking the lower posterior border of rectus sheath is known as the *arcuate line* (of Douglas) and at this level the inferior epigastric vessels enter the rectus sheath.

Contents of the rectus sheath

- The rectus abdominis and pyramidalis muscles.
- The anterior rami of lower six thoracic nerves.
- The superior and inferior epigastric vessels.

The inguinal canal

Oblique slit-like space above and parallel to the medial half of the inguinal ligament, bounded:

- Laterally by the deep (internal) inguinal ring, a defect in the transversalis fascia, at the midpoint of the inguinal ligament.
- Medially by the superficial (external) inguinal ring, a triangular aperture in the external oblique aponeurosis, 1–2cm above the pubic tubercle.
- Inferiorly (floor): the upper surface of the inguinal ligament and lacunar ligament medially.
- Superiorly (roof): Internal oblique and transversus abdominis fibres.
- Anterior wall: external oblique aponeurosis, reinforced laterally by internal oblique fibres.
- Posterior wall: Transversalis fascia, reinforced medially by the conjoint tendon.
- Contents: Ilioinguinal nerve and spermatic cord in males or the round ligament of the uterus in females.

Three layers of fascia
Internal spermatic fascia (from transversalis fascia)
Cremasteric fascia (from internal oblique and transversus abdominis)
External spermatic fascia (from external oblique muscle)
Three arteries
Testicular (from aorta)
Cremasteric (from inferior epigastric)
Artery of the vas (from the inferior vesical artery)
Three nerves
Nerve to the cremaster (from genitofemoral)
Sympathetic fibres and
The ilioinguinal nerve (runs on the cord, it is not part of it)
Three other structures
Vas deferens
Pampiniform plexus of veins (right vein drains into IVC, left into left renal vein)
Lymphatics draining into aortic lymph nodes

Table 1.23. Contents of the spermatic cord

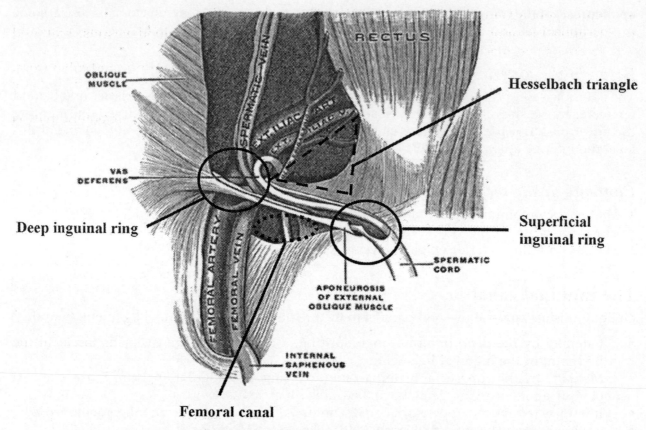

Figure 1.18. Basic anatomy of the groin area
Based on Gray H (1918) Anatomy of the Human Body, 20th edition, Lea & Febiger, Philadelphia
(*This image is in the public domain because its copyright has expired. This applies worldwide.*)

The gastrointestinal tract

The gastrointestinal (GI) tract is divided into three regions during its embryologic development, the foregut, midgut, and hindgut.

	Borders	Organs	Arterial supply
Foregut	From the pharynx, to the ampulla of Vater	Oesophagus, stomach, upper duodenum, liver, gallbladder, and pancreas	Coeliac artery
Midgut	From ampulla of Vater to the proximal two-thirds of the transverse colon	Lower duodenum, jejunum, ileum, caecum, appendix, ascending colon, and proximal two-thirds of the transverse colon	Superior mesenteric artery
Hindgut	From the distal third of the transverse colon, to the upper part of the anal canal	Distal third of the transverse colon, descending colon, sigmoid colon, rectum, and upper part of the anal canal	Inferior mesenteric artery

Table 1.24. Classification of abdominal GI tract based on embryologic development

The oesophagus

Morphology

The oesophagus is a muscular tube 20–25 cm in length, starting in the neck at the lower border of the cricoid cartilage (C6 vertebra) and ending by opening in the stomach (T11 vertebra). It is divided into a cervical, a thoracic and an abdominal portion. The oesophagus consists of the following layers:

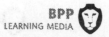

- Mucosa: non-keratinised stratified squamous epithelium.
- Lamina propria: a loose network of connective tissue with blood vessels, scattered lymphocytes, macrophages and plasma cells.
- Muscularis mucosae: a thin layer of circular muscle between lamina propria and submucosa.
- Submucosa: a dense network of connective tissue containing blood vessels, lymphatic channels, Meissner's nerve plexus and oesophageal glands.
- Muscularis propria: an inner circular layer containing the Auerbach's myenteric plexus and outer longitudinal layer of muscles.
- Adventitia/Fibrous coat – the oesophagus lacks a serosal layer.

Blood supply

The arterial supply, venous and lymphatic drainage is summarised below (Table 1.25).

Oesophageal portion	Arterial supply	Venous drainage	Lymphatic drainage
Cervical	Inferior thyroid artery	Brachiocephalic vein	Deep cervical nodes
Thoracic	Oesophageal branches of aorta	Azygous vein	Posterior mediastinal nodes
Abdominal	Oesophageal branches of left gastric artery	Left gastric vein	Left gastric nodes (this drains in coeliac nodes)

Table 1.25. Blood supply and lymphatic drainage of the oesophagus

Submucosal oesophageal tumours have a substantial risk of lymph node metastases. Local lymph node invasion occurs early and quickly because the lymphatics in the oesophagus are located in the lamina propria, in contrast to the rest of the gastrointestinal tract, in which they are located in the submucosa.

The stomach

The stomach is a muscular, hollow, dilated part of the alimentary canal involved in the digestion of food, following mastication. It secretes protein-digesting enzymes (pepsin) and acid (hydrochloric acid with pH ranging between 1 and 2) that are mixed with food; this mixture of partially digested food (*chyme*) is then transferred to the duodenum.

Morphology

The stomach has three parts. The uppermost part is the cardia; the middle and largest part consists of the body and fundus; and the distal portion, the pylorus, connects to the duodenum. These anatomic zones have distinct histologic features. The cardia contains predominantly mucin-secreting cells. The fundus contains mucoid cells, chief cells, and parietal cells. The pylorus is composed of mucus-producing cells and endocrine cells. The stomach wall consists of five layers: the mucosa, submucosa, the muscularis layer, the subserosal layer, and the serosal layer.

Important relations

The peritoneum of the greater sac covers the anterior surface of the stomach. A portion of the lesser sac drapes posteriorly over the stomach. The gastroesophageal junction has limited or no serosal covering. The right portion of the anterior gastric surface is adjacent to the left lobe

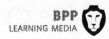

of the liver and the anterior abdominal wall. The left portion of the stomach (anteriorly to posteriorly) is adjacent to the diaphragm, spleen, the left adrenal gland, the superior portion of the left kidney, the ventral portion of the pancreas, and the transverse colon. The lesser omentum extends from the lesser curve of the stomach to the liver and the greater omentum is connected to the greater curve of the stomach.

Blood supply

The arterial supply of the stomach is from:

* The left gastric artery (from the coeliac axis)
* The right gastric artery (from the common hepatic artery)
* The right gastro-epiploic (from the gastroduodenal artery)
* The left gastro-epiploic (from the splenic artery)
* The short gastric arteries (from the splenic artery)

Venous drainage: the stomach drains either directly or indirectly into the portal vein.

* Short gastric veins from the fundus to the splenic vein
* Left gastroepiploic along greater curvature to superior mesenteric vein
* Right gastroepiploic from the right end of greater curvature to superior mesenteric vein
* Left gastric vein from the lesser curvature of the stomach to the portal vein
* Right gastric vein from the lesser curvature of the stomach to the portal vein

The lymphatic drainage takes place into four groups of nodes, the hepatic group, the subpyloric group, the gastric group and the pancreaticolienal group. The final group of nodes that receive lymph from the stomach is the preaortic (coeliac) nodes located around the coeliac trunk.

Innervation

Parasympathetic:

* Preganglionic neurons from right (posterior vagal trunk) and left (anterior vagal trunk) vagus nerves.
* Postganglionic neurons are very short and lie within the wall of the stomach.

Sympathetic:

* Preganglionic fibres: mainly from the thoracic splanchnic nerves.
* Postganglionic fibres arise in the ganglia of the coeliac plexus.

The small bowel

The small bowel is the longest part of the alimentary canal and consists of the duodenum, jejunum and ileum.

The duodenum

Morphology

It is C-shaped and approximately 25cm long. Morphologically it is divided into four parts, all but the first part, retroperitoneal.

1. First part or duodenal bulb: It is the continuation of the pylorus and runs transversely.
2. Second part: It runs vertically in front of the hilum of the right kidney and contains the duodenal papilla which is the site of entry of the common bile duct and pancreatic duct at the ampulla of Vater.

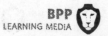

3. Third part: It runs horizontally below the pancreas.
4. Fourth part: It runs upward to the duodenojejunal junction (DJ flexure) which is connected to the right crus of the diaphragm by the ligament of Treitz.

Blood supply

Arterial supply from:
- The superior pancreaticoduodenal artery (from the gastroduodenal artery).
- The inferior pancreaticoduodenal artery (from the superior mesenteric artery).

Venous drainage: into the portal and superior mesenteric vein.
Lymphatic drainage: to the coeliac and superior mesenteric nodes.

The jejunum and ileum
Morphology

The total length of jejunum and ileum is about 6.5m, of which the proximal 2.5m is the jejunum and the distal 4m is the ileum. The jejunum begins at the duodenojejunal junction and the ileum ends at the ileocaecal valve. They are slung by the mesentery that arises from the posterior abdominal wall (root of the mesentery) and are very mobile.

Blood supply

Arterial supply: from branches (vasa recta) arising from arterial arcades within the mesentery which originate from the superior mesenteric artery. The lower part if the ileum is supplied by the ileocolic artery.

Venous drainage: into the superior mesenteric vein.
Lymphatic drainage: into the superior mesenteric nodes.

Main function of the small bowel: chemical digestion and absorption of nutrients

Absorption of the majority of nutrients takes place in the jejunum, except from iron (absorbed in the duodenum), vitamin B12 and bile salts (absorbed in the terminal ileum). Water and lipids are absorbed by passive diffusion throughout the small intestine. Sodium bicarbonate is absorbed by active transport and glucose and amino acid co-transport, whereas fructose is absorbed by facilitated diffusion.

The large intestine

The large intestine extends from the ileocaecal valve to the anus and is about 1.5m long. The intestinal wall has three longitudinal muscle bands, the *taeniae coli* that converge on the base of appendix. Along the sides of the taeniae, there are tags of peritoneum filled with fat, called epiploic appendages (or appendices epiploicae).

The large intestine comprises the caecum and appendix vermicularis, the ascending, transverse, descending and sigmoid colon and the rectum.

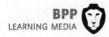

The caecum

The caecum is a blind cul-de-sac, about 6cm long, that lies in the right iliac fossa below the level of ileocaecal valve. It is covered by peritoneum, with the peritoneal folds creating the superior ileocaecal fossa, inferior ileocaecal fossa and the retrocaecal fossa. Its arterial supply originates from the anterior and posterior caecal arteries, branches of the ileocolic artery of the superior mesenteric artery.

The vermiform appendix

It hangs off the caecum and opens into it about 2cm below the ileocaecal opening, with average length about 10cm. It is covered in peritoneum and has a short mesentery known as the mesoappendix. It contains a large amount of lymphoid tissue and its base is attached to the postero-medial surface of the caecum, whereas the tip can be found in various positions including:

- Into the pelvis related to the right pelvic wall.
- Behind the caecum in the retrocaecal fossa.
- Projecting upward along the lateral side of the caecum.
- In front or behind the terminal ileum.

Its arterial supply is from the appendicular artery, a branch of the posterior caecal artery.

Blood supply of the large intestine

Arterial supply

- Caecum: from the anterior and posterior caecal arteries, branches of the ileocolic artery.
- Appendix: from appendicular artery, branch of the posterior caecal artery.
- Ascending colon: from the ileocolic and right colic arteries.
- Proximal transverse colon: from the middle colic artery.
- Distal transverse colon: from the superior left colic artery.
- Descending and sigmoid colon: from the inferior left colic artery.
- The ileocolic, right and middle colic arteries are branches of the superior mesenteric artery.
- The superior and inferior left colic arteries are branches of the inferior mesenteric artery.
- Anastomosis of branches of all the above arteries forms a vascular arcade running close to the bowel wall, the *marginal artery*.

Venous and lymphatic drainage

They follow the arterial supply, with the veins eventually draining into the portal venous system.

Good knowledge of the blood supply to the colon is necessary for optimum surgical and oncological results in colon resections (see also Chapter 2 – *Surgical Pathology – Colorectal Pathology – Colorectal cancer*). A successful anastomosis with minimal risk of anastomotic leak largely relies on adequate blood supply to the approximated segments of the bowel. Moreover, in cancer surgery the aim is to achieve regional lymphadenectomy; at least 12 nodes must be assessed in the surgical specimen for optimum staging and determination of the need for adjuvant therapy, which also relies on good knowledge of the lymphatic drainage of the bowel.

The rectum
Morphology

The rectum is the final straight portion of the large intestine, approximately 15cm long. It begins at the confluence of the three taeniae coli of the sigmoid colon (at about the level of third sacral vertebra) and ends at the anal canal. It is intraperitoneal at its proximal and anterior end, and extraperitoneal at its distal and posterior end. It has an outer longitudinal and inner circular muscle coat. Its mucous membrane forms three transverse folds.

Blood supply

The arterial supply of the rectum derives from the:

- Superior rectal artery, from the inferior mesenteric artery.
- Middle rectal artery, from the internal iliac artery.
- Inferior rectal artery, from the internal pudendal artery.

Its venous drainage corresponds to arterial supply:

- Superior rectal vein drains into inferior mesenteric vein.
- Middle rectal vein drains into internal iliac vein.
- Inferior rectal vein drains into internal pudendal vein.

The lymphatic drainage of the rectum is served by the pararectal nodes.

Important relations

Important relations of the rectum:

- Anteriorly: the rectovesical pouch and bladder in males. Uterus, cervix and vagina in females.
- Laterally: the ischial tuberosity and spine.
- Posteriorly: the sacrum and coccyx.

The liver
Morphology and topography

Wedge-shaped, weighing about 1.5kg, the liver is the largest solid organ in the body. It occupies the right hypochondrium, is protected by ribs and costal cartilages, and extends into the epigastrium. It is supported in this position by the inferior vena cava, the suprahepatic veins,

Caudate lobe	I
Left lateral superior	II
Left lateral inferior	III
Left medial	IV
Right anterior inferior	V
Right anterior superior	VIII
Right posterior inferior	VI
Right posterior superior	VII

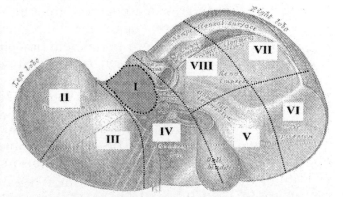

Figure 1.19. Liver segment anatomy (interior surface of liver) modified according to Couinaud, 1957
Based on Gray H (1918) Anatomy of the Human Body, 20th edition, Lea & Febiger, Philadelphia
(This image is in the public domain because its copyright has expired. This applies worldwide.)

the round and coronary ligaments, peritoneal folds and the positive intra-abdominal pressure. It is surrounded by the fibrous Glisson's capsule.

The peritoneal attachments of the liver are:

1. The falciform ligament ascends from the umbilicus, contains the ligamentum teres (round ligament), remnant of the obliterated umbilical vein.
2. The left and right triangular ligaments secure the two sides of the liver to the diaphragm.
3. The coronary ligaments extend from the triangular ligaments anteriorly on the liver; the right coronary ligament also extends from the right undersurface of the liver to the peritoneum overlying the right kidney, thereby anchoring the liver to the right retroperitoneum.
4. The area devoid of peritoneum is known as the 'bare area'.
5. Centrally and just to the left of the gallbladder fossa, the liver attaches via the hepatoduodenal and the gastrohepatic ligaments.
6. The hepatoduodenal ligament contains the common bile duct, hepatic artery, and portal vein and extends upwards to the porta hepatis.

The porta hepatis is found on the posterior-inferior surface, with free edge of lesser omentum attaching to its margins and contains the right and left hepatic ducts, the right and left branches of hepatic artery, the portal vein and hepatic lymph nodes.

The anatomy of the liver is classified into morphological and functional.

- Morphologically, the liver is divided into right and left lobes by the falciform ligament. The right lobe is further divided into the quadrate lobe and caudate lobes.
- Functionally, it is divided into eight segments based on the branching of the portal triads and hepatic veins, described by Couinaud (French surgeon and anatomist) in the early 1950s and bearing his name (Figure 1.19). The 'functional' right and left hemilivers are separated by an imaginary line running from the medial aspect of the gallbladder fossa to the inferior vena cava, running parallel with the fissure of the round ligament (Cantlie line) that marks the course of the middle hepatic vein.

Blood supply

- The blood supply to the liver is dual; from the hepatic artery proper (25%) and the portal vein (75%).
  - The hepatic artery proper arises from the common hepatic artery, branch of the coeliac axis, although in 25% of individuals the anatomy is variable.
  - Portal vein (normal pressure 3–5 mmHg): formed by the confluence of the splenic vein and the superior mesenteric vein, with the inferior mesenteric vein usually draining into the splenic vein before the confluence. It traverses the porta hepatis before dividing into the left and right portal vein branches and drains the splanchnic blood from the stomach, pancreas, spleen, small intestine, and majority of the colon to the liver before returning to the systemic circulation.
- Venous drainage: by three hepatic veins (right, middle, and left) that pass obliquely through the liver to drain the blood to the suprahepatic IVC and eventually the right atrium.
- Biliary drainage: within the hepatoduodenal ligament lies the common bile duct (CBD, about 8cm long) that drains into second part of duodenum at the ampulla of Vater, with its terminal part surrounded by the sphincter of Oddi. The CBD gives off the cystic duct to the gallbladder and becomes the common hepatic duct (about 4cm long) before dividing into the right and left hepatic ducts. In general, the hepatic ducts follow the arterial branching pattern inside the liver.

- Lymph drainage: Via the perisinusoidal space of Disse and periportal clefts of Mall to larger lymphatics that drain to:
  - The hilar cystic duct lymph node (Calot's triangle node)
  - The common bile duct nodes
  - Hepatic artery nodes
  - Retropancreatic nodes
  - Coeliac lymph nodes
  - Cephalad to the cardiophrenic lymph nodes

Innervation

- Parasympathetic: from the left vagus, which gives off the anterior hepatic branch, and the right vagus, which gives off the posterior hepatic branch.
- The sympathetic: from the greater thoracic splanchnic nerves and the coeliac ganglia (the function of these nerves is poorly understood, the denervated liver transplant allograft functions with normal capacity).

The gallbladder
Morphology and topography

A pear-shaped sac, about 7 to 10cm long, with an average normal capacity of 30 to 50ml, the gallbladder lies on the visceral surface of the liver. It is divided into fundus, body, infundibulum (Hartmann's pouch) and neck. The fundus projects from the inferior margin of the liver and comes into contact with the abdominal wall at level of tip of the ninth costal cartilage. The neck is funnel-shaped, continuous with the cystic duct. The fundus and the inferior surface of the gallbladder are covered by peritoneum, although, occasionally the gallbladder has a complete peritoneal covering, and is suspended in a mesentery off the inferior surface of the liver or, rarely, it is embedded deep inside the liver parenchyma (an intrahepatic gallbladder).

Blood supply

The arterial supply is from the cystic artery, a branch of the right hepatic artery. The course of the cystic artery may vary, but it nearly always is found within the hepatocystic triangle (triangle of Calot), bound by the cystic duct, common hepatic duct, and the liver margin. The cystic vein drains directly into the portal vein. Lymph drains into nodes at the neck of the gallbladder. Frequently a visible lymph node overlies the insertion of the cystic artery into the gallbladder wall.

Innervation

- Parasympathetic: from the vagus that supplies cholinergic fibres to the gallbladder, bile ducts, and the liver. The vagal branches also have peptide-containing nerves containing agents such as substance P, somatostatin, enkephalins, and vasoactive intestinal polypeptide.
- Sympathetic: from the coeliac plexus. Impulses from the liver, gallbladder, and the bile ducts pass by means of sympathetic afferent fibres through the splanchnic nerves and mediate the pain of biliary colic.

The pancreas
Morphology, topography and important relations

It is a gland with both exocrine and endocrine functions. The pancreas lies in the retroperitoneum, at L2 level, its length is 12–15cm, and it weighs 70–100g.

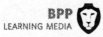

It is divided into:

- The head of pancreas that includes the uncinate process. This is a flattened structure, 2–3cm thick, attached to the second and third portions of the duodenum on the right. It emerges into the neck on the left. The border between head and neck is determined by insertion of the gastroduodenal artery. The superior and inferior pancreaticoduodenal arteries anastomose between the duodenum and the right lateral border.
- The neck of pancreas. Measuring 2.5 cm in length, this straddles the superior mesenteric vein (SMV) and portal vein. Its antero-superior surface supports the pylorus. The superior mesenteric vessels emerge from the inferior border. Posteriorly, SMV and splenic vein confluence to form the portal vein.
- The body of pancreas. This is an elongated, long structure. The anterior surface is separated from the stomach by the lesser sac. The posterior surface is related to the aorta, left adrenal gland, left renal vessels and the upper third of the left kidney. The splenic vein runs embedded in the posterior surface. The inferior surface is covered by transverse mesocolon.
- The tail of pancreas. A narrow, short segment, lying at the level of the T12 vertebra, ending within the splenic hilum. It lies in the splenophrenic ligament and is related anteriorly to the splenic flexure of colon.

The pancreas has two pancreatic ducts:

- The main duct (Wirsung) runs the entire length of the pancreas and joins the CBD at the ampulla of Vater. It is 2–4mm in diameter, with 20 secondary branches.
- The lesser duct (Santorini) drains the superior portion of the head and empties separately into the second portion of the duodenum.

Blood supply

Arterial supply by the:

- Superior pancreaticoduodenal artery (SPDA, which divides into anterior and posterior branches), branch of the gastroduodenal artery (from the common hepatic artery).
- Inferior pancreaticoduodenal artery (IPDA, which divides into anterior and posterior branches) of the superior mesenteric artery.
- Anterior collateral arcade between the anterosuperior and anteroinferior PDA.
- Posterior collateral arcade between posterosuperior and posteroinferior PDA.
- The body and tail are supplied by splenic artery by about ten branches, the three biggest of which are:
  - Dorsal pancreatic artery
  - Pancreatica Magna (midportion of body)
  - Caudal pancreatic artery (tail)

Venous drainage of the pancreas: It follows the arterial supply ultimately draining into the portal vein.

Lymphatic drainage: There is a rich periacinar network that drain into five nodal groups; the superior, anterior, inferior, posterior and splenic nodes.

Innervation

- Parasympathetic fibres: from the vagus, they stimulate both exocrine and endocrine secretion.
- Sympathetic fibres from the splanchnic nerves have a predominantly inhibitory effect.
- Peptidergic neurons that secrete amines and peptides (somatostatin, vasoactive intestinal peptide, calcitonin gene-related peptide, and galanin).
- There is a rich afferent sensory fibre network transmitting pancreatic pain; ganglionectomy or coeliac ganglion blockade is used to interrupt these somatic fibres aiming to treat chronic pain.

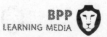

Histology and function
Exocrine pancreas

It consists of two major components, the acinar cells and ducts, and constitutes 80% to 90% of the pancreatic mass.

- The acinar cells secrete the digestive enzymes. A total of 20 to 40 acinar cells coalesce into a unit called the acinus. The centroacinar cell is responsible for fluid and electrolyte secretion by the pancreas.
- The ductular system is a network of conduits that carry the exocrine secretions into the duodenum. The interlobular ducts contribute to fluid and electrolyte secretion along with the centroacinar cells.

Endocrine pancreas

It accounts for only 2% of the pancreatic mass. It consists of nests of cells, the islets of Langerhans that contain four major cell types:

- Alpha (A) cells secrete glucagon
- Beta (B) cells secrete insulin
- Delta (D) cells secrete somatostatin
- F cells secrete pancreatic polypeptide

The pancreas secretes 500–800ml of digestive juices per 24 hours containing *amylase, lipase and proteases (trypsinogen, chymotrypsin, elastase, carboxypeptidase, and phospholipase)*. The amylase is the only pancreatic enzyme secreted in an active form. Lipases emulsify and hydrolyse lipids in the presence of bile salts. Proteases are secreted as pro-enzymes that are activated in the intestinal lumen. The pancreatic juice also contains *water* and *electrolytes* (especially *bicarbonate*) secreted by the centroacinar and intercalated duct cells.

Secretion of enzymes by pancreatic gland cells is stimulated by the hormone *cholecystokinin* (released from the wall of the duodenum). The hormone *secretin* (released from the duodenal mucosa in response to a duodenal luminal pH < 3) results in the pancreas making bicarbonate rich fluid.

The spleen
Morphology, topography and important relations

The spleen lies in the left hypochondrium between the fundus of the stomach and the diaphragm, opposite the 9th, 10th and 11th ribs, with the long axis parallel to the 10th rib.

It weighs 100–150g and usually cannot be palpated. It consists of the white pulp (lymphatic tissue) and the red pulp (reticular cells and sinuses).

It has two ends (medial and lateral), two borders (superior with a notch and inferior) and two surfaces:

- Diaphragmatic: Convex and related to the diaphragm which separates it from the left pleura, lung , 9th, 10th, 11th ribs and intercostal muscles.
- Visceral: Directed towards the abdominal cavity and carries four impressions:
  - Gastric impression: related to the back of the upper part of the stomach. The hilum is in its lower part and presents a linear series of 5–6 holes which transmit the terminal branches of the splenic artery with the corresponding veins, nerves and lymphatics.

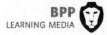

- Renal impression: related to the upper part of the left kidney, close to the inferior border.
- Colic impression: related to the splenic flexure of the colon close to the lateral end.
- Pancreatic impression: related to the tail of the pancreas, below the lateral part of the hilum.

Ligaments of the spleen:

- Gastrosplenic ligament: transmits the *vasa brevia* (short gastric vessels).
- Leinorenal ligament: transmits the splenic vessels, nerves, lymphatics and tail of the pancreas.
- Phrenocolic ligament: between the left colic flexure and the diaphragm.
- Colicosplenic ligament.

Blood supply

Arterial supply: by the splenic artery and short gastric arteries.

Venous drainage: via the splenic vein that receives the inferior mesenteric vein and then the superior mesenteric vein behind the neck of the pancreas to form the portal vein.

Splenic functions

1. Immune function:
   a. Processes foreign antigens.
   b. IgM production.
   c. Produces opsonins such as tuftsin and properdin that make bacteria more susceptible to phagocytosis.
2. Filter function for bacteria.
3. Culling: Removal of effete platelets and red cells.
4. Pitting: Removal of particulate inclusions from the red cells.
5. Iron reutilisation: Return iron to plasma during culling.
6. Pooling: 30–40% of platelets are sequestered normally. In splenomegaly, up to 80% are sequestered (thrombocytopenia).
7. Reservoir function of blood in animals.
8. Haematopoiesis: up to 5th month of intrauterine life.

The abdominal aorta

The abdominal aorta is the largest artery in the body, originating from the left ventricle of the heart and extending down to the abdomen, where it branches off into the common iliac arteries. It distributes oxygenated blood to all parts of the body through the systemic circulation.

The aorta is usually divided into three segments / sections:
- Ascending aorta (between the heart and the arch of aorta).
- Arch of aorta (inverted 'U' shape).
- Descending aorta (from the aortic arch to the point where it divides into the common iliac arteries), further subdivided into:
  - Thoracic aorta – the half of the descending aorta above the diaphragm
  - Abdominal aorta – the half of the descending aorta below the diaphragm

Branches of the abdominal aorta (Figure 1.20 and Tables 1.26, 1.27, 1.28)

The branches of the abdominal aorta are classified into unpaired visceral, paired visceral, parietal (paired) and terminal (Tables 1.26, 1.27, 1.28).

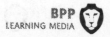

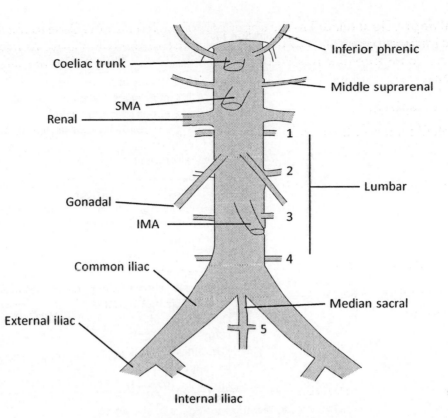

Figure 1.20. Branches of the abdominal aorta

Coeliac axis	Superior mesenteric artery	Inferior mesenteric artery
Left gastric • Oesophageal branches	**Inferior pancreaticoduodenal**	**Left colic**
Splenic • Pancreatic branches (greater, dorsal) • Short gastric • Left gastro-epiploic	**Intestinal** • Jejunal • Ileal • Arcades • Vasa recta	**Sigmoid** **Superior rectal**

Common hepatic
• Proper hepatic
  – Cystic
• Right gastric
• Gastroduodenal
  – Right gastro-epiploic
  – Superior pancreaticoduodenal
  – Supraduodenal
	Ileocolic
	• Colic
	• Anterior caecal
	• Posterior caecal
	• Ileal branch
	• Appendicular
	Right colic
	Middle colic
		Marginal

Table 1.26. Unpaired visceral branches of the aorta

Paired visceral branches	Parietal branches
Middle suprarenal **Renal** • Inferior suprarenal • Ureteral **Gonadal**	**Inferior phrenic** • Superior suprarenal **Lumbar branches (4)** **Median sacral** **Coccygeal**

Table 1.27. Paired visceral and parietal branches of the aorta

Common iliac arteties	
External iliac	**Internal iliac**
Inferior epigastric • Cremasteric (male) • Round ligament (female) **Deep circumflex iliac** **Femoral**	**Obturator** (gives anterior and posterior branches) **Middle rectal** (gives a vaginal branch) **Uterine** (female) **Vaginal** (female) **or inferior vesical** (male) **Inferior gluteal** **Internal pudendal** • Inferior rectal • Perineal − Posterior scrotal (male) or labial (female) • Artery to the bulb of penis (male) or vestibule (female) • Urethral • Deep artery of the penis (male) or clitoris (female) • Dorsal artery of the penis (male) or clitoris (female) **Iliolumbar (lumbar, iliac)** **Lateral sacral** **Superior gluteal** **Umbilical** • Superior vesical • Artery to ductus deferens (male)

Table 1.28. Terminal branches of the aorta

The urogenital tract

The reproductive and urinary systems are grouped together because of their proximity to each other, their common embryological origin (from the intermediate mesoderm) and the use of common pathways (like the male urethra).

The kidneys

Morphology and topography

The kidneys are paired solid organs, sized 11cm × 6cm × 3cm, usually situated within the retroperitoneum on either side of the spine, largely covered by costal margins, with their position changing during respiration. The right kidney lies slightly lower than left (levels of L1–L3 and T12–L3 vertebrae respectively). They are surrounded by perinephric fat and fascia (Gerota's fascia). A thin fibroelastic capsule encases the renal parenchyma.

The hilum of the kidney is a depression on the medial surface of each kidney, which opens into the renal sinus, a central space surrounded by the renal parenchyma that contains the urinary collecting structures and renal vessels.

Histology and function of kidneys

The kidney has a pale outer region (cortex) and a darker inner region (medulla). The medulla is divided into 8–18 conical regions (renal pyramids). The base of each pyramid starts at the corticomedullary border, and the apex ends in the renal papilla which merges to form the renal pelvis and then on to form the ureter.

In humans, the renal pelvis is divided into two or three major calyces, which in turn divide into further minor calyces. The walls of the calyces, pelvis and ureters are lined with smooth muscle that can contract to force urine towards the bladder by peristalsis.

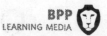

The cortex and the medulla are made up of nephrons, the functional units of the kidney (1.3 million nephrons in each kidney), responsible for ultrafiltration of the blood and reabsorption or excretion of products in the subsequent filtrate.

Each nephron is made up of:

- The glomerulus: A filtering unit, forming 125ml/min of filtrate as blood is filtered through this sieve-like structure (uncontrolled).
- The proximal convoluted tubule: Controlled absorption of glucose, sodium, and other solutes.
- The loop of Henle: Responsible for concentration and dilution of urine by utilising a counter-current multiplying mechanism.
- The distal convoluted tubule: Responsible, along with the collecting duct that it joins, for absorbing water back into the body.

Right kidney	Left kidney

Anterior
    Suprarenal gland
    Liver
    Second part of duodenum
    Hepatic flexure of colon
	Anterior
	    Suprarenal gland
	    Spleen
	    Stomach
	    Pancreas
	    Splenic flexure of colon

Posterior
    Diaphragm
    Costodiaphragmatic recess of pleura
    Twelfth rib
    Psoas muscle
	Posterior
	    Diaphragm
	    Costodiaphragmatic recess of pleura
	    Twelfth rib
	    Psoas muscle

Table 1.29. Important relations of the kidneys

Blood supply

- Arterial supply is by the renal artery arising directly from the aorta.
- Venous drainage is via the renal vein into the inferior vena cava.
- Lymph drains to the para-aortic lymph nodes.

Innervation

The nerve supply is the renal sympathetic plexus. The afferent fibres that travel through the renal plexus enter the spinal cord in the 10th, 11th, and 12th thoracic nerves.

The suprarenal glands (adrenals)

The suprarenal glands are paired glands lying superomedial to the kidneys, surrounded by perirenal fat and contained within the Gerota's fascia. The right suprarenal gland lies between the superior pole of the right kidney and the IVC and the left suprarenal gland on the superomedial border of the left kidney.

Blood supply

The arterial supply stems from branches of the renal arteries, the inferior phrenic arteries and the aorta. Regarding the venous drainage, the left suprarenal vein drains into the left renal vein, whereas the right suprarenal vein drains directly into the IVC. Lymph drains to the para-aortic lymph nodes.

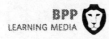

Right ureter	Left ureter
Anterior	**Anterior**
Duodenum	Pelvic colon
Terminal ileum	Left colic vessels
Right colic and ileocolic vessels	Left testicular / ovarian vessels
Right testicular/ovarian vessels	
Posterior	**Posterior**
Psoas muscle	Psoas muscle
Bifurcation of right common iliac artery	Bifurcation of left common iliac artery

Table 1.30. Relations of ureters (very important in colonic resections)

The ureters

Morphology and topography (course)

The ureters are paired, hollow smooth muscular conduits lined by transitional epithelium, about 25cm long. They actively transport urine into the bladder.

They lie in the retroperitoneum, descending from the pelvi-ureteric junction (PUJ) on psoas major (in the line of the tips of the transverse processes of the lumbar vertebrae) down to the pelvic brim; there they cross the bifurcation of the common iliac artery over the sacro-iliac joint. In the pelvis they run over the external iliac artery and then continue down the pelvic sidewall anterior to the internal iliac artery and anteriorly at the level of the ischial spine to enter the base of the bladder.

Each ureter has three constrictions along its course: at the pelvi-ureteric junction (PUJ), at the level where ureter crosses the pelvic brim and at the vesico-ureteric junction (VUJ).

Blood supply

Arterial supply:

- Proximal ureter: from the ureteric branch of the renal artery.
- Mid portion: from an anastomosis of the gonadal artery with branches from the common iliac.
- Distal ureter: from branches of the inferior and superior vesical arteries.

Venous drainage follows the arterial supply.

The bladder

Morphology and topography

The bladder is a hollow muscular organ, pyramidal in shape, consisting of:

- An apex, anteriorly, lying behind the pubis bone, attached to the umbilicus by the median umbilical ligament (remnant of the foetal urachus).
- A triangular base, posteriorly, related to the vagina and cervix (female) or the rectum, vas deferens and seminal vesicles (male).
- A superior surface, covered by pelvic peritoneum.
- Two inferolateral surfaces, supported by the levator ani.
- The bladder neck, where the inferolateral surfaces meet the base.

The two ureters each insert obliquely into the bladder postero-inferiorly, approximately 5cm apart, and the ureteric orifices are joined by the interureteric ridge. With the urethral orifice this forms a triangular area known as the trigone. The bladder neck fuses with the prostate in men.

The bladder has two sphincters:

- Internal sphincter – smooth muscle at bladder neck
- External sphincter – voluntary muscles distal to the internal sphincter

Blood supply

Arterial supply:

- From the superior, middle and inferior vesical arteries, from the hypogastric branch of the internal iliac artery.
- From the obturator and inferior gluteal arteries.
- From the uterine and vaginal arteries (females).

Venous drainage into the corresponding veins.

Lymphatic drainage is to the paravesical, hypogastric (internal iliac), the iliac and para-aortic nodes.

Innervation

1. Motor supply, autonomic:
   - Sympathetic: from T10–L2 (inhibitory). They relax the detrusor smooth muscle and contract the smooth muscle of the involuntary sphincteric mechanisms at the bladder neck.
   - Parasympathetic: from S2–S4 (motor to the detrusor muscle). They contract the detrusor muscle and relax the involuntary sphincteric mechanisms.
2. Sensory supply, parasympathetic.

Functions of the bladder

- A low-pressure reservoir for the storage of urine (capacity in the adult is approximately 500 ml).
- To expel the urine at high pressure at an appropriate time and under voluntary control via the urethra.

The prostate

Morphology and topography

It is a fibromuscular and glandular organ, ovoid in shape, of walnut-size (weighing 20g). The prostate lies behind the pubic symphysis, enclosed within a capsule of strong connective tissue. It surrounds the beginning of the urethra in men and has five lobes (anterior, posterior, middle and two lateral lobes).

Relations

- Above: Continuous with the base of the bladder.
- Below: The apex sits on the sphincter urethrae in the deep perineal pouch.
- Posteriorly: It is separated from the rectum by Denonvillier's fascia.
- Anteriorly: It is separated from the pubis by extraperitoneal fat.

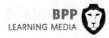

- The ejaculatory ducts formed by the fusion of the vas deferens and seminal vesicles enter the upper posterior part of the prostate and open into the urethra.

Blood supply

Arterial supply: From the inferior vesical artery.

Venous plexus: Surrounded by prostatic venous plexus.

Lymphatic drainage: The primary lymphatic vessels from the prostate gland drain into the regional lymph nodes of the true pelvis, including the internal iliac (hypogastric), obturator, sacral, peri-vesical, and external iliac lymph nodes. (Occasionally, in prostate cancer, metastases go beyond regional lymph nodes and involve distant lymph nodes outside the true pelvis, such as the deep and superficial inguinal, common iliac, retro-peritoneal (aortocaval nodes), supra-clavicular, cervical and scalene nodes.)

The male urethra

The male urethra is about 20cm in length and is divided into three parts.

- The prostatic urethra (about 4cm in length): the longitudinal elevation on the posterior wall is the urethral crest; in the middle there is an elevation, the verumontanum (the prostatic utricle opens into it and the ejaculatory ducts are on each side of it).
- The membranous urethra (about 2cm in length): the narrowest part of the urethra; it traverses the external urethral sphincter.
- The spongy urethra (about 15cm in length): traverses the corpus spongiosum of the penis. Its narrowest part is the external urethral orifice.

Further reading

- Gastrotraining (2011): Website managed by UK-based gastroenterology Consultants directed at Gastroenterology trainees and professionals. Available at: www.gastrotraining.com
- The Anatomy Lesson (2011): *Study of human anatomy*. Available at: www.wesnorman.com
- California State University (2011) *Dept of Anth: Skull Module*. Available at: www.csuchico.edu/anth/Module/skull.html
- Gateway Community College (2011) *Skull Anatomy Tutorial*. Available at: www.gwc.maricopa.edu/class/bio201/skull/skulltt.htm
- Wesley Norman (2011) *Skeleton of the Larynx*. Available at: www.wesnorman.com/lesson11.htm
- The Electronic Textbook of Hand Surgery (2007). Available at: www.eatonhand.com

Chapter 2
Surgical pathology

Overview

In the stations of surgical pathology the clinical background knowledge of candidates is examined. Emphasis is on the understanding of basic epidemiology, aetiology and clinical manifestations of common surgical diseases, along with the ability of candidates to compile a list of differential diagnoses and formulate a diagnostic work-up plan. Although the new MRCS Part B (OSCE) does not contain a separate operative surgery section, sound knowledge of operative procedures relevant to the management of common surgical conditions is required. Revision of basic principles of histopathology and immunology is also important for this station, particularly of those subjects related to surgical malignancy, inflammation and infection. Please note that the surgical pathology content of this book is not exhausted in this chapter only. We chose to attach more topics elsewhere in the text, wherever appropriate, such as in the *Clinical examinations* chapter, in order to ensure meaningful continuity of the subjects and also simulate potential exam conditions. Candidates should not be surprised, for instance, if a brief anatomy question arises in the clinical examination station and vice versa!

Acute inflammation

Acute inflammation is the physiological response of the body to local injury, usually lasting as long as the stimulus is present.

Aetiological factors

- Endogenous, including hypersensitivity reactions (tuberculosis, parasites) and autoimmune conditions.
- Exogenous, including infections (pyogenic bacteria or viruses), chemical agents (such as acids), physical agents (such as ionising radiation or heat) and tissue necrosis following ischaemic infarction.

Clinical features of inflammation

- Local signs were initially described by Celsus with further signs added over time:
  - Calor – heat produced due to increased blood flow through the tissue.
  - Dolor – pain caused by stretching tissues and release of mediators such as bradykinin.
  - Rubor – redness caused by capillary dilatation.
  - Tumour – swelling resulting from excess interstitial fluid.
  - Functio laesa – loss of function due to oedema.

- Systemic signs: they are results of the overall acute phase response:
  - Pyrexia caused by the released endogenous pyrogens (macrophages and polymorphs).
  - Constitutional symptoms – weight loss, anorexia, malaise and nausea.
  - Reactive hyperplasia of reticuloendothelial system, lymphadenopathy, splenomegaly.
  - Anaemia – haemorrhagic inflammation, anaemia of chronic disease.
  - Secondary amyloidosis in long standing inflammation.

Phases of inflammation

Vascular phase

There is a triple response that correlates to the 'flush, flare and wheal' seen. Initially there is a transient *vasoconstriction*, followed by a prolonged period of *vasodilatation* of arterioles and venules, and finally with increased vascular permeability a zone of *oedema* develops due to accumulation of fluid within the extravascular space.

Exudative phase

With increased vascular permeability and an increase in the capillary hydrostatic pressure in inflammation, there is increased fluid transfer into the extravascular space. An *exudate* is a protein rich fluid (>30g/l) containing both immunoglobulins and factors of the coagulation system. Various cells and systems are stimulated by a cascade of events. Neutrophils initially emigrate into the interstitium by *margination* along the vessel wall, *adhesion* to the endothelial surface and *transmigration* between the endothelial cells (stimulated by leukotrienes and tumour necrosis factor). *Chemotaxis* (stimulated by leukotriene B and interleukin-8) directs the neutrophils to the initial injury site. At the site a process of degranulation releases lysosome granules (containing collagenase and elastase) which aid in phagocytosis of debris and micro-organisms. Lymphatics also aid in the removal of oedema fluid of the inflammatory exudate, thereby presenting specific antigens for recognition by lymphocytes at regional lymph nodes.

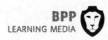

Mediators of inflammation

These are molecules participating in the processes of acute inflammation and are classified based on their source into *cellular* and *plasma-derived*. A summary of the mediators of inflammation and their origin is presented in Figure 2.1 and of the immune system cells and their function in Table 2.1.

The plasma-derived mediators of inflammation are made up of four major systems:

- Complement system: Enzymatic cascade of 20 proteins, activated during inflammation by cell necrosis and infection aiding with chemotaxis (C5a), opsonisation and phagocytosis (C3b, C4b).

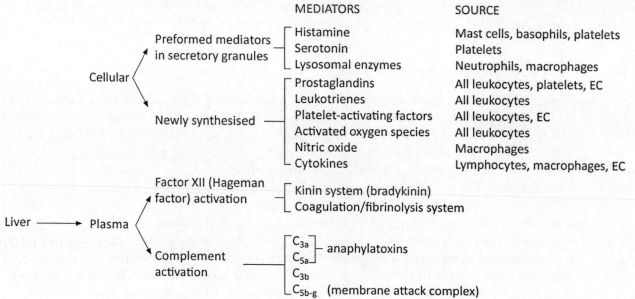

Figure 2.1. Mediators of inflammation, and source

- Coagulation system: This cascade of proteins leads to platelet aggregation and clot formation by the conversion of fibrinogen to fibrin. Activation of factors within this system in turn also activates the other kinin, complement and fibrinolytic systems.
- Kinin system: Stimulated by coagulation factor XII, causing conversion of prekallikrein to kallikrein which causes bradykinin to be released (from kininogen) responsible for vascular permeability and pain mediation.
- Fibrinolytic system: This negative feedback system releases plasmin which cleaves fibrin into degradation products, thereby limiting coagulation.

Specific forms of inflammation

- Serous: This form includes acute inflammation of serous cavities with substantial protein-rich (low cells) fluid.
- Suppurative: This form develops pus, a thick fluid containing liquefied tissue, organisms and dead neutrophils. Fibrous tissue can develop walling off the pus to form an *abscess*, or if develops within a hollow viscus an *empyema*.
- Haemorrhagic: This form accompanies either coagulopathy or a vascular injury. Acute haemorrhagic pancreatitis involves proteolytic digestion of the vessel wall.
- Fibrinous: Fibrinogen is found within the exudate and a layer of fibrinous coating develops within the cavity eg peritoneum, pericardium. The fibrin can develop into a membrane containing inflammatory cells as seen in *membranous inflammation* (diphtheria).

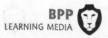

Cell type	Function and characteristics
Leukocytes	White blood cells. These are the cells which provide immunity, and they can be subdivided into three classes: Lymphocytes, Granulocytes and Monocytes.
Lymphocytes	Small white blood cells which are responsible for much of the work of the immune system. Lymphocytes can be divided into three classes: B cells, T cells and null cells.
B cells	B cells spend their entire *early* life in the bone marrow. Upon maturity, they travel throughout the blood and lymph looking for antigens with which they can interlock. Once a B cell has identified an antigen, it starts replicating itself. These cloned cells mature into antibody-manufacturing *plasma cells*.
Plasma cells	Specialised B cells which churn out antibodies – more than 2,000 per second. Most of these die after four to five days; however, a few survive to become *memory cells*.
Memory cells	Specialised B cells which grant the body the ability to manufacture more of a particular antibody as needed, in case a particular antigen is ever encountered again.
T cells	Unlike B cells, these cells leave the marrow at an early age and travel to the *thymus*, where they mature. Here they are imprinted with critical information for recognising 'self' and 'non-self' substances. Among the subclasses of T cells are *helper T cells* and *cytotoxic (or killer) T cells*.
Helper T cells	These cells travel through the blood and lymph, looking for antigens (such as those captured by *antigen-presenting cells*). Upon locating an antigen, they notify other cells to assist in combating the invader. This is sometimes done through the use of cytokines (or specifically, lymphokines) which help destroy target cells and stimulate the production of healthy new tissue (eg interferon).
Cytotoxic T cells	They are capable of inducing the death of infected somatic or tumour cells; they kill cells that are infected with viruses (or other pathogens), or are otherwise damaged or dysfunctional. Most cytotoxic T cells express T-cell receptors (TCRs) that can recognise a specific antigenic peptide bound to Class I MHC molecules, present on all nucleated cells, and a glycoprotein called CD8.
Granulocytes	Leukocytes (white blood cells) containing granules in the cytoplasm. They seem to act as a first line of defence, as they rush toward an infected area and engulf the offending microbes. Granulocytes kill microbes by digesting them with killer enzymes contained in small units called lysosomes.
Antigen-presenting cells	Cells with no antigen-specific receptors. They capture and process antigens, present them to T cell receptors. These cells include macrophages, dentritic cells and B cells.
Macrophages	Literally, 'large eaters.' These are large, long-lived phagocytes which capture foreign cells, digest them and present protein fragments (peptides) from these cells and manifest them on their exterior. In this manner, they present the antigens to the T cells. Macrophages are strategically located in lymphoid tissues, connective tissues and body cavities, where they are likely to encounter antigens. They also act as effector cells in cell-mediated immunity.
Mast cells	Cells concentrated within the respiratory and gastrointestinal tracts, and within the deep layers of the skin. These cells release histamine upon encountering certain antigens, thereby triggering an allergic reaction.
Basophils	Similar to mast cells, but distributed throughout the body. Like mast cells, basophils release histamine upon encountering certain antigens, thereby triggering an allergic reaction.
Dendritic cells	Mostly found in the skin and mucosal epithelium, where they are referred to as Langerhan's cells. Unlike macrophages, dendritic cells can also recognise viral particles as non-self.
Monocytes	Large, agranular leukocytes with relatively small, eccentric, oval or kidney-shaped nuclei.

Table 2.1. Summary of the cellular immune system

- Pseudomembranous: This specific form is mostly associated with *Clostridium difficile* infection causing superficial ulceration and inflammation and mucosal sloughing.
- Necrotising: Thrombosis and vascular occlusion can develop causing septic necrosis in cases such as gangrenous appendicitis.

Sequelae of acute inflammation

- Resolution: This describes complete restoration of the involved tissue and is more likely in cases of early removal of the causative agent and minimal injury, particularly in organs with good regenerative capacity.
- Suppuration: This is the formation of pus. Pus consists of both living and dead bacteria, cellular debris, neutrophils and liquefied tissue. The commonest causative organisms are from the Staphylococcus group. The collection of pus can become surrounded by a pyogenic membrane forming an abscess. Antibiotics can be ineffective at penetrating these abscesses and therefore drainage is the preferred method of treatment.
- Organisation: This describes replacement of the involved tissue with granulation tissue. This is more common in cases of large amounts of necrotic tissue or fibrin production. Capillaries grow into the inflammatory area and fibroblast proliferation is stimulated by tumour growth factors leading to fibrosis.
- Chronic inflammation: If the causative agent is not removed progression to chronic inflammation occurs.

Chronic inflammation and granulomatous disease
Differences between acute and chronic inflammation

The time over which inflammation occurs and *the type of cellular infiltrate* are the main distinguishing factors between acute and chronic inflammation. In chronic inflammation the predominant cells involved are lymphocytes, plasma cells and macrophages. Chronic inflammation may develop primarily, secondarily following an acute inflammatory process (persistent or recurrent), or, as a specific form of allograft rejection in transplantation.

Primary chronic inflammation

This can be caused by a number of sources. In infective causes this may be attributed to resistance of the organism to phagocytosis (tuberculosis). Other causes include reactions to foreign bodies (endogenous or exogenous) or autoimmune disease (Hashimoto's thyroiditis). Crohn's disease and sarcoidosis are examples of granulomatous diseases which demonstrate signs of chronic inflammation.

Secondary chronic inflammation

Episodes originating from acute inflammatory processes may involve persistent suppurative inflammation with inadequate drainage of abscesses leading to chronic disease (osteomyelitis) or granulomatous reactions (foreign bodies). Other examples exist with recurrent episodes of acute inflammation and healing as seen in chronic gallstone cholecystitis.

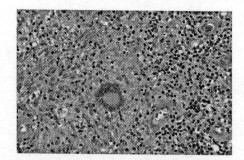

Figure 2.2. A multinucleate giant cell of the Langhans type in a patient with a healing mycobacterial infection of the skin (M. ulcerans).

Granulomas are aggregates of epithelioid histiocytes. Aetiological agents include infective sources (mycobacteria, fungi), foreign bodies (silica, talc), drugs (allopurinol causing hepatic disease) or idiopathic (Crohn's disease). Epithelioid histiocytes produce angiotensin converting enzyme (ACE) and may be converted into multinucleate giant cells (Langhans cells).

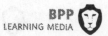

Gallstone disease

Epidemiology

Gallstones are found in 10–20% of patients at post mortem. They are responsible for 1–2% of deaths. An estimated 1.5% of men and 6.1% of women will have gallstones by the age of 40 years. Approximately 50,000 cholecystectomies are performed in England and Wales per year.

Pathology

Gallstones are classified into *cholesterol* and *pigment* stones. Cholesterol stones make up approximately 70–80% of all gallstones. Cholesterol is poorly soluble in water and held in solution in bile in mixed micelles comprising *cholesterol, phospholipids* and *bile salts*. Patients with *cholesterol stones* secrete bile supersaturated with cholesterol, related to reduced secretion of bile salts and increased cholesterol secretion. These stones are generally solitary, large and yellow in colour. *Pigment stones* are formed of calcium salts of unconjugated bilirubin deposited in a glycoprotein matrix. Risk factors for these stones include chronic haemolysis and cirrhosis. The stones are usually smaller and darker in colour (black/brown).

Risk factors

- Familial: There is a two-fold increase in gallstones in first-degree relatives.
- Age: Prevalence increases with age.
- Gender: Gallstones are more common in females of all ages.
- Obesity: This increases supersaturated bile.
- Diabetes: Associated with altered cholesterol metabolism and gallbladder dysfunction.
- Inflammatory bowel disease: Terminal ileum disease leads to altered enterohepatic circulation of bile salts. Reduced absorption of bile salts and acids leads to a smaller total bile acid pool.
- Haemolytic anaemia: Leads to increased formation of pigment stones.
- Geographical: Higher prevalence in certain Native American communities.
- Total parenteral nutrition: Lengthy periods of treatment lead to pigment stone formation.
- Gastric surgery: Fundoplication may be associated with an increase in gallstone disease due to damage to the hepatic branches of the vagus nerve.

Clinical presentations

Asymptomatic

Patients with gallstones found during screening examinations have a 2% risk per year of developing symptoms. The presenting symptoms depend on the location of obstruction in the biliary tree, if present. Common sites of obstruction include Hartmann's pouch of the gallbladder, the cystic duct and the common bile duct.

Biliary colic

This is associated with an intermittent visceral pain in the epigastrium and right upper quadrant of the abdomen, radiating to the back and scapula. The symptoms last for between 20 minutes and several hours. Other associated symptoms include nausea and anorexia. Examination will reveal some tenderness within the right upper quadrant of the abdomen, with normal inflammatory markers. The pain may be relieved by spontaneous disimpaction of Hartmann's pouch or migration of the stone into the distal biliary tree.

Acute cholecystitis

Persistent right upper quadrant pain with associated pyrexia indicates a cholecystitis. This is associated with the impaction of a stone within Hartmann's pouch leading initially to a sterile inflammation followed by secondary bacterial infection. Symptoms commence as severe right upper quadrant pain which becomes constant and progresses to signs of localised peritonism. Examination findings include tenderness in the right upper quadrant with cessation of breathing on deep inspiration (Murphy's sign). Investigations commonly reveal raised inflammatory markers with or without derangement of liver function tests. Findings on ultrasound examination include a thickened oedematous gallbladder wall ± pericholecystic fluid. Acute cholecystitis is more common in diabetics, and often patients describe a previous history of biliary symptoms. Approximately 5–10% of patients develop complications from acute cholecystitis. These include empyema, gangrene, and perforation (rarely cholecysto-colic fistula).

Empyema of gallbladder

Stone impaction within the gallbladder and persistent infection can lead to the development of a pus filled abscess within the gallbladder. Patients often present toxic with high swinging temperatures. A palpable mass may be found on examination due to adherence of omentum. Management includes broad spectrum antibiotics and percutaneous ultrasound/CT-guided drainage of the gallbladder (cholecystostomy). In cases of co-morbid or elderly patients this may be the sole procedure performed.

Mucocele of gallbladder

In cases of a persistent episode of biliary colic or cholecystitis impaction of a stone without the presence of infection can lead to the development of a tense, large gallbladder. Although the bile pigment is absorbed, mucus continues to be secreted filling the gallbladder. Management involves either a cholecystectomy or percutaneous cholecystostomy.

Mirizzi syndrome type 1

A stone impacting the Hartmann's pouch may compress the common bile duct causing obstructive jaundice.

Mirizzi syndrome type 2

With time the stone may erode through the wall of the gallbladder into the common bile duct creating a cholecysto-choledochal fistula.

Cholangitis

Stones leave the gallbladder to impact within the common bile duct initially causing obstruction with secondary infection by gram negative organisms (E. coli, K. pneumoniae). Ascending cholangitis typically presents with epigastric pain, fever with rigors and jaundice (Charcot's triad). This is often associated with systemic upset and may lead to the development of septicaemia and hepatic abscesses. Management includes broad spectrum antibiotics and early ERCP to decompress the biliary tree. Stents may be placed in certain circumstances (pus within the biliary tree).

Acute pancreatitis

If the stone becomes impacted within the terminal part of the common bile duct it can cause compression of the pancreatic duct at the ampulla of Vater causing pancreatitis. (See Chapter 4: *Critical Care – Acute pancreatitis* and *Chronic pancreatitis*).

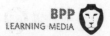

Investigations

Ultrasound scan

Simple, non invasive, sensitive test with 97% sensitivity and 95% specificity for diagnosing gallstones within the gallbladder, and 88% sensitivity and 80% specificity for acute cholecystitis. Its sensitivity for identifying stones within the distal biliary tree is low due to the presence of the overlying gaseous colon or small bowel. The test is best performed in a fasted state to ensure full distension of the gallbladder.

> **Ultrasonographic signs of gallbladder abnormalities**
>
> - Gallbladder wall thickening is defined as > 3mm, typically with a layered appearance.
> - Acute cholecystitis: Gallbladder wall thickening, an obstructing gallstone (for calculus cholecystitis), hydropical dilatation of the gallbladder, a positive sonographic Murphy's sign (pain elicited by pressure over the sonographically located gallbladder), pericholecystic fat inflammation or fluid and hyperaemia of the gallbladder wall at power Doppler.
> - Gallstones appear with a thin, echogenic rim and pronounced shadowing obscuring the tissues behind, often are mobile and 'roll' to the most dependent portion of the gallbladder.
> - The normal width of the CBD is 4–6mm. Older patients may have a normally dilated duct up to 1mm for every decade past the age of 40. The CBD may be dilated up to 1cm normally after cholecystectomy.

CT scan

This can identify biliary tree dilatation (intra/extrahepatic), calcifications and relation of any biliary abnormalities to the local viscera. In malignant causes of obstruction, CT is also used for staging.

MRCP (Magnetic Resonance CholangioPancreatography)

Non invasive and involves no radiation. It remains the best test to assess the biliary tree for the presence of stones, duct dilatation, and strictures. Its sensitivity is similar to ERCP (see below) in identifying the level of obstruction within the biliary tree. It requires the use of contrast agent (gadolinium) and can be used as a staging tool for biliary malignancies. It is contraindicated in patients with ferrous metal clips and cardiac pacemakers.

ERCP (Endoscopic Retrograde CholangioPancreatography)

This investigation involves the insertion of a side-viewing duodenoscope orally into the second part of the duodenum and cannulation of the papilla. Contrast is then injected to visualise the biliary and pancreatic ducts. This therapeutic procedure can be used to relieve obstruction in jaundiced patients by retrieval of stones, placement of stents and sphincterotomy. Cytological and histological specimens can also be obtained from the bile duct, duodenum and pancreas. Complications of this procedure include acute pancreatitis (5% of cases), perforation and haemorrhage (most commonly from the sphincterotomy site) and failure to complete cannulation of ducts or extraction of stones.

Endoscopic ultrasound (EUS)

Under sedation an ultrasound probe is passed orally to the duodenum allowing visualisation of the porta hepatis and extrahepatic biliary tree. This is a useful test for identifying smaller ductal calculi, for investigation of patients with idiopathic pancreatitis and for staging of

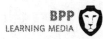

pancreatobiliary malignancies. Small abnormalities can be detected, with variable sensitivity in distinguishing between benign and malignant lesions. Fine needle aspiration cytology can be performed to aid assessment of local nodes in suspicious lesions.

PTC (Percutaneous Transhepatic Cholangiography) ± drainage

This procedure consists of the insertion of a thin needle into an intrahepatic biliary duct between the 7th/8th intercostal spaces under local anaesthesia and with image guidance, most commonly ultrasonography. Contrast is injected and the biliary tree entered. From here stents can be inserted to decompress the biliary tree, draining into the duodenum or externally. Complications include bacteraemia/sepsis, haemorrhage and peritoneal bile leaks.

HIDA (hydroximinodiacetic) scan

A test reserved to assess functional gallbladder disease.

Management of symptomatic gallstones

Laparoscopic cholecystectomy is the gold standard treatment for gallstones. It can be performed as a day case surgery in selected patients.

Patient selection for day surgery laparoscopic cholecystectomy

- No previous upper abdominal surgery
- No gallstone complications, ie no jaundice, pancreatitis or acute cholecystitis
- BMI <35 kg/m^2 and appropriate shape
- No significant co-morbidities (ASA ≤ II)
- Motivated patients with organised discharge plans

(Adapted from British Association of Day Surgery, 2004. Also see Chapter 3 *Applied Surgical Science – Day Surgery*.)

Early v late cholecystectomy

In cases of acute gallstone disease treatment options include acute cholecystectomy ('hot') or conservative therapy with late elective cholecystectomy. Proponents for conservative management discuss the higher conversion and complication rate in acute surgery; the other side justify acute surgery quoting the potential risk of repeat admissions to hospital and the associated morbidity and costs. Ideally an acute cholecystectomy for gallstone disease necessitating hospital admission should be performed within three to four days to minimise risks and complications. Two systematic reviews and meta-analyses comparing early versus delayed laparoscopic cholecystectomy for biliary colic (Gurusamy *et al*, 2008) and acute cholecystitis (Lau *et al*, 2006) reported a shorter total hospital length of stay with no statistically significant difference in the outcomes.

Laparoscopic cholecystectomy – procedure

Patient preparation includes fasting and venous thromboembolic prophylaxis. Pneumoperitoneum is established via either the Veress needle or open Hasson technique in the peri-umbilical region (above or below the umbilicus). A 10mm port is inserted here and the intra-abdominal pressure kept between 10–12 mmHg. Further ports are placed just below the xiphisternum in the midline (10mm), in the subcostal region (5mm) and right flank (5mm). Following an initial laparoscopic examination of the abdomen, the fundus of the gallbladder is grasped and pushed

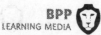

cephalad. Hartmann's pouch is then pulled laterally to expose and open the Calot's triangle, which is bounded by the cystic duct inferiorly, the edge of liver superiorly and the common hepatic duct medially. Within this lies the cystic artery and node. Both the cystic duct and artery are divided between clips and then retrograde dissection of the gallbladder from the liver bed is performed using diathermy. Once the gallbladder is freed, the camera can be moved to the epigastric port and the gallbladder removed through the umbilical port.

(See also video-link for standard Laparoscopic Cholecystectomy by WeBSurg: www.websurg. com/ref/Standard_laparoscopic_cholecystectomy-vd01en1608e.htm)

Intra-operative cholangiogram can be performed to identify previously undetected stones within the biliary tree. It offers better definition of the anatomy of the biliary tree and minimises the risk of iatrogenic CBD injury. It can identify asymptomatic ductal stones in up to 10% of cases and can limit unnecessary exploration of the biliary system. On the other hand, it incurs additional costs, albeit minimal, requires longer operative time and if performed routinely, most of the examinations are negative. The procedure involves the initial introduction of a thin catheter (14Fr) into the abdomen in the subcostal region. The cystic duct is opened partially and carefully with scissors and any obvious stones are milked out. A small feeding tube or similar (flushed with saline) is then passed through the catheter into the cystic duct and fixed in place with a metal clip. Contrast is injected and an image intensifier is used to obtain images. Reviewing of images must confirm the entry position of the catheter, good flow of contrast in both directions (cephalad and caudally), no obvious obstruction or filling defects and free flow of contrast into the duodenum. Obstructing stones can be managed in various ways as described below.

> **Specific complications of cholecystectomy**
>
> - Early: Common bile duct injury (prevalence for the laparoscopic approach 0.3–0.6% and 0.1% for the open method), bile leak, injury to viscera, haemorrhage, retained gallstones, abscess formation and conversion to open.
> - Late: Biliary strictures, cystic duct clip stones, chronic post cholecystectomy pain.

Management of common bile duct stones (choledocholithiasis)

There are two main options, ERCP or exploration of the common bile duct, either via the open approach or laparoscopically:

ERCP

For patients unfit for surgery this may be the sole procedure required if ductal clearance is successful. For fit patients ERCP can be performed pre/postoperatively or even intra-operatively.

Exploration of common bile duct (either via the open approach or laparoscopically)

Generally this is reserved for cases where ERCP has failed, although in specialist centres laparoscopic CBD exploration can also be performed during the laparoscopic cholecystectomy. The procedure involves passing a choledochoscope or Dormia basket through the bile duct to extract the stone(s). In cases of small stones a laparoscopic exploration can be performed transcystically which can then be easily clipped shut. The recovery of the patient is then not different from a routine laparoscopic cholecystectomy. In cases of larger stones within the bile

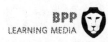

duct a choledochotomy is performed and choledochoscopy/Dormia basket are used for retrieval. The opening can then be sutured closed. In cases of incomplete clearance of the bile duct a T tube can be left in situ. A T tube cholangiogram is performed a week later and if the CBD is clear of stone, the tube is ligated and the patient discharged; the tube can be removed three weeks later in the outpatients clinic.

A Cochrane review performed (Martin *et al*, 2006) comparing surgical and endoscopic treatment of bile duct stones reported just as efficient stone clearance with laparoscopic exploration of the bile duct as with either preoperative or postoperative ERCP with no significant difference in morbidity or mortality.

Upper gastrointestinal pathology

Oesophagogastric cancer

Gastric cancer worldwide mostly affects the distal stomach. A significant migration of tumours towards the oesophago-gastric junction has been noted in the last two decades reflecting on certain aetiological factors such as gastro-oesophageal reflux disease and obesity. Tumours at the gastro-oesophageal junction are classified into three types:

- Type I – true oesophageal tumours associated with columnar cell metaplasia.
- Type II – true carcinomas arising from the cardia.
- Type III – subcardial tumours spreading across the junction.

Gastric cancer

Epidemiology

Gastric cancer is the fourth most common cancer behind lung, breast and colorectal cancer. The disease is more common in Japan, with lower rates in Western Europe and USA. It is more prevalent in males with a peak incidence in the 70s. Early screening investigations in high risk populations (especially in countries with higher incidence), improvements in staging methods and centralisation of surgical expertise have improved survival outcomes.

Risk factors

Inherited predisposition

About 10% of gastric cancer cases are familial; there is higher predisposition for patients with hereditary non-polyposis colorectal cancer, Li-Fraumeni syndrome, familial adenomatous polyposis, and Peutz-Jeghers syndrome.

Environmental factors

- Diet rich in pickled vegetables, salted fish, salt, and smoked meats.
- Smoking (1.5- to 1.6-fold increase in risk).
- Chronic bacterial infection with Helicobacter pylori.
- Epstein-Barr virus (lymphoepithelioma-like carcinoma).
- Pernicious anaemia associated with advanced atrophic gastritis and intrinsic factor deficiency.
- Helicobacter pylori infection and associated chronic atrophic gastritis.
- Previous gastric surgery, adenomatous polyps.
- Obesity (gastric cardia cancer).
- Radiation exposure.

Histology

Most gastric cancers (around 95%) are adenocarcinomas which may be further classified into 'intestinal' and 'diffuse' type. 'Intestinal' adenocarcinomas are associated with a history of atrophic gastritis, have better survival and are associated with older patients, whereas the 'diffuse' adenocarcinomas are more common, with poorer survival and occur more frequently in women and people with blood group 'A'. Other stomach malignant histologic types include lymphomas and leiomyosarcomas.

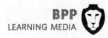

Precancerous lesions

- Polyps: These arise in the gastric mucosa and may be either hyperplastic or adenomatous. Hyperplastic polyps are covered with well differentiated glands and have a low risk of malignant change. Adenomatous polyps can have dysplastic epithelium and the risk of malignant change is 18–75%, increasing if the polyp is > 2cm.
- Gastric ulcer: It is now believed the incidence of malignant change in a gastric ulcer is extremely rare.
- Chronic gastritis: Approximately 94% of superficial cancers are found in the areas of gastritis, and cancers are identified in 10% of patients with chronic gastritis and intestinal metaplasia.
- Autoimmune gastritis is associated with pernicious anaemia. It mostly affects the body and fundus of the stomach. Intestinal metaplasia commonly accompanies this form of gastritis, thus there is a high risk of malignancy.
- Hypersecretory gastritis: This form of gastritis commonly accompanies an ulcer. There is no significant metaplasia or association with malignant change.
- Environmental chronic gastritis is present in certain parts of the world. It has a characteristic multifocal distribution. Its development commences with acute gastritis, leading to atrophy of the mucosa and progressive loss of gastric glands. Regeneration leads to an intestinal type of mucosa which can undergo dysplastic changes.

Clinical presentation

Symptoms

Early disease is asymptomatic. Most symptoms of gastric cancer reflect advanced disease. Patients may complain of new onset dyspepsia which may be worsening or resistant to therapy, nausea or vomiting, dysphagia, post-prandial fullness, loss of appetite, melaena, haematemesis, and weight loss. Late complications include peritoneal and pleural effusions; obstruction of the gastric outlet, gastroesophageal junction, or small bowel; bleeding from oesophageal varices or at the anastomosis after surgery; intrahepatic or extrahepatic jaundice and inanition or cachexia.

Physical signs

They are usually late events: an epigastric mass (spread to the omentum), palpable enlarged stomach with succussion splash, hepatomegaly, ascites and jaundice (distant spread). The presence of a Virchow's node (left supraclavicular node) is diagnostic of advanced gastrointestinal disease as is the metastatic nodule of the umbilicus, known as Sister Mary Joseph's sign.

Differential diagnosis

It includes peptic ulcer disease, oesophageal cancer, Crohn's disease of the stomach, pancreatic cancer, gastric lymphoma, leiomyosarcoma.

Diagnostic work up and staging

- Oesophagogastroduodenoscopy (OGD): The first line investigation, with diagnostic accuracy of 95%. It allows visualisation of the tumour and obtaining multiple biopsies (four, one from each quadrant around the lesion). Brush cytology can also improve the diagnostic yield. Endoscopic reports should include the size of the tumour, site with limits from the incisors, relationship to specific anatomical landmarks, and evidence of any possible complications. (See NICE guidelines: *Referral for suspected upper GI malignancy* below.)
- Double-contrast study and barium swallow, when endoscopy is not feasible.
- CT scan (chest/abdomen/pelvis) for staging (metastatic spread).

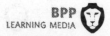

- Endoscopic ultrasound: Useful in assessing early gastric cancers, the depth of invasion, the peri-gastric lymph node status, and local invasion.
- Laparoscopy: CT scanning is limited by the inability to detect tumour deposits of < 5mm. Biopsies can be taken at laparoscopy from the liver and peritoneal surface, sometimes with the use of intraoperative ultrasound to increase the diagnostic yield of liver disease.
- Blood tests: FBC count (anaemia), LFTs (liver dysfunction, or poor nutrition) electrolyte and renal function tests also are essential to characterise the patient's clinical state. Regarding tumour markers, carcinoembryonic antigen (CEA) is increased in 45–50% of cases and the cancer antigen (CA) 19-9 is elevated in about 20% of cases, used mainly to monitor response to therapy.

Management

Appropriate treatment planning is based on staging of tumours (Table 2.2) and the assessment of the patient's co-morbidities. This requires input from various specialties and all cases must be discussed in a multidisciplinary meeting.

Endoscopic

This method can be used for excision of early gastric cancers, recanalisation of neoplastic obstruction, managing bleeding lesions and palliative procedures such as stent insertion or laser ablation.

Surgery

A major determining factor for the outcome of surgical resection is the preoperative physiological state of the patient. Co-morbidities such as cardiorespiratory disease and diabetes must be evaluated and optimised thoroughly preoperatively. Investigations should include baseline blood tests, pulmonary function tests, arterial blood gases, echocardiograms and ECGs. Many patients will be malnourished and cachectic and preoperative input from the dietician is essential. Preoperative nutritional support either at home or as an inpatient is common. The curative resection rate is approximately 30% and the following procedures are indicated.

- Carcinoma of the cardia: Total gastrectomy and resection of lower oesophagus.
- Carcinoma of the middle third: Subtotal gastrectomy for early or well circumscribed T2 lesions if the proximal edge is > 2cm from the oesophagogastric junction (OGJ), or total gastrectomy for infiltrative lesions < 5cm from the oesophagogastric junction.
- Antral carcinoma: Subtotal gastrectomy and resection of the first part of the duodenum.

In all cases excision of the greater and lesser omentum with the anterior leaf of the omental bursa is taken. The duodenum is divided at least 2cm beyond the pylorus. The preferred method of reconstruction of gastrointestinal continuity is by a Roux-en-Y jejunal loop.

Extended lymphadenectomy should also be performed to reduce the chances of locoregional recurrence, and allow a more accurate staging of the disease and better prediction of survival.

Chemotherapy

There may be a role for neoadjuvant chemotherapy in selective patients. Other uses for chemotherapy are in cases of locoregional relapse following resection.

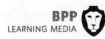

Radiotherapy

This has a palliative role in controlling bleeding.

TO – No evidence of tumour			N0 – no regional lymph node involvement	
Tis – Carcinoma in situ (no invasion of the lamina propria)			N1 – 1–6 regional lymph nodes involvement	
T1 – Invasion of mucosa/submucosa			N2 – 7–15 regional lymph nodes involvement	
T2 – Invasion of muscularis propria			N3 – >15 regional lymph nodes involvement	
T3 – Penetration of serosa			M0 – no distant metastases present	
T4 – Invasion of adjacent structures			M1 – distant metastases present	
	T1	**T2**	**T3**	**T4**
N0	Ia	Ib	II	IIIa
N1	Ib	II	IIIa	IV
N2	II	IIIa	IIIb	IV

Five-year survival according to stage	
Stage	**Five-year survival (%)**
Ia	99
Ib	88–90
II	69–79
IIIa	46–52
IIIb	16–23
IV	10

Table 2.2. TNM staging system for gastric cancer, stage grouping and five-year survival

Oesophageal cancer

Oesophageal cancer remains a challenging condition with only one-third of patients suitable for surgical resection due to advanced disease at presentation or co-morbidities.

Epidemiology

It is the sixth leading cause of cancer deaths worldwide accounting for 3.5% of newly diagnosed cancers per year in the UK. There has been an increase in adenocarcinoma to the predominant histological type. Eighty per cent of patients are over 60 years at diagnosis, with a male: female ratio of 2:1.

Oesophageal adenocarcinoma

These account for 65% of all oesophageal cancers in the UK, with an incidence of 5 per 100,000 in the UK. It is seen in younger patients (> 40 years). The most common aetiological factor in its development is the presence of metaplasia of oesophageal mucosa (Barrett's oesophagus). The chronic acid and bile reflux leads to dysplastic changes and eventually adenocarcinoma that is therefore found mainly in the lower third of the oesophagus.

Risk factors

- Gastroesophageal reflux, triggering the sequence:
  reflux → metaplasia (Barrett's) → low grade dysplasia → high grade dysplasia → adenocarcinoma.
- Vitamin and nutritional deficiencies (Riboflavin).
- Obesity, high dietary fat intake.
- High alcohol intake, smoking.

(See also Chapter 6 *History Taking – Dysphagia.*)

Squamous cell carcinoma of the oesophagus

The incidence in the UK is 2.5 per 100,000 population and is gradually decreasing. It is twice as common in men and commonly seen in elder patients (> 65 years). These can occur at any level within the oesophagus, although are most commonly found in the middle third.

Risk factors

- Alcohol consumption
- Tobacco use
- Diet rich in nitrosamines (Japan/Russia)
- Achalasia of cardia
- Coeliac disease
- Hereditary tylosis
- Low vitamin intake (A,B,C)

Clinical features

Small superficial lesions are often associated with non-specific symptoms. The most common presenting symptom is dysphagia, which usually represents transmural disease. The dysphagia is typically progressive, initially for solids and worsening to liquids with time. Patients also often present with dyspepsia and retrosternal pain not controlled with commonly used acid suppressors. Atypical chest pain is another early presentation that may cause difficulty. Other symptoms include general malaise (iron deficiency anaemia), acute haemorrhage and weight loss. Features of loco-regional spread include hoarseness (recurrent laryngeal nerve invasion), jaundice (liver involvement), recurrent cough (oesophagotracheal fistula).

NICE: Referral guideline for suspected upper gastrointestinal cancer (Adapted from NICE, 2005)

An urgent referral for endoscopy or to a specialist upper gastrointestinal cancer unit should be made for the following patients;

- Patients of any age with dyspepsia and any of the following signs/symptoms:
  - Chronic gastrointestinal bleeding.
  - Dysphagia.
  - Progressive unintentional weight loss.
  - Persistent vomiting.

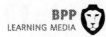

- Iron deficiency anaemia.
- Epigastric mass.
- Suspicious barium meal result.
- Patients aged ≥ 55 years with persistent new-onset dyspepsia should be referred for endoscopic eva luation. In younger patients in the absence of red flag symptoms endoscopy is not indicated.
- Patients with dysphagia (symptoms commence within 5 seconds of initiating swallowing).
- Patients with persistent vomiting and weight loss without dyspepsia.
- Patients with unexplained weight loss and upper abdominal pain.
- Patients with obstructive jaundice, depending on clinical presentation. Urgent ultrasound scan recommended.

Helicobacter pylori status does not alter the indication for referral.

Diagnostic work up and staging

- Blood tests: FBC (anaemia), renal function, liver function tests.
- OGD with biopsies +/- stenting for obstruction, as appropriate.
- Barium swallow: If OGD is not feasible. Not as comprehensive or accurate for diagnosis as endoscopy, biopsies are not possible and involves radiation exposure; however it is useful for functional assessment of motility, reflux and oesophageal distention.
- Endoscopic ultrasound (EUS): To assess the depth of tumour invasion and presence of lymph node spread (accuracy of 80% in assessing lymph node status).
- Diagnostic laparoscopy: Indicated in certain infra-diaphragmatic cases to assess for small volume peritoneal deposits, which will affect decision-making regarding surgery.
- Liver US/ MRI: Assess for possible metastatic spread.
- Bronchoscopy: This can be performed in cases of respiratory complications.
- Bone scintigraphy / CT PET: To assess the patient for metastatic spread.

Tx Cannot be assessed	Nx Cannot be assessed
T0 No evidence of tumour	N0 No regional lymph node metastases
Tis Carcinoma in situ	N1 Regional lymph node metastases
T1 Invades submucosa	Mx Cannot be assessed
T2 Invades muscularis propria	M0 No distant metastases
T3 Invades up to adventitia	M1 Distant metastases
T4 Invades adjacent structures	

Stage	Tumour	Nodes	Metastasis	5-year survival rates
0	In situ	0	0	70% (Stages 0–1)
1	1	0	0	
2a	2/3	0	0	33% (Stage 2)
2b	1/2	1	0	
3	3/4	1	0	8%
4a	Any	Any	1a (coeliac node metastasis)	
4b	Any	Any	1b (non regional lymph node or distant metastasis)	

Table 2.3. TMN staging for oesophageal carcinoma and five-year survival

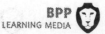

Treatment
Surgery

Resection is reserved for patients with:

- Loco-regional disease (no metastatic spread, no other nodal disease other than peri-tumour) and fit enough to tolerate such treatment, offering a chance of long term survival for 20% of patients.
- High grade dysplasia within Barrett's oesophagus. This is considered an indication for resection due to the progression to adenocarcinoma and a 40% risk of undetected foci of invasive carcinoma.

Approximately 60–70% of tumours have involved lymph nodes at the time of surgery. In order to perform a potentially curative procedure for carcinoma of the middle and lower third of the oesophagus, dissection of mediastinal and abdominal lymph nodes is recommended. The aims of the procedure are to resect the tumour and loco-regional lymph nodes with full restoration of gastrointestinal tract continuity.

Procedures include:

- Two or three-stage subtotal oesophagectomy
- Transhiatal subtotal oesophagectomy without thoracotomy
- Transhiatal total oesophagectomy with Roux-en-Y jejunal reconstruction
- Minimally invasive approaches are being performed in specialist centres with the advantages of shorter recovery period, reduced respiratory complications and earlier return to preoperative function.

Specific complications of surgery are:

- Pleural effusion, pneumonia
- Anastomotic leak
- Recurrent laryngeal nerve injury
- Benign anastomotic stricture
- Chylothorax

Neo-adjuvant therapy

Adjuvant therapy is poorly tolerated following resection and not been associated with a survival benefit. Neo-adjuvant chemotherapy is offered to most cases except early stage disease. Randomised controlled trials have found a significant improvement in progression free survival and a 13% increase in five-year survival. Similarly, preoperative chemo-radiotherapy has been associated with good clinical response rates.

Palliative therapy

Palliative procedures are offered to patients with advanced loco-regional disease, distant metastatic spread, those unfit for surgical resection or recurrent disease following resection.

- Metal stents: Expandable stents are widely used for malignant dysphagia. They are covered with a polymer to prevent tumour ingrowth and are inserted at endoscopy or under radiological guidance. They can be used in conjunction with radiotherapy. Stents are not inserted in tumours of the upper third of the oesophagus due to patient discomfort.
- Ablation: Both laser and argon beam plasma coagulation is effective in recanalisation of the lumen of the oesophagus. A disadvantage of this approach is that often repeated therapies are required.

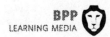

- Palliative chemotherapy: This has been associated with a survival benefit. The most commonly used regime is epirubicin, cisplatin and 5-fluorouracil.
- Radiotherapy: Both external beam and intraluminal therapy can be offered to reduce pain, swallowing difficulties and haemorrhage. This technique is more effective for squamous cell carcinoma. A potential complication is oesophagotracheal fistula formation.

Peptic ulcer disease (PUD)

Epidemiology

Peptic ulcer is the presence of an established defect within the columnar mucosa of the lower oesophagus, stomach or duodenum. The incidence of PUD (currently 0.8% of the population per annum) has decreased in the last 20–30 years due to a significant improvement in its medical management. Evidence from autopsies suggest approximately 20% of men and 10% of women have suffered from peptic ulcers at some point in their life. Surgery has now been reduced to mostly emergency cases e.g. haemorrhage, perforation.

Risk factors

- Infection: Helicobacter pylori
- Tobacco smoking
- Alcohol intake
- Drugs: NSAIDs, steroids, immunosuppressants, bisphosphonates
- Stress: Psychological, Curling's ulcer (burns), Cushing's ulcer (head injury)
- Zollinger-Ellison syndrome
- Male sex (3:1)

Helicobacter pylori is a gram negative, helical, microaerophilic flagellated bacterium, responsible for approximately 95% of duodenal and 70% of gastric ulcers. Its prevalence increases with age, with almost half the population over 60 years showing evidence of infection. Infection is believed to be acquired in childhood via the faecal-oral route. The bacteria colonises the gastric mucosa in the antrum and pyloric regions. *H. Pylori* produces the enzyme urease converting urea to ammonia and carbon dioxide. Initially, infection leads to a period of hypogastrinaemia. Subsequently, the *H. Pylori* produces an alkaline environment, reducing the secretion of somatostatin, thereby preventing inhibition of gastrin and causing a hypergastrinaemic state. Metaplasia of duodenal mucosa to ectopic gastric mucosa allows *H. Pylori* colonisation and causes ulceration. Other effects include a release of cytokines and recruitment of inflammatory mediators.

NSAID use is the most common cause of mucosal injury in the Western population. This occurs by inhibition of *cyclo-oxygenase 1*, preventing prostaglandin formation, resulting in a reduction in the normal protective mechanism of the mucosa.

Classification of ulcer types (modified Johnson)

- Type I: proximal ulcer, commonly found at the lesser curvature and antrum.
- Type II: distal ulcer / duodenal.
- Type III: prepyloric ulcer.
- Type IV: proximal gastroesophageal.
- Type V: NSAID-related, throughout the stomach.

Clinical presentation

Common presenting symptoms include pain which may either be a long history of upper abdominal discomfort or a severe exacerbation. The pain is often described as a gnawing sensation felt in the back. It may follow an intermittent course. Eating may affect the discomfort in certain cases. The pain associated with type II ulcers is described as worse on fasting, and relieved by food. Type I ulcers on the other hand present with epigastric pain on eating. Associated symptoms include vomiting, anorexia and heartburn. Other presentations consist of waterbrash and complications such as bleeding, from erosion into a vessel, which may be occult leading to iron deficiency anaemia or overt causing haematemesis or melaena. Patients may also present with an acute abdomen due to peritonitis from perforation of the ulcer.

Differential diagnosis

- Myocardial infarction
- Gallstones / cholecystitis
- Lower lobe pneumonia
- Acute pancreatitis
- Pulmonary embolus
- Gastro-oesophageal reflux disease

Diagnostic work up

- Blood tests: Haemoglobin, ferritin and urea and electrolytes.
- OGD: This will allow inspection of the mucosa of the upper gastrointestinal tract. Ulceration of the duodenum is more common (often first part) with stomach ulceration often found in the lesser curvature.
- *Helicobacter pylori* can be detected using a variety of tests:
  - Using endoscopic biopsy samples; the organism can be detected on histological examination, culture, polymerase chain reaction or a positive rapid urease test performed on the sample. Histological diagnosis via tissue sample is considered the gold standard, although costly. Similarly microbiological culture of the tissue sample is 100% sensitive. The most commonly performed investigation at the time of endoscopy is the rapid urease test (CLOtest). This involves a small tissue sample from the gastric antrum being placed in a pH sensitive gel containing urea. If positive the urea will be broken down to ammonium causing a rise in the pH and change in colour.
  - Serological tests for *H. pylori* antibodies performed on blood or less commonly saliva ^{13}C or ^{14}C urea breath test: Non-invasive investigation, where the patient is given a radiolabelled solution to drink. If positive the labelled carbon dioxide in exhaled breath can be measured by mass spectrometry or scintillation.
  - Faecal antigen testing.
  - *H. pylori* serum antibodies.

Management

Most uncomplicated disease can be managed conservatively.

- H_2 receptor antagonists are effective at suppressing acid secretion and ulcer healing in 80-90% of cases. However, some acid secretion can still be induced by vagal and gastrin stimulation.
- Proton pump inhibitors block the H+/K+-ATPase pump found in the apical membrane of the gastric parietal cell irreversibly giving faster ulcer healing (80–90% healing at eight weeks).
- Eradication therapy for *H. pylori*, if present, according to the following regimes (Table 2.4).

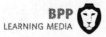

Antibiotics		PPI
Amoxicillin 1g BD	Clarithromycin 500mg BD or Metronidazole 400mg BD	Esomeprazole 20mg BD or Lansoprazole 30mg BD or Omeprazole 20mg BD or Pantoprazole 40mg BD or Rabeprazole 20mg BD
Clarithromycin 250mg BD	Metronidazole 400mg BD	

Table 2.4. Triple therapy for Helicobacter pylori eradication

- Also assessment of long term ulcerogenic medication and lifestyle modification (smoking cessation, alcohol intake reduction and weight loss).

Complications of peptic ulcer disease

Eradication treatment of *H. pylori* and antisecretory treatment have decreased the incidence of complications, which most commonly include:

- Perforation
- Bleeding
- Obstruction secondary to pyloric stenosis or duodenal oedema
- Penetration through to neighbouring structures (pancreas, gastrocolic fistula)
- Refractory ulcer
- Increased risk of gastric malignancy, in association with *H. pylori* infection

Management of complications

Bleeding ulcer (management as per management of upper GI bleeding)

Active resuscitation to maintain haemodynamic stability is the priority. Patients should undergo urgent OGD. This will allow diagnosis and the opportunity to treat the cause with injection of vasoconstrictors (adrenaline), application of haemostatic clips, argon photocoagulation or laser / heater probes. Proton pump inhibitors are also essential in reducing further bleeds, with some supporting evidence in the use of tranexamic acid. In approximately 70–80% of cases, bleeding will stop spontaneously. Surgery is indicated in cases of continued bleeding despite endoscopic intervention (particularly with visible vessels / ulcers) or large transfusions. With the benefit of information from endoscopy, the vessel can be ligated by suture under-running in minimal time.

Cause of bleeding	Relative frequency
Peptic ulcer	44
Oesophagitis	28
Gastritis / erosions	26
Erosive duodenitis	15
Varices	13
Portal hypertensive gastropathy	7
Malignancy	5
Mallory Weiss tear	5
Vascular malformation	3

Table 2.5. Causes of upper GI bleeding (% abnormalities identified at endoscopy)

In approximately 20% of patients presenting with apparent acute upper gastrointestinal bleeding, endoscopy does not reveal a cause.

Perforation

Commonly seen in elderly patients, it is often associated with use of NSAIDs. The incidence of perforation is approximately 0.5% per year, in comparison to 2.8% per year for bleeding. Patients present with sudden onset of severe upper abdominal pain and signs of sepsis and shock. In cases of posterior perforation into the lesser sac the signs can be more subtle. Free air under the diaphragm is noted in an erect chest radiograph in 75% of perforations. If there is diagnostic difficulty in a stable patient, a CT scan of the abdomen should be performed. Active resuscitation followed by surgery is the best management. Frail patients with high perioperative risk can be managed by nasogastric tube drainage and IV antibiotics alone.

The two main principles of surgery are to cover or close the ulcer defect and achieve thorough lavage of the peritoneal cavity. The commonly used method is the omental patch via a small upper midline laparotomy incision and thorough peritoneal lavage followed by eradication and antisecretory therapy. Complications of the procedure include intra-abdominal abscess formation, prolonged ileus and haemorrhage. At surgery gastric ulcers should be biopsied to exclude malignancy. This procedure is now being performed more often laparoscopically.

A Cochrane review (Sanabria *et al*, 2005) measured the effect of laparoscopic vs open surgical treatment in patients with a diagnosis of perforated peptic ulcer in relation to abdominal septic complications, surgical wound infection, extra-abdominal complications, hospital length of stay and direct costs. Three randomised controlled studies including a total of 315 patients were included in the analysis. The results showed a tendency to a decrease in septic intra-abdominal complications, surgical site infections, postoperative ileus, pulmonary complications and mortality with laparoscopic repair compared with open surgery although none of these were statistically significant.

Chronic ulceration and gastric outlet obstruction

Prior to the introduction of proton pump inhibitors/H_2-antagonists, many patients underwent the following surgical procedures for chronic or obstructing ulcers.

* Pyloroplasty and vagotomy (truncal or hyperselective)
* The Bilroth I: Distal gastric resection and gastroduodenal anastomosis
* The Bilroth II: Gastric resection with a gastrojejunostomy, in cases where a gastroduodenal anastomosis was not possible.

Complications associated with these procedures include:

* Diarrhoea: Caused by rapid gastric emptying and large volumes of liquid chime.
* Dumping: Early dumping (10%) is due to large volumes of osmotically active food moving rapidly into the small bowel causing palpitations, faintness and abdominal discomfort. Late dumping is caused by hypoglycaemia causing similar symptoms.
* Bile reflux: Procedures affecting the function of the pylorus can lead to bile reflux.
* Iron deficiency anaemia: Stomach acid is required for the conversion of ferric iron to ferrous iron enabling uptake within the terminal ileum. Resection may lead to iron deficiency anaemia.

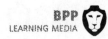

Lower gastrointestinal pathology

Acute appendicitis

Epidemiology

Appendicitis is the most common acute surgical condition of the abdomen. Approximately 7% of the population will have appendicitis in their lifetime, with the peak incidence occurring between the ages of 10 and 30 years.

Aetiology and pathogenesis

Obstruction of the narrow appendiceal lumen initiates acute appendicitis, potentially caused by lymphoid hyperplasia (related to viral illnesses, including upper respiratory infection, mononucleosis, gastroenteritis) faecaliths, parasites, foreign bodies, Crohn's disease, primary or metastatic cancer and carcinoid syndrome. Lymphoid hyperplasia is more common in children and young adults, accounting for the increased incidence of appendicitis in these age groups.

Clinical manifestations

Abdominal pain is the most common symptom of appendicitis (~100% present), with anorexia (~100%), nausea (90%), vomiting (75%) and pain migration (from the periumbilical area to the right lower quadrant 50%). Duration of symptoms exceeding 24 to 36 hours is uncommon in non-perforated appendicitis.

Diagnostic work up

- A thorough review of the history of the abdominal pain, of the patient's recent genitourinary, gynaecologic and pulmonary history and co-morbidities should be obtained.
- Common signs of appendicitis include:
  - Right lower quadrant pain on palpation (the single most important sign)
  - Low-grade fever (38°C), although absence of fever or high fever can occur
  - Peritoneal signs
    - Localised tenderness to percussion
    - Guarding
  - Other confirmatory peritoneal signs (absence of these signs does not exclude appendicitis)
    - Psoas sign – pain on extension of right thigh (retrocaecal appendix)
    - Obturator sign – pain on internal rotation of right thigh (pelvic appendix)
    - Rovsing's sign – pain in right lower quadrant with palpation of left lower quadrant
    - Dunphy's sign – increased pain with coughing
    - Flank tenderness in right lower quadrant (retroperitoneal retrocaecal appendix)
    - Patient maintains hip flexion with knees drawn up for comfort (See also Chapter 7: Clinical examinations – *Examination of the abdominal system.*)
- Laboratory tests including FBC, assessing the leukocyte and neutrophil count; U&E and clotting (fitness for surgery); LFTs (differential from gallbladder pathology) and inflammatory markers (C-reactive protein, Erythrocyte Sedimentation Rate). Also a urine dipstick (differential from urine infections) and b-HCG test in women of reproductive age (to exclude pregnancy-related pain) are essential.
- Imaging: Ultrasonography (US) and computed tomographic (CT) scans are helpful in evaluating patients with suspected appendicitis, with US more appropriate for paediatric and female patients with right lower quadrant or pelvic pain. Their comparison, advantages and disadvantages are presented in Table 2.6.

Management

The standard for management of appendicitis remains surgical: appendicectomy. Because prompt treatment of appendicitis is important in preventing further morbidity and mortality, a margin of error in over-diagnosis is acceptable.

	Ultrasound scan	CT scan
Sensitivity	85%	90 to 100%
Specificity	92%	95 to 97%
Use	Evaluate patients with equivocal diagnosis of appendicitis	Evaluate patients with equivocal diagnosis of appendicitis
Advantages	Safe Relatively inexpensive Can rule out pelvic disease in females Better for children	More accurate Better identification of phlegmon and abscess Better identification of normal appendix
Disadvantages	Operator dependent Technically inadequate studies due to gas Pain	Cost Ionising radiation Contrast

Table 2.6. Comparison between US and CT in the diagnosis of acute appendicitis

Appendicectomy – procedure

- Antibiotics are given immediately if there are signs of sepsis, otherwise a single dose of prophylactic intravenous antibiotics is given immediately prior to surgery.
- General anaesthesia is induced, with full muscle relaxation, and the patient is positioned supine.
- The full abdomen is prepared and draped and is examined under anaesthesia; if a mass is present, the incision is made over the mass; otherwise, the incision is made over McBurney's point, one-third of the way from the anterior superior iliac spine (ASIS) and the umbilicus; this represents the position of the base of the appendix (the position of the tip is variable). Alternatively, a Lanz incision (made along skin creases over the McBurney point) can be chosen for better cosmetic result. A lower midline incision should be considered in the middle aged or elderly patient or if the diagnosis is in doubt.
- The various layers of the abdominal wall are then opened, aiming to preserve the integrity of the abdominal wall; the external oblique aponeurosis is slitted along its fibres, and the internal oblique muscle is split along its length, not cut. As the two run at right angles to each other, this prevents later the formation of an incisional hernia.
- Once the peritoneum is reached, it is grasped between two artery forceps and opened to ensure no abdominal organ (bowel) is injured.
- On entering the peritoneum, the appendix is identified, mobilised, preferably with delivering the caecum through the wound for better control.
- The mesoappendix containing the appendiceal artery (branch from the ileocolic) is then divided between ligatures.
- The appendix is then ligated and divided at its base and the specimen is sent to histology.
- Some surgeons choose to bury the stump of the appendix by inverting it so it points into the caecum.
- Each layer of the abdominal wall is then closed in turn and haemostasis is ensured.
- The skin may be closed with staples or stitches and the wound is dressed.

- The same principles are followed during laparoscopic appendicectomy. The pneumoperitoneum is established according to the standard method (see the chapter on *Applied Surgical Science*). The ports used are: one at the umbilicus, one suprapubic and one either at the left iliac fossa or the right upper quadrant to allow instrument triangulation. After laparoscopic examination of the abdominal cavity and confirmation of diagnosis the sequence of steps follows those of open appendicectomy (mesoappendix ligated using clips/diathermy and base of appendix ligated using endoloop suture). The specimen is delivered either in a bag or through a port; finally the ports are closed according to standard technique. (See Further Reading webSurg video-link for lapaoscopic appendicectomy).

Colorectal polyps

Epidemiology

Over 70% of colorectal cancers arise from adenomatous polyps which are benign precursors of malignancy. The adenoma-carcinoma sequence describes a continuum by which a sequence of genetic abnormalities alters the normal colonic epithelium through hyperproliferation, dysplasia and ultimately invasive carcinoma. The process is believed to take five years. The size of the polyp affects the chance of developing malignancy, with lesions < 1cm having a 2% risk and those of 1–2cm a 10% risk. The prevalence of colonic adenomas is 30%–40% at age 60 years.

Aetiological factors
Genetic

- Familial adenomatous polyposis (FAP): This genetic abnormality affecting the APC (tumour suppressor) gene leads to the development of widespread adenomas which can inevitably progress into malignant disease. By the age of 30, over 100 polyps have usually developed. Together with these lesions other extra-gastrointestinal lesions such as desmoid tumours and tumours of the thyroid and adrenal glands may develop. The condition is inherited by autosomal dominant pattern and surveillance via colonoscopy is offered to family members. Given the significant risk of developing malignancy many patients are offered prophylactic colectomy.
- Hereditary non-polyposis colon cancer (HNPCC): This heterogeneous group accounts for up to 5% of all colorectal cancer. Patients display polyps in smaller number but with accelerated progression to malignancy. Some patients are also predisposed to develop other malignancies such as endometrial, ovarian, urothelial and gastric.
- Peutz-Jeghers syndrome: This autosomal dominant condition involves the development of numerous hamartomatous polyps within the gastrointestinal tract together with mucocutaneous pigmentation. There is a lifetime risk of developing colorectal cancer of 20%.
- Juvenile polyposis: This autosomal dominant condition involving an abnormality in the tyrosine kinase gene is characterised by numerous hamartomatous polyps within the gastrointestinal tract with a high lifetime risk of malignancy.

Lifestyle

- Dietary: The colonic mucosa is continuously exposed to dietary carcinogens. There is some evidence to suggest that diets with less red meat and higher amounts of fruit and vegetables are associated with a reduced risk of developing colorectal cancer.
- Smoking and alcohol: High intake of alcohol is believed to increase the risk of cancer.
- Obesity: The risk of developing cancer is increased by 15% in the overweight and 33% in the obese.

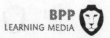

- Drugs: NSAIDs have been found to inhibit adenoma growth by suppressing *cyclo-oxygenase 2*. Also the oral contraceptive pill and hormone replacement therapy have been attributed to decreasing polyp formation and growth.

Histopathological classification

- Hyperplastic (90% of all polyps): They are benign protrusions, usually less than 0.5cm in diameter. They possess some malignant potential in the setting of hyperplastic polyposis syndrome.
- Adenomas (10% of polyps): Those larger than 1cm approach a 10% chance of containing invasive cancer. These neoplastic lesions may show high, moderate or low levels of dysplasia. Those without a stalk (sessile) pose more challenges compared to those with a stalk (pedunculated) as they have shorter pathway for migration of invasive cells from the tumour into submucosa and complete endoscopic removal is more challenging and more difficult to ascertain. The adenomas are further classified histologically into:
  - Tubular (75%), found anywhere in the colon.
  - Villous, found most common in the rectum and associated with higher morbidity and mortality of all polyps (mucous discharge, hypersecretory state with hypokalaemia, in situ/invasive carcinoma).
  - Tubulovillous.
- Hamartomata: These tumour-like lesions are made up of a mixture of tissue types. They are seen in certain genetic conditions (see above).
- Inflammatory polyps: These lesions are also called benign lymphoid polyps and can be seen in ulcerative colitis and occasionally Crohn's disease.
- Metaplastic: These lesions are characterised by a change in the colonic epithelium to an alternative form.

Complications of polyps

- Malignant change (higher risk if size > 1cm, high grade dysplasia, and villous form)
- Intussusception
- Protein loss
- Haemorrhage and ulceration

Management of colonic polyps

Polypectomy

Small polyps can be removed during colonoscopy (pedunculated easier to remove). Removal of a solitary colonic polyp is usually curative for that lesion. Complete colonoscopic examination is necessary to rule out development of others. Repeat colonoscopy at 3–12 months is sometimes advocated if there is substantial doubt whether a colonic polyp has been completely resected and/or contains high-grade dysplasia.

Colonic resection

Colonic resection is indicated in the cases of:

- Multiple intestinal polyps associated with FAP.
- Patients with long-standing ulcerative colitis who have developed high-grade dysplasia or a dysplasia-associated lesion or mass.
- Large, sessile polyps that are difficult to remove.
- Advanced colonic polyps that recur despite adequate initial endoscopic treatment.
- Malignant polyps with involved margins.

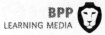

Several surgical options should be discussed with the patient, including total colectomy, subtotal colectomy with rectal sparing, or segmental resection.

Surveillance

The British Society of Gastroenterology guidelines (Atkins and Saunders, 2002) recommend that further follow-up of patients diagnosed with colorectal polyps in a baseline colonoscopy is determined by their risk stratification:

*   Low risk: Patients with only 1–2, small (< 1cm) adenomas.
    Recommendation: no follow up or five-yearly until one negative examination.
*   Intermediate risk: Patients with 3–4 small adenomas or at least one > 1cm.
    Recommendation: three-yearly until two consecutive negative examinations.
*   High risk: If either of the following are detected at any single examination (at baseline or follow up): ≥ 5 adenomas or ≥ 3 adenomas at least one of which ≥ 1cm.
    Recommendation: An extra examination should be undertaken at 12 months before returning to three-yearly surveillance.

Colorectal cancer

Epidemiology

Colorectal cancer is the second most common malignancy in the West and the second leading cause of cancer-related death. There are approximately 100 new cases diagnosed each day in the UK, with a lifetime risk for men of 1 in 16 and 1 in 20 for women. Of the cancers within the colon and rectum, 98% are adenocarcinomas, with carcinoids and squamous cell carcinomas making up the rest. Most patients present between the sixth and eighth decades, with approximately 250 cases below the age of 35 years diagnosed in the UK per year, although this figure continues to increase. Rectal cancer is more common in males, while colon cancer is equal between male and female patients.

Aetiological factors

Both genetic and environmental factors are identified in the pathogenesis of colorectal cancer.

*   Dietary factors: Lack of fibre, increased fat, bile acids.
*   Inflammatory bowel disease: Increased incidence in patients with ulcerative colitis and Crohn's disease.
*   Irradiation: Pelvic irradiation increases the risk of developing rectosigmoid tumours.
*   Previous ureterosigmoidostomy.
*   Familial adenomatous polyposis.
*   Hereditary non-polyposis colorectal cancer.

Histology

Approximately 40% of cancers are present within the rectum, 30% in the descending/sigmoid colon, 20% in the caecum and ascending colon and 10% in the transverse colon. Synchronous tumours (present at the time of primary carcinoma) are found in 3% of cases and metachronous carcinomas (develop subsequently to primary lesion) occur in 10% of cases. The tumours are either polypoid or ulcerating and can spread around the circumference of the colon to form an annular, obstructing lesion. Approximately 10% of tumours are colloid, producing excessive mucus. Almost two thirds of all cancers are moderately differentiated with the remaining third split equally between well differentiated and poorly differentiated.

Modes of cancer spread

- Direct: Lateral spread is more common than longitudinal spread.
- Haematogenous: Up to 30% of patients have occult liver metastases at the time of presentation, with pulmonary lesions identified in 5% of cases. Spread can also be seen in the adrenal glands, kidneys and bone.
- Lymphatic: Rectal cancers usually spread via the lymphatics proximally.
- Transperitoneal: This occurs in 10% of cases after resection. Spread to the ovaries may be seen, developing Krukenberg tumours.
- Implantation: An uncommon form, possibly a mechanism for port site recurrences seen following laparoscopic resection.

Clinical features

In the early stages of development patients are mostly asymptomatic. As the lesions grow, symptoms are often dictated by the site of the tumour.

- Right sided tumours (including transverse colon): Tumours are often soft and friable and therefore bleed easily. This is often occult and can lead to iron deficiency anaemia. Other presenting symptoms may include right sided abdominal pain or even a mass.
- Left sided tumours: These tumours are more likely to obstruct. Patients commonly present with a change in bowel habit and associated left sided abdominal pain. Intermittent episodes of bloating and distension can also be reported, as can rectal bleeding (dark blood can be mixed with stools).
- Rectal tumours: Patients with these tumours often present with rectal bleeding which may be bright red or even darker. There is often associated mucus discharge. A significant change in bowel habit is also described with many suffering from urgency and increased frequency. Some complain of the painful need to repeatedly pass a stool (tenesmus), and the feeling of incomplete evacuation. Other symptoms related to local invasion may also be present such as back pain/sciatica (sacral nerves), urinary tract symptoms or anal pain.
- As the tumour advances, other systemic upset such as anorexia and weight loss can also be apparent.

Investigations

- Blood tests: FBC (anaemia), U&Es (renal function, electrolytes), LFTs (metastatic spread), CEA (for monitoring postoperative recurrence).
- Flexible sigmoidoscopy / Colonoscopy with biopsy.
- CT Pneumocolon: A useful test for frail patients; it has lower sensitivity for identifying smaller polyps, does not offer biopsy option, and involves radiation.
- CT scan chest / abdomen / pelvis: For staging.
- MRI Pelvis: Staging of rectal tumours to assess local extension, and follow up after neoadjuvant therapy.
- Transrectal ultrasound: For assessing depth of invasion.
- Double contrast barium enema: Now superseded by above tests.

Referral guidelines for suspected colorectal cancer (Adapted from NICE, 2005)

An urgent referral to specialist colorectal cancer unit should be made for:

- Patients aged ≥ 40 years, suffering from rectal bleeding together with a change of bowel habit (loose/increased frequency) persisting for ≥ 6 weeks.
- Patients aged ≥ 60 years, with rectal bleeding persisting for ≥ 6 weeks without altered bowel habit or anal symptoms.
- Patients aged ≥ 60 years, with a change in bowel habit (loose / increased frequency) persisting for ≥ 6 weeks without rectal bleeding.
- Patients of any age presenting with a right lower abdominal mass (colonic), or a palpable rectal mass (intraluminal).
- Men of any age with iron deficiency anaemia of unknown cause (haemoglobin ≤ 11 g/100 ml).
- Non-menstruating women with iron deficiency anaemia of unknown cause (haemoglobin ≤ 10 g/100 ml).

Staging of tumour (Table 2.7)

The two commonest staging systems used for colorectal cancer are the Dukes' staging and TMN classification system.

Dukes' staging:

Stage A – Tumour confined to bowel wall with no involvement of local lymph nodes
Stage B – Tumour extends through the bowel wall without spreading to lymph nodes
Stage C – Lymph node metastases; if apical node is involved C2, otherwise stage C1
Stage D – Distant metastases

T0 – No evidence of tumour	N0 – No regional lymph node involvement
Tis – Carcinoma in situ; intraepithelial	N1 – Metastasis in one to three regional lymph nodes
T1 – Tumour invades the submucosa	N2 – Metastases in four or more regional lymph nodes
T2 – Tumour invades the muscularis propria	M0 – No distant metastases
T3 – Tumour invades through the muscularis propria into subserosa	M1 – Distant metastases present
T4 – Tumour invades other organs or structures, perforates visceral peritoneum	
Dukes' stage	**Corrected five-year survival (%)**
A	92
B	71
C1	40
C2	26
D	16

Table 2.7 TMN and Dukes' classification of colorectal cancer and five-year survival

Management

All cases must be discussed in a multidisciplinary team including an oncologist, pathologist, radiologist, gastroenterologist, colorectal nurses and surgeons. The standard treatment is surgical resection with some improvements in survival rates seen with adjuvant or neoadjuvant therapy. Curative resection aims to eradicate the disease and remove regional lyphovascular drainage.

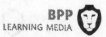

Neoadjuvant therapy

For rectal tumours found to be locally advanced (invading mesorectal fascia) on MRI scanning. The radiotherapy can be given as a short course – five fractions over five days or a long course – twenty five fractions over five weeks. Additional chemotherapy with agents such as 5-flourouracil is administered. Such therapy leads to downsizing of the tumour in a majority of patients. Further MRI scans can be used to plan the appropriate timing of surgery, usually 6–12 weeks post completion of therapy in most units.

Surgical resection

Surgery aims to remove the primary lesion with all locally involved tissue and its related vascular and lymphatic drainage to obtain a clear resection margin. Resection can be performed open via a midline incision or now more commonly laparoscopically. The National Institute for Health and Clinical Excellence (NICE) have recommended the use of laparoscopic surgery as an alternative to open surgery for colorectal cancer in suitable cases in the hands of appropriately trained and experienced surgeons. Together with the introduction of an enhanced recovery programme (Enhanced Recovery After Surgery – ERAS) the short-term outcomes regarding hospital stay, postoperative pain and return to bowel function are significantly shorter. No significant difference in long term oncological outcomes has been identified between the two approaches.

The operation types vary according to the site of the tumour.

- Right hemicolectomy: For tumours of the caecum, ascending colon, hepatic flexure and proximal transverse colon. The ileocolic and right colic arteries are ligated and an ileocolic anastomosis is performed. In cases of distal transverse colon tumours an extended right hemicolectomy can be performed. In this case the middle colic artery is also ligated.
- Left hemicolectomy: Reserved for lesions of the splenic flexure and descending colon. The left colic and in certain cases sigmoid arteries are ligated and a colo-colic anastomosis is performed. A segmental sigmoid colon resection can also be performed in specific instances (sigmoid colectomy).
- Anterior resection: Resection for the lower two-thirds of the rectum should include a total mesorectal excision (TME). The mesorectum is a layer of fatty tissue enveloped in fascia surrounding the posterolateral aspects of the rectum. The lesion can spread into this layer either directly or via lymphatic spread to the mesorectal nodes. The common vessels involved are the inferior mesenteric artery and superior rectal artery. The anastomosis is usually performed by a circular stapler and can be combined with a defunctioning loop ileostomy (reversed in 6–8 weeks).
- Abdominoperineal resection: For tumours invading the anal sphincter or too low for a safe anastomosis to be performed. Dissection is performed via an abdominal and perineal incision. Vessels involved include the inferior mesenteric and pudendal arteries. A permanent end colostomy is created in the left iliac fossa and the perineal incision is closed.

Emergency surgery

Up to 30% of patients present as emergencies, commonly with intestinal obstruction, perforation or haemorrhage. Left sided obstruction leads to colonic dilatation, which in the presence of a functioning ileocaecal valve will cause a closed loop obstruction. This may result in a right sided caecal perforation. All patients should be repeatedly examined for right sided tenderness. The majority of patients requiring emergency surgery due to a left-sided perforation (faecal contamination) undergo a Hartmann's procedure, where the tumour is resected, the rectum oversewn and an end colostomy is formed. The procedure can be reversed in the future. In selected circumstances a primary anastomosis can be performed with on table lavage ± defunctioning stoma. An alternative in emergency situations is to manage left sided obstructions endososcopically by placing a stent and operating semi-electively.

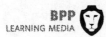

Adjuvant therapy

Adjuvant chemotherapy has shown to have a role in improving prognosis. Indicated for patients with node positive disease, the regime is based on 5-flourouracil (or the oral less toxic form – capecitabine) for up to six months. Results have shown a 13% increase in five-year survival. Other regimes based around oxaliplatin are also administered. Palliative therapy for incurable disease can be offered in the form of certain chemotherapeutic schemes or endoscopic stenting to relieve obstructing symptoms for left sided lesions.

Complications of surgery for colorectal cancer

General complications

Cardiac (arrhythmias or myocardial infarction), respiratory (infections or pulmonary embolism), deep vein thrombosis, bleeding or urinary tract infections.

Local / specific complications

- Anastomotic leak: This dangerous complication can cause generalised peritonitis if leaking occurs into the abdominal cavity or a pelvic abscess if there is a localised distal leak. In cases of localised leaks, some patients can be managed by radiological drainage and intravenous antibiotics. An alternative is laparoscopic washout of localised abscess and surgical drainage. In cases of generalised peritonitis further surgical intervention is the mainstay of treatment.
- Urinary complications: Denervation of the bladder or injury can cause retention of urine, injury to the ureters (left sided dissection) causes hydronephrosis or even a fistula.
- Sexual dysfunction: Pelvic nerve damage can cause impotence (nervi erigentes) or failure to ejaculate (presacral nerves).
- Intestinal obstruction: Small bowel obstruction can develop due to either herniation of a loop next to a colostomy (para-stomal hernia) or with time due to intra-abdominal adhesions.
- Wound infection: This is the most frequent complication of the wound which can lead to abscess formation, secondary haemorrhage or even incisional hernia, more commonly in the perineal wound of APR.
- Stoma complications: Bleeding, prolapse, retraction, para-stomal herniation, excoriation of skin (ileostomy) or stenosis. (See Chapter 7, *Clinical examination – stoma.*)

NHS Bowel Cancer Screening Programme (NHS BCSP)

Randomised controlled trials in the UK in the nineties reported a 16% reduction in mortality associated with colorectal cancer in a population undergoing screening. The NHS BCSP commenced in 2006. The programme screens people of ages 60–69 years on a two-yearly basis (upper limit to be extended to 75 years). The test used is the guaiac faecal occult blood test (gFOBT), which tests for the presence of blood within the stools, by using the peroxidase activity of the haem component of haemoglobin. Limitations of the test include the inability to detect low concentrations of blood, false positives with other gastrointestinal conditions such as inflammatory bowel disease or even dietary causes (raw steaks or black pudding). Patients that are found to be positive on are invited for a nurse appointment and colonoscopy. If the FOBT is negative or the colonoscopy is normal the patient is offered a repeat faecal occult test within two years time if < 70 years. If the colonoscopy identifies polyps, patients will be treated and followed up with surveillance colonoscopy. If other pathology is detected, patients are treated accordingly and if cancer is diagnosed, an urgent referral is made. More sensitive tests are in development and being trialled in other countries. An alternative immunochemical FOBT has a higher sensitivity and specificity than the guaiac form but can be unstable at certain temperatures. Other tests such as faecal DNA testing are still under trial.

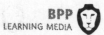

Principles of screening test (Adapted from World Health Organisation, 1968)

The condition should be an important health problem for the individual and community.

There should be an acceptable treatment or intervention for patients with the disease.

Facilities for diagnosis and treatment should be available.

There should be a recognisable latent or early symptomatic stage.

There should be a suitable screening test for the population.

The natural history of the disease should be adequately understood.

There should be an agreed policy for referral for further examination and for whom to treat as patients.

The cost should be economically balanced in relation to possible expenditure on medical care as a whole.

Case finding should be a continuing process and not a once-only project.

Colonic diverticulosis

Diverticulosis is the presence of small outpouchings (pseudo-diverticulae) from the colonic lumen due to mucosal herniation through the colonic wall at sites of vascular perforation. The most common site for diverticulosis is the sigmoid colon, although any part can be affected; in developed countries there is 90% involvement of sigmoid colon and 15% of the right side.

Epidemiology

There has been a significant increase in prevalence over the last few decades, which increases with age, although complications occur in only 10–30% patients. The prevalence is less than 10% in individuals below 40 years, approximately 30% above 60 years, and more than 50% prevalence above 80 years of age.

Aetiology

- Results from increase in intraluminal pressure from straining to pass stool (caused by deficiency in dietary fibre) resulting in mucosal blowouts through weak points in muscle.
- Hypertrophy of circular muscle and taeniae coli also occur.
- Age-related structural changes in the bowel, such as decrease in collagen, reduce the overall tensile strength, thus facilitating formation of diverticulae.
- Connective tissue disorders can also be responsible in younger patients.

Uncomplicated diverticular disease

- Patients with diverticulosis are asymptomatic (incidental finding).
- Symptomatic diverticular disease manifests with episodic lower abdominal pain, associated with a change in bowel habit and abdominal bloating.
- The inflammatory markers are normal.
- Anti-spasmodic agents may be beneficial in some patients.
- Some patients report dietary links.

Complicated diverticular disease

Complicated diverticular disease comprises a spectrum of conditions including acute diverticulitis, bleeding, perforation, abscess, fistula, and intestinal obstruction.

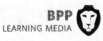

Acute diverticulitis

- It is the most common complication of diverticular disease (affects up to 25%), characterised by inflammation of one or more diverticulae.
- It is likely caused by stool obstructing the narrow-necked diverticulae, rubbing the mucosa, which may be breached by bacteria, leading to inflammation.
- Symptoms include abdominal pain (left iliac fossa most commonly, as sigmoid colon is most commonly affected), fever, lethargy, anorexia, altered bowel habit. Rectal bleeding is rare.
- Examination reveals localised tenderness ± palpable mass and pyrexia.
- Raised inflammatory markers, with patients showing signs of sepsis.
- Necessary investigations include an erect CXR (to exclude free air) and AXR (may show signs of intestinal obstruction, soft tissue densities/abscesses).
- Urinalysis to rule out urinary infection (common differential) or confirm colovesical fistula.
- Ultrasound of the abdomen may be useful, although it is operator-dependent.
- Optimum investigation is a CT scan of abdomen/pelvis with contrast (intravenous, oral and possibly rectal) (Figure 2.3).
- Colonoscopy is contraindicated in the acute phase (high risk of perforation).
- Treatment includes bowel rest (clear fluids), antibiotics (for aerobic and anaerobic bacteria) and analgesia. If symptoms do not settle within 72 hours, further investigations (CT) are required to exclude the presence of an abscess.
- 33% patients with confirmed diverticulitis will have recurrent episodes, which are less likely to respond to conservative treatment (70% first episode, 10% third episode). Prophylactic elective resection is recommended by some centres, after confirmed episodes of recurrent uncomplicated diverticulitis.
- Acute diverticulitis in patients < 40 years is more aggressive with response rates falling to below 50%.

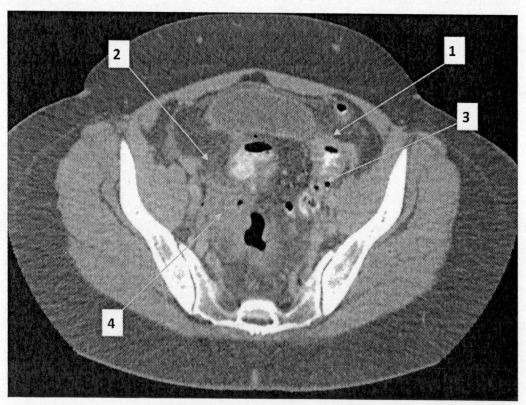

Figure 2.3. CT findings in diverticulitis
Reproduced with permission from Maidstone Hospital

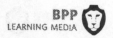

CT findings in diverticulitis: Localised mural thickening (> 5mm in 70% of cases), usually asymmetric (1); stranding of nearby mesenteric fat (seen in 98% of cases) (2); diverticulae are present in 84% of cases (an inflamed diverticulum is frequently seen at the epicentre of inflammatory change) (3); a soft tissue mass, phlegmon (4), pericolic fluid collection, or abscess, seen in 35% of cases. Peritonitis, fistula formation, and obstruction can also be noted on CT.

Diverticular bleeding

- One of the most common causes of lower GI haemorrhage.
- Changes in the lumen of the arteries within diverticulae predispose to rupture.
- Bleeding is often painless, of sudden onset and consists of either fresh bright red blood or maroon in colour, sometimes with associated clots.
- 70–80% of cases settle spontaneously, re-bleeding occurs in one-third.
- Management includes initial fluid resuscitation, routine blood tests including clotting studies, and discontinuation of agents predisposing to bleeding.
- OGD should be performed to exclude an upper gastrointestinal cause in certain cases.
- Flexible sigmoidoscopy or colonoscopy may identify the source (anorectal cause must be excluded), although the optimum time for the examination is debatable.
- Scintigraphy is a simple non-invasive test that may identify the site of bleeding, but requires haemorrhage to be active during the examination.
- Angiography (advantage of therapeutic ability via embolisation or intra-arterial vasopressin).
- Surgery: In cases of significant persistent bleeding, a selective hemicolectomy if site identified; alternatively, total colectomy with ileostomy if the source cannot be identified.

Diverticular perforation

- One of the most common causes of death from benign disease in the UK.
- Usually due to rupture of a previously localised abscess.
- Small perforations are contained by fat and mesentery forming *pericolic abscesses*.
- Large perforations cause extensive abscess formation with the development of an *inflammatory phlegmon*.
- Intraperitoneal perforation causes purulent or faecal peritonitis.
- Patients often present shocked and need urgent resuscitation.
- Management includes fluid resuscitation, antibiotics, analgesia and surgery.
- Surgical options include Hartmann's procedure or primary anastomosis with / without covering ileostomy, or laparoscopic washout.

Stage	Features
I	Pericolic / mesenteric abscess
II	Pelvic / retroperitoneal abscess
III	Purulent peritonitis
IV	Faecal peritonitis

Table 2.8. Hinchey classification of complicated diverticulitis

In a systematic review by Toorenvliet *et al* (2010), two prospective cohort studies, nine retrospective case series and two case reports reporting 231 patients were selected for data extraction. Most (77%) patients had purulent peritonitis (Hinchey III). Laparoscopic peritoneal lavage successfully controlled abdominal and systemic sepsis in 95.7% of patients. Mortality was 1.7%, morbidity 10.4% and only four (1.7%) of the 231 patients received a colostomy.

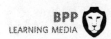

Diverticular abscess

- Perforations may be contained locally as pericolic, mesenteric abscesses or walled off as pelvic or retroperitoneal abscesses.
- Patients present as acute diverticulitis with localised peritonism and signs of sepsis.
- Abdominal or pelvic masses may be palpable.
- Investigations include routine blood tests, erect CXR and AXR, as above.
- Ultrasound may be useful, contrast CT scan is the optimum imaging modality.
- Management of small pericolic abscesses includes bowel rest, fluid resuscitation, analgesia and antibiotics.
- Larger abscesses may be drained either percutaneously under ultrasound or CT guidance, or surgically (laparoscopically).
- Resection can then be appropriately planned.

Diverticular fistulas

- Fistulas develop if a phlegmon or abscess ruptures or extends into an adjacent organ.
- Colovesical fistulas more commonly affect males than females.
- Colovaginal fistulas are more common after hysterectomy.
- Patients may present with pneumaturia, recurrent urinary tract infections, vaginal discharge or the passage of faeces per vagina.
- The differential diagnosis includes Crohn's disease, carcinoma of the colon, uterus or bladder or radiation damage.
- The anatomy of the fistula can be outlined by flexible sigmoidoscopy, cystoscopy, contrast enemas and contrast CT scans.
- Surgical options include defunctioning colostomies for patients unfit for major resection, or an elective single stage resection of diseased segment with closure of the fistula. A urinary catheter should be left in situ for at least ten days postoperatively if the bladder has been involved with some units advocating a cystogram before removal.

Intestinal obstruction

- Obstruction may involve the small bowel as part of an inflammatory mass. Colonic obstruction may be caused by narrowing of the lumen due to inflammation or extrinsic compression from an abscess. Recurrent diverticulitis can cause progressive fibrosis and stricturing of the colon leading to subacute obstruction.
- Contrast enemas or CT scans can be used to distinguish between mechanical obstruction and pseudo-obstruction.
- Differentiating between a benign diverticular and malignant stricture is not always possible.
- Conservative treatment options include endoscopic balloon dilatation or metal stent insertion, which could be used as a bridge to surgery, or permanently for unfit patients.
- Surgical options include resection with primary anastomosis (with / without covering ileostomy) or Hartmann's procedure.

Indications for elective surgery (open or laparoscopic) for diverticular disease

- Recurrent acute inflammatory episodes
- Recurrent chronic symptoms
- Symptomatic fistula
- Symptomatic stricture

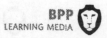

In a meta-analysis by Purkayastha et al (2006) comparing open and laparoscopic surgery for diverticular disease, twelve non-randomised studies were included, incorporating 19,608 patients. Laparoscopic surgery resulted in reduced infective, pulmonary, gastrointestinal tract, and cardiovascular complications with no significant heterogeneity. Operative time was longer with laparoscopic surgery, and length of stay was significantly shorter. Laparoscopic surgery for diverticular disease performed by appropriately experienced surgeons in the elective setting was shown to be safe and feasible.

Urogenital pathology

Benign Prostatic Hyperplasia (BPH)

Epidemiology

Western men are more prone to develop BPH due to complex interplay of hormonal and dietary influences. Approximately 25% will present with lower urinary tract (LUTS) symptoms, increasing to 43% for those above 60 years of age. The mean prostatic volume increases with age from 25ml in men in their thirties to 45ml in men in their seventies.

Development of the prostate gland

Male and female embryos develop identically in the initial stage. Both have undifferentiated gonads and Wolffian ducts (develops into male genitals) and Mullerian ducts (develops into female genitals). Male phenotype develops under the influence of testicular androgens and the Mullerian inhibiting substance, which is a peptide hormone that acts on type I and II receptors and causes regression of the Mullerian duct. Testicular androgens act on the Wolffian duct which develops to form the epididymis, vas deferens and seminal vesicles and the urogenital sinus develops into the prostate, the urethra, and periurethral glands. Testicular androgens bind to androgen receptors expressed on the urogenital sinus mesenchymal cells, which then signals morphogenesis of prostatic epithelial ducts and acini. This pivotal role of mesenchyme continues in adult life influencing the development of BPH.

Function of the prostate gland

(See also Chapter 1, *Anatomy – the prostate gland*.)

The prostate gland is responsible for fertility (contributing to most of the ejaculation volume). The secretions are rich in fructose and provide substrate for oxidative metabolism of spermatozoa and prostate specific antigen (easily measured marker), which liquefies the viscous seminal fluid, facilitating spermatozoa's motility.

Risk factors for development of BPH

- Age is associated with increasing prostate enlargement related to BPH. Approximately 40% of men with age above 50 years and 90% above 80 years have microscopic histopathological evidence of BPH.
- Genetics: Males who have first-degree relatives with BPH are at increased risk.
- Racial: BPH prevalence and surgical intervention is lower in Asian men. The Olmsted County cohort showed higher prevalence of moderate to severe urinary tract symptoms in Afro-Caribbean than Caucasians. Other studies also showed similar results in Afro-Caribbean.
- Diet: BPH has been associated with intake of higher total energy and animal protein. Western diet seems to be a risk factor for BPH and prostate cancer.

Histology and pathogenesis

The pathogenesis of BPH is multifactorial and poorly understood because of the great variation in microscopic, macroscopic and molecular changes seen in BPH. BPH consists of 50% connective tissue, 25% smooth muscle and 25% epithelium. Hyperplasia of the epithelial component is at least partially linked to age-related changes within the cells. The cells are regularly lost or replaced by replication of stem cells hence, with differentiation, identical cell layers are created. The evidence suggests that this process changes gradually with increasing age.
The process initiates with proliferation of fibroblast-like stromal cells in the periurethral region.

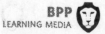

These form micronodules near the bladder neck. Epithelial buds in the transitional zone form new glands taking on a nodular form. The micronodules eventually coalesce. Common findings on endoscopic examination are enlarged lateral lobes kissing in the midline (transitional zone enlargement), with an enlargement of the median lobe at the 6 o'clock position (periurethral stromal proliferation).

Clinical manifestations

Men usually present with lower urinary tract symptoms (LUTS) or a complication from unrelieved bladder outflow obstruction (BOO). Severe life threatening urinary infection and renal failure is unusual in western countries.

During history taking it is important to establish the oral intake of dietary fluids; the frequency of urine; the input and output balance; the drug history; (vasoactive agents, as found in various cold and cough remedies, can cause voiding difficulties or retention by stimulation of a-adrenoceptors); the presence and quality of sexual functions; the presence of normal ejaculation or fertility.

Many patients are asymptomatic and a diagnosis is made by identifying a palpable bladder on examination, an incidentally raised PSA or abnormal renal function, or finding an enlarged prostate on digital rectal examination. Lower urinary tract symptoms include nocturia, voiding symptoms such as hesitancy, slow flow, terminal dribbling and feeling of incomplete emptying, or storage symptoms, such as urgency and urge incontinence.

The clinical examination should include: a urine dipstick to exclude infection and haematuria; looking for an obviously distended or palpable bladder and signs of renal impairment; digital rectal examination (DRE) to assess the anal tone, prostate consistency and size (a simple assessment of 'normal', 'big' or 'very big' is sufficient for choosing therapy). DRE detailing the shape, consistency or irregularities of a gland, can reveal up to 20% of palpable abnormalities.

Diagnostic work up

- Serum Prostate-Specific Antigen (PSA) measurement.
- Flow studies: Uroflowmetry is a useful tool to assess bladder outflow obstructions. A flow rate of > 15ml/second excludes bladder outflow obstruction (BOO) while flow rate < 10ml/second is more suggestive of BOO. As men with poor functioning bladder detrusor muscle do not tolerate surgery well, some urologists suggest all patients should undergo pressure flow studies to prove obstruction and functioning detrusor muscle before surgery.
- The transrectal ultrasound (TRUS) is valuable if digital rectal examination and PSA are abnormal and provides useful information of prostate volume facilitating accurate placing of the biopsy needle in the prostate (TRUS biopsy).
- Other tests: There is little evidence to suggest examination of upper urinary tract by radiology or ultrasound unless there is a large residual urine, palpable bladder or raised creatinine.

Management

- Lifestyle changes including stopping smoking, and alerting the nature, volume, timing of fluid intake may help considerably.
- Medical: Pharmacotherapy is commonly used to relieve excessive smooth muscle tone within the lower urinary tract or reduce prostatic size.

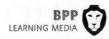

- *Alpha-blockers* block alpha adrenoreceptor sites based at the bladder neck and trigone and within the prostate. They act quickly on all sizes of prostate and are usually well tolerated apart from postural hypotension causing dizziness. Younger men often complain of interference with ejaculation and nasal stuffiness. Patients with CCF should require extra care. Overall the failure rate with alpha-blockers has been reported at 38% in three years, increasing to 54% in five years.
- *5-alpha reductase* inhibitors work slowly on established BPH to achieve symptomatic improvement over four to six months by blocking the enzymes metabolising testosterone to much more potent DHT. It can shrink the prostate by 30% and halve PSA levels. They are safe agents with expected hormonal side effects such as altered libido and sexual functions in all age groups.

Minimally invasive procedures

This usually involves heating the prostate gland by various means (electrical, microwave, laser). It is inserted directly into the prostate via a catheter, probe or endoscope. Heating can be relatively low energy and effects are thought to be due to alpha-adrenoreceptor blockade avoiding anaesthesia. A more direct high energy thermal coagulating or vaporising effect on prostatic tissue with the intention of destroying obstructing prostatic tissue, but with less bleeding than conventional surgery can also be administered under anaesthesia. Retreatment rate appears to be higher than conventional surgery thus reducing the cost effectiveness of this procedure.

Surgical procedures

Surgical procedures involve incision and removal of obstructing tissue. It requires anaesthesia, a catheter and at least a short stay in hospital.

(1)   Transurethral Resection of Prostate (TURP)

The obstructing prostatic tissue is removed with the help of diathermy with a fine cutting loop. It offers low re-operation rate and is the gold standard in BPH management relieving symptoms of obstruction. Complications include mortality (0–0.5%), septicaemia (1.5%), significant blood loss (0.4–6.4%), erectile dysfunction (0–10%), retrograde ejaculation in 70% and incontinence in 1%. Between 1–2% of patients per year require re-operation. Intravascular absorption of irrigating fluid causing cardiovascular and neurological symptoms occurs in 0.5–2% of patients. This leads to intracellular oedema and extracellular sodium and water depletion. Patients develop profound hyponatraemia needing careful correction and monitoring (Post TURP syndrome).

(2)   Transurethral Incision of the Prostate (TUIP; bladder neck incision)

It is commonly used in patients with a small prostate and bladder neck muscular problem. In sexually active men an endoscopic incision is used to reduce the incidence of retrograde ejaculation, although not guaranteed. If fertility is important then medical therapy should be considered and surgery should be avoided. TUIP is a minimal invasive therapy and can be suitable for up to 40% of men.

(3)   Open retropubic prostatectomy

For very large prostate > 100ml open retropubic prostatectomy remains an option.

Bladder outflow obstruction (BOO) secondary to bladder neck obstruction

This is commonly seen in with smaller prostates, often in younger men with low PSA (< 1.4ng/ ml). The choices are lifestyle modification, alpha-blockers, minimally invasive treatments and TUIP based on the severity of the symptoms. TUIP is chosen often in younger men with severe symptoms and clear evidence of bladder neck obstruction. If the symptoms are severe and medical treatment has failed or the patient prefers surgery, TUIP should be offered to small prostate and TURP should be offered to large prostate.

Complications of BOO

- Urinary tract infections
- Bladder stones
- Urinary retention
- Renal impairment

Retention of urine

This is defined as the inability to pass urine and can be classified accordingly:

Acute painful retention

This is associated with suprapubic pain and a tender palpable bladder. The risk of developing painful retention increases with age, severity of LUTS and a family history of BPH. It may be precipitated by excess fluid consumption, forcible delayed micturition and anticholinergic medication. BPH accounts for about 50%, with urethral strictures and prostate cancer accounting for 7.5% and 7% respectively. A majority of recurrent retention episodes occur within one week of the initial trial without catheter.

Acute painless retention

Usually the result of an acute neurological event such as a central disc prolapse or trauma. Urgent assessment including MRI of the spine is required.

Postoperative urinary retention

This is usually multi-factorial in origin. Bladder outflow obstruction by an enlarged prostate is rarely the cause. Normal voiding usually returns within days unless an iatrogenic injury has occurred.

Low pressure chronic retention

This is typically painless and characterised by a large residual volume (> 1L). It is caused by detrusor failure and may be associated with long standing bladder outflow obstruction from BPH or an atonic bladder.

High pressure chronic retention

In this case the resting pressure of the bladder remains high after micturition, causing impaired drainage, hydronephrosis and obstructive uropathy. Patients commonly present with dribbling and overflow incontinence, particularly at night. Transurethral resection of the prostate can lead to normal voiding in a majority of cases.

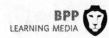

Cancer of the prostate gland

Epidemiology

Prostate cancer is diagnosed in approximately 30,000 men in the UK each year. The figures have increased over the years due to early detection and availability of Prostate-Specific Antigen estimation. Prostate cancer kills > 9,000 men in the UK each year. The geographical incidence varies considerably; it is higher in Northern Europe and North America, intermediate in Southern Europe and South America and lowest in the Far East and Asia. It is more common in Afro-American men and lowest in Chinese men. The lifetime risk for a western male of developing prostate cancer is 30% with a risk of dying from the disease only 3%. A routine screening programme does not currently exist in the UK, but an informed choice programme, Prostate Cancer Risk Management has been introduced.

Risk factors

Age

It is one of the strongest predetermining factors of prostate cancer and rarely develops < 50 years of age. It is very common in advancing age. The probability of developing cancer in men aged 60–79 years is 1 in 8 and in those below 40 years of age is 1 in 10,000.

Genetic

A family history of prostate cancer is one of the strongest known risk factors for this disease. 5–10% of all prostate cancer cases and 30–40% of early-onset cases (men diagnosed < 55 years) are caused by inherited susceptibility genes. Risk increases two to three times for men with a first-degree relative diagnosed with prostate cancer. If the relative is < 60 years old at diagnosis or more than one relative is affected (at any age), the individual's risk is four times the average. These factors combine so that if more than one relative is affected by early-onset prostate cancer, the risk is increased by seven-fold. A strong family history of breast cancer may also affect a man's risk of prostate cancer, particularly if the family members were diagnosed under the age of 60. In particular, germline mutations in the breast cancer susceptibility genes, BRCA1 and BRCA2, can predispose men to prostate cancer.

Diet

It plays a significant role in the risk of developing and preventing prostate cancer. A diet rich in fat, high in dairy products and red meat plays a major role in the higher incidence of prostate cancer.

Testosterone

Testosterone and its metabolite DHT (dihydrotestosterone) are responsible for regulating the growth and function of the prostate gland. High concentrations of testosterone have been identified in Afro-American men explaining higher incidence of prostate cancer in comparison to Caucasian men.

Differential diagnosis

- Benign prostatic hyperplasia
- Prostatitis
- Prostatic calculi

Histopathology

Adenocarcinoma is responsible for > 95% of prostate cancers; the remainder are neuroendocrine tumours or sarcomas. The cytological characteristics of prostate adenocarcinomas include hyperchromatic, enlarged nuclei with prominent nucleoli and abundant cytoplasm. The basal cell layer is absent in prostate cancer, but present in normal glands and the glands of benign prostatic hyperplasia. The areas of prostate adenocarcinoma within the prostate gland are often multifocal. About 70% are found in the peripheral zone, 20% originate in the transition zone, and 10% are within the central zone.

Prostatic intraepithelial neoplasia is the precursor of prostate cancer and cells show similar characteristics, but the basal cell layer is present. Prostatic intraepithelial neoplasia is often found adjacent to prostate cancer areas and biopsy is required to confirm the diagnosis.

Tx – Tumour cannot be assessed
T0 – No evidence of primary tumour
T1 – Not palpable, diagnosed following biopsy for raised PSA or in TURP chips
T2 – Palpable or radiologically confirmed disease (2a – one lobe, 2b – two lobes)
T3 – Tumour extends through prostate capsule (3b – invasion of seminal vesicles)
T4 – Tumour fixed to adjacent structures
N0 – No regional lymph node involvement
N1 – Regional lymph nodes involved
M0 – No distant metastases
M1 – Distant metastases (1a – non regional lymph nodes, 1b – bone, 1c – other)

Table 2.9. TMN classification of prostate cancer

Grading and staging

Gleason grading system is used to grade the cancer based on the microscopic appearance of the glandular architecture of the prostate (grade 1–5). The two commonest Gleason grades are added together to give a score ranging from 2–10 and is usually annotated (eg 3+4 = 7). The grade indicates the degree of glandular differentiation: grade 1 indicates a well-differentiated tumour, whereas grade 5 is a poorly differentiated tumour. The Gleason score gives an indication of prognosis and tumour progression.

The staging of prostate cancer is assessed using a number of tools, digital rectal examination, MRI scan and bone scintigraphy. Most decisions are based on the PSA concentration, clinical examination and Gleason score.

Diagnostic work up

Prostate-specific antigen (PSA) in the serum

Advantages offered:

- Earlier detection of the disease and decrease in mortality from advanced disease.
- Increase in relative survival rate, compared to other causes of death.
- Detection of disease at a younger age and at lower concentrations of PSA.

Disadvantages:

- False high PSA serum levels, because of other causes, such as infection (prostatitis), prostatic hyperplasia, acute urinary retention, vigorous digital rectal examination).

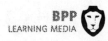

The upper limit of PSA is 4ng/ml; this value will include some patients with BHP and some with prostate cancer. The PSA increases with age, therefore further refinement is required. The speed of rise of PSA during the year before the diagnosis of cancer is strongly associated with risk of death from prostate cancer. The ratio of free : total concentration of PSA is due to BPH or cancer. A value of less than 18 is suggestive of cancer and biopsy should be performed.

The digital rectal examination (DRE)

This is an essential part of the urological examination helping to assess the size, texture, nodularity of the gland, also helping to determine the need for further examinations.

Transrectal ultrasound and biopsy

These are indicated if cancer is suspected due to raised PSA and digital rectal examination. The procedure is done under local anaesthesia and biopsies are taken via a transrectal ultrasound probe allowing more accurate staging than DRE and also the volume of the prostate gland to be measured. The biopsies usually have low morbidity and are taken with a Tru-Cut needle and 6–12 cores are removed. Complications include infection (< 5%) and significant bleeding (< 2%). Anticoagulation should be stopped before biopsy and prophylactic antibiotics are given.

MRI or CT scan of the pelvis for staging

They provide anatomical information about local extension of the cancer and involvement of lymph nodes which assist in decision-making, if radical prostatectomy is being considered.

Whole body bone scintigraphy

This is performed if the PSA > 10ng/ml, evaluates for bony metastases.

New molecular studies

A specific urine sample assay can detect PCA3, a gene that has been over expressed in prostate cancer tissues. A prostate massage is done to shed the prostate cells in the urine.

Management of Localised prostate cancer
Active surveillance

The method should be adopted for men > 70 yrs with multiple co-morbidities with low volume cancer and a low Gleason score. Careful regular follow up with DRE and PSA monitoring is essential.

Radical prostatectomy, to remove the whole prostate

Radical prostatectomy significantly improves the mean patient survival and reduces by 50% the risk of metastases. The procedure is commonly carried out via a horizontal or vertical abdominal incision, although increasingly surgeons prefer the laparoscopic or robotic method. Particular attention is required to preserve the nerves on either side of the prostate and reduce the risk of impotence. The seminal vesicles are removed, urethra is anastomosed to the base of the bladder and the obturator lymph nodes are sampled. A catheter is left for two weeks while the urethra and bladder heal.

Early complications include a mortality of 0.1% and small risks of myocardial infarction, pulmonary embolism and haemorrhage. Late complications include early incontinence in up to one-third of patients and erectile dysfunction in at least one-half, many responding well to

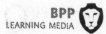

early treatment with phosphodiesterase 5-inhibitors. Significant stress incontinence is seen in 5% of men by 12 months and can be effectively treated by inserting an artificial sphincter.

External beam radiotherapy

This provides a definitive approach for localised and locally advanced disease including pelvic lymph nodes. The recent advances in radiotherapy have helped to focus the beam radiation to the prostate gland with fewer side effects, but proctitis, rectal bleeding, haematuria and 1–3% risk of incontinence have been noted. Erectile dysfunction develops in approximately one third of patients. An overall 15-year survival is similar to that seen in radical prostatectomy, although in cases of recurrence surgery cannot be offered.

Brachytherapy

This involves deployment of radioactive seeds into the prostate gland by one or two stages. It is most suitable for men with small or medium-sized prostate glands with lower risk of cancers. This can also be combined with external beam therapy in patients with a high risk of recurrence. In the one stage procedure 15–20 needles are inserted under anaesthesia into the prostate gland through the perineum under transrectal ultrasound guidance. The field of radiation is calculated to avoid radiation to the urethra and the rectum. This one stage technique has been recorded to have the same outcome as radical prostatectomy and external-beam radiotherapy. Complications include urinary retention in 6–8% and incontinence in 13–18%. Cystitis, proctitis and urethritis affect approximately 10% of patients, with erectile dysfunction in a half.

Cryotherapy

This less commonly used technique involves passing liquid nitrogen down needles that have been inserted into the prostate gland via the perineum, creating an ice ball destroying cancer cells. The side effects are urinary retention, pain and erectile dysfunction. The urethra is protected by a warming urethral catheter. A colovesical fistula is a serious potential complication.

Locally advanced prostate cancer
Hormonal therapy

This can be used on its own or with external beam radiotherapy. Cancer of the prostate is dependent on or stimulated by testosterone, 95% of which is derived from testicles; 70–80% of prostate cancers respond to various forms of androgen deprivation.

The therapy aims to block the production of testosterone at different levels.

- Analogues of luteinizing hormone (LH)-releasing hormone (goserelin) are usually given as a depot injection three-monthly. They stimulate luteinizing hormone receptors in the pituitary gland via negative feedback, and stop the release of LH from the pituitary gland. They produce castrate levels of testosterone within two weeks. The main side effects are reduced sex drive and impotence, which are reversible on stopping the medication. These agents slow the progression of the cancer but do not eradicate the disease.
- Anti-androgens (cyproterone) block the effect of testosterone on the prostate gland and have no profound effect on potency and libido. They cause breast enlargement, soreness and mild GI and liver impairment. They also slow the progression but do not cure the disease.

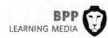

Management of Metastatic prostate cancer

The five-year survival rate for metastatic prostate cancer is 30%. The progression can be delayed by the treatments mentioned below.

- Bilateral orchidectomy stops the production of testosterone. Prostheses can be placed for cosmetic appearance. The main side effects are hot flushes, loss of libido and impotence. Approximately 80% men respond to treatment and it slows disease progression for about 18 months.
- Analogues of luteinizing hormone (LH) releasing hormone. They have a response in 80% of patients, lasting for 18-36 months. Initially they increase the circulating testosterone causing pain and even spinal stenosis; anti androgens are given to protect that. Ultimately a subset of prostate cancer cells proliferate without the need for androgens, causing standard anti-androgen treatment to fail. Alternative anti-androgen medication, oestrogens and steroids can lead to temporary remission, however usually life expectancy is less than one year.

Complications of prostate cancer

- Pain from bony metastases: Individual sites can be given radiotherapy or hemi-body treatment for more extensive disease. It can be given systemically with an infusion of strontium.
- Ureteric obstruction, causing loin pain and renal failure. Patients who have not previously undergone hormone therapy should be treated with a nephrostomy, urinary diversion and androgen deprivation.
- Spinal cord compression: Symptoms may be acute or progressive, consisting of sensory or motor deficits, bladder dysfunction or radicular pain. MRI of the spine should be performed for diagnosis. Immediate treatment with systemic steroids and androgen deprivation by orchidectomy are indicated, followed by urgent radiotherapy and surgical decompression.

Follow up

Most patients have regular serum PSA measurement, which after radical prostatectomy should remain at zero. In patients treated with hormonal therapy, prostate cancer eventually becomes insensitive to hormone ablation and the PSA begins to rise. Whole body scintigraphy must be carried out to exclude metastatic spread. If the PSA rises, therapeutic options include modification of existing hormonal therapy, cytotoxic chemotherapy, oestrogen therapy, bisphosphonates and palliative radiotherapy.

Prognosis

The natural history of prostate cancer is highly dependent on stage, grade of the disease and patient co-morbidity. The ten-year survival rate may be as high as 90% for a well-differentiated, localised prostate cancer; for poorly differentiated tumours it drops to $\leq$ 60%. On the whole, prostate cancer progression is slower than for most other cancers and treatment is not required in many cases. Prostate cancer is one of the few solid cancers that are readily curable, providing it is detected early.

Bladder and ureteric tumours

Epidemiology

Bladder cancer is the commonest tumour of the urinary tract. It is the fifth commonest malignancy in Europe, accounting for 6–8% of all malignancies in males and 2–3% in females. There is a peak incidence in the sixth and seventh decades.

 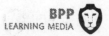

Aetiology and risk factors

- Abnormalities in chromosome 9 are common in superficial bladder cancer, and chromosome 17 in invasive bladder cancer.
- Bladder cancer is strongly linked to environmental and occupational exposure. Disease development is linked to excretion of carcinogenic metabolites in the urine. Long latency periods are often seen.
- Smoking: Aromatic amines and nitrosamines contained in cigarette smoke. Smokers have a fourfold increase in the risk of developing bladder cancer. It is believed that approximately one-third of bladder cancers are related to cigarette smoking.
- Occupational factors: An increased prevalence is noted in aniline dye workers, associated with B naphthylamine and benzidine exposure.
- Infections: Chronic urinary tract infections and cystitis can predispose to bladder cancer. Endemic areas of schistosomiasis show a higher incidence of squamous cell carcinoma.
- Cyclophosphamide treatment and pelvic radiotherapy are also associated with an increased prevalence of bladder cancer.

Histopathology

Approximately 90% of all bladder cancers are transitional cell carcinomas (TCC), ranging from small solitary lesions to metastatic disease. Over 70% are superficial tumours limited to the lamina propria and mucosa. Although there is a high recurrence rate of such mucosal lesions, very few progress (2–4%). Those involving the lamina propria have a much higher chance of progression (30–50%). Superficial tumours are commonly papillary in appearance, while invasive tumours more solid. Approximately 5–10% of lesions are squamous cell carcinomas, although much higher in endemic areas of schistosomiasis. Adenocarcinomas are found in 1% of cases. Carcinoma in situ are flat poorly differentiated epithelial changes which may progress into invasive carcinoma. Tumours are graded according to the degree of cellular abnormality (G1 – well differentiated, G2 – moderately differentiated, G3 – poorly differentiated).

Clinical manifestation and assessment

The commonest presenting symptom is haematuria, which may be macroscopic or microscopic. Of patients presenting with painless macroscopic haematuria approximately 20% will have an underlying malignancy (90% of these with bladder cancer), as opposed to 5% of cases of microscopic haematuria. Other presenting symptoms are those of urinary tract infections, or those relating to advanced disease, such as bony pain or shortness of breath. A thorough history and examination is essential to look for other symptoms and signs of malignancy. (See Chapter 6: *History taking-Haematuria*.)

Diagnostic work up

- Mid-stream urine: Microscopy and culture (to exclude infection) and cytology (malignant cells).
- Intravenous urography, which can detect most upper tract urothelial and bladder tumours.
- Ultrasound KUB: Safe and easy to use, can detect renal and bladder tumours.
- Flexible cystoscopy: Under local urethral anaesthesia, this allows direct visualisation of the lower tract and bladder mucosa. An estimation of the stage of the disease can be made, and cases of carcinoma in situ can be identified. In cases of positive findings, a further (rigid) cystoscopy under general anaesthesia can be performed, with endoscopic excision of the tumour including detrusor muscle (TURBT – Transurethral resection of bladder tumour).

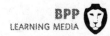

Transitional cell carcinoma of the bladder

Patient management depends on the disease stage (Table 2.10) and histology.

Superficial lesions and carcinoma in situ

Over two-thirds of patients with superficial tumours develop recurrent disease. Risk factors for recurrence include large tumours, poor differentiation, multifocal lesions and carcinoma in situ.

All patients initially undergo transurethral excision to allow full staging. Those found to have solitary low grade (Ta) lesions can be managed by regular cystoscopies, usually three-monthly, then six-monthly and annually. Higher risk patients with either multiple lesions, recurrence, carcinoma in situ or G3T1 lesions should receive some form of intravesical adjuvant therapy. Such therapy can include a chemotherapeutic drug, such as mitomycin or epirubicin. This is administered as a single instillation after excision in superficial cases or by weekly instillation for six weeks in cases of recurrent disease. Alternatively, an immunotherapeutic agent such as BCG can be used at weekly instillation for six weeks. Responders can have maintenance therapy every six months. There are more side effects following BCG instillation, such as cystitis and systemic toxicity. Both types of agents reduce recurrence rates.

T0 – No evidence of tumour	N0 – No regional lymph node involvement
Tis – Carcinoma in situ	N1 – Metastasis in a single node < 2cm
Ta – Non invasive papillary carcinoma	N2 – Metastases in a single node 2–5cm or multiple lymph nodes < 5cm
T1 – Superficial tumour invading subepithelial connective tissue	N3 – Metastases in single or multiple lymph node > 5cm
T2 – Tumour invading muscle	
T3 – Tumour invading prevesical fat	M0 – No distant metastases present
T4 – Invasion of adjacent structures (prostate, uterus, vagina)	M1 – Distant metastases present

Table 2.10. TMN classification of bladder cancer

Muscle invasive tumours (pT2)

In this group of patients the following options are available:

- Radical cystectomy with pelvic lymph node dissection with ileal conduit diversion or orthotopic bladder reconstruction for tumours that have not extended beyond the bladder. The procedure consists of anterior pelvic exenteration including the perivesical and pelvic lymph nodes. The ureters are anastomosed to an ileal conduit or a reservoir constructed of bowel as an orthotopic bladder or the anterior abdominal wall. In males the prostate is also excised and in females the ovaries, fallopian tubes and uterus. Urethral recurrence can develop in up to one-fifth of cases. In cases of urethral involvement, orthotopic diversion or preservative procedures cannot be performed. The five-year survival rates range between 63–83% for T2 lesions, 53–71% for T3a lesions and 0–28% for T4 tumours.
- Radical radiotherapy with salvage cystectomy for those who fail to respond. The duration of treatment is four to six weeks, delivering a total dose of 60–65 Gy to the tumour, with minimal damage to the surrounding structures. Complications include haematuria, bladder contracture and damage to the bowel. One-third of patients with invasive tumours can be managed by this method with up to 50% of this group requiring a salvage cystectomy at some point. There is no obvious difference in survival for the radical radiotherapy group compared with those undergoing a radical cystectomy.

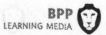

- Chemotherapy is used as adjuvant therapy to conservative surgery, to radical cystectomy or radical radiotherapy or as a sole treatment option. Commonly used regimes include methotrexate, vinblastine, doxorubicin and cisplatin (MVAC). MVAC can achieve a response rate in up to 20% of patients with metastatic disease.
- Palliative therapy in cases of advanced metastatic disease.

Squamous carcinoma of the bladder

It makes up 5% of all bladder tumours, except in endemic areas of schistosomiasis. These tumours are related to chronic bladder irritation due to persistent infection, stones or urinary stasis. They tend to be more aggressive than transitional cell carcinomas with a more infiltrative pattern and higher frequency of muscle invasion at presentation. The treatment of choice is a radical cystectomy. These tumours are not radiosensitive; some success has been shown with chemotherapeutic regimes.

Adenocarcinoma of the bladder

A majority of these lesions are found in the location of the dome of the bladder and may be of urachal origin. Primary lesions tend to infiltrate early and the prognosis is poor. The treatment of choice is surgery as they are also radioresistant. In some cases secondary adenocarcinomas from the colon or prostate can be found within the bladder.

Malignant tumours of the skin

The skin is a large structurally complex organ with many diverse functions. Any of the skin components ie epidermis and dermis including sweat glands, hair follicles and appendageal structures can give rise to malignant tumours. The commonest tumours arise from epidermal squamous cells. The malignant tumours of sweat glands and hair follicles are rare. Malignant tumours of the skin are heterogeneous group, and mostly caused by the exposure to ultraviolet light; immunosuppressive or genetic causes are less often recognised. The most common malignant skin tumours are discussed below and their study is best combined with a Dermatology atlas (see Further Reading at the end of this chapter).

Basal cell carcinoma (rodent ulcer)

Epidemiology and risk factors

This is the most common skin malignancy, usually occurring in the elderly, on hair bearing surfaces of the body. The estimated lifetime risk is 33–39% for men and 23–28% for women. They are most commonly found on sun-exposed areas such as the face, arms and trunk (80%). They originate from pluripotent stem cells within the epidermis. Early onset of multiple lesions could reflect a genetic abnormality such as xeroderma pigmentosum (an autosomal recessive condition involving an inability to repair deoxyribonucleic acid damaged by ultraviolet light). In Gorlin's syndrome, an autosomal dominant condition due to a mutation on chromosome 9, multiple lesions develop from adolescence. The majority of lesions can be treated with local excision with narrow margins.

Classification

Various clinical subtypes are recognised:

*   Nodular (up to 60%).
    This is the commonest subtype, usually displaying clear margins making them easy to remove. As they enlarge, a central focus of ulceration can develop. The classic description of a rolled edge is seen with some surface telangiectasia. An element of melanin deposition can also be found. A micronodular type is described which resemble nodular lesions with not so well defined margins, and are more infiltrative.
*   Infiltrative (5%)
    These lesions are often flat with poorly defined margins and excision can be incomplete; can be dangerous due to possible extension particularly in certain areas of the face (orbit).
*   Superficial
    These lesions occur on the trunk, presenting as erythematous scaly patches which gradually increase in size (10%–30%).
*   Sclerosing / morpheaform (5%).
*   Less common forms such as micronodular, metatypical, infundibulocystic, nodulocystic, adenoid, clear cell, follicular, sebaceous and perineurally invasive.

Histology

Microscopically, lesions consist of islands of basaloid cells in the dermis, similar to the epidermis basal layer. Peripheral pallisading of nests of cells is also seen, with some ulceration of the epidermis. Basal cell carcinomas are locally invasive, with metastatic spread extremely rare (< 0.1%).

Management

Best treatment constitutes local excision with adequate margins (see also Table 2.11). The risk of local recurrence depends on the anatomical location, tumour subtype and adequacy of treatment and in certain cases further surgery is necessary. Overall basal cell carcinoma is associated with an excellent prognosis.

Lesion	Treatment options
Actinic keratosis	• Cryosurgery- Commonest modality using liquid nitrogen. Cure rates of 75-99% reported • Curettage- Highly effective with local anaesthesia. Can be used with electrosurgery • Photodynamic therapy- Application of a photosensitising agent (aminolevulinic acid) followed by exposure to a light of specific wavelength (blue) after a short incubation period (1 hour) has reported cure rates of between 69-93% • Topical diclofenac- 3% diclofenac in 2.5% hyaluronan has demonstrated a 50% complete resolution after 3 months treatment • Topical 5-Flourouracil- a highly effective topical treatment but with some cosmetic side effects necessitating lower dose preparations. Can also be used as neoadjuvant treatment before cryotherapy • Topical Imiquimod- Stimulates the immune system to produce interferon. Up to 57% complete response rates have been reported with 5% cream use
Basal cell carcinoma (BCC)/ Squamous cell carcinoma (SCC)	• Excisional surgery- Under local anaesthesia cure rates of approximately 90% can be achieved • Moh's surgery- Microscopically controlled surgery aiming to obtain complete margin control during removal of a skin cancer using frozen section histology. Samples are repeatedly analysed during the procedure to ensure the highest cure rate and taking the minimum amount of normal tissue. Cure rates of approximately 94%-99% are reported (BCC/SCC) • Curettage and desiccation- A useful technique for smaller lesions, but not as effective for more aggressive/ high risk tumours • Laser surgery- Using carbon dioxide or YAG laser. Can be utilised as secondary therapy • Radiation- Complete destruction of the tumour can require multiple sessions (25-30) achieving cure rates of 90% (BCC/SCC). Repeated therapy has associated risks (cosmetic and radiation) • Cryosurgery • Intralesional interferon (BCC)- Up to 30% failure rates reported with side effects including 'flu' like symptoms and localised inflammation • Topical treatment- Both 5-Flourouracil and Imiquimod are utilised for superficial BCCs only

Table 2.11. Treatments and outcomes for non-melanoma skin cancer

Squamous cell carcinoma

Epidemiology

This is the second commonest skin malignancy and develops from epidermal keratinocytes. In comparison to basal cell carcinoma, it has significant risk of metastasis and associated mortality. Lesions may develop in an area of Bowen's disease or de novo, with multiple lesions developing in immunosuppressed patients.

Risk factors

These include sun exposure, radiation therapy, chronic cutaneous ulceration – Marjolin's ulcers (venous), chronic unhealed burns, genetic conditions (xeroderma pigmentosum, dystrophic epidermolysis) and actinic keratosis (precursor lesion).

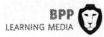

Clinical manifestations

They present as enlarging keratotic nodules with a heaped up border. As the lesion continues to enlarge a central portion of ulceration appears. Microscopically there are irregular areas of dysplastic squamous epithelium arising from the base of the ulcer. The tumour may be well differentiated with keratin production, moderately differentiated or poorly differentiated. These are locally destructive tumours and can metastasise to local lymph nodes (5–10%).

Differential diagnosis

This includes basal cell carcinoma, keratoacanthoma and amelanotic melanoma.

Management and outcomes (also Table 2.11)

As the local recurrence rate is twice as that of basal cell carcinoma, a wider excision margin must be planned at surgery. Lymph node spread is higher in mucosal or irradiated areas (up to 20%), requiring regional block dissection ± radiotherapy.

The outcome depends on tumour grading. A well differentiated lesion has a better outcome than poor differentiated lesions with severe cytonuclear atypia and scant keratinisation.

Factors affecting prognosis

- Stage pT2 tumours (> 20mm in diameter) are three times more likely to metastasise compared to pT1 lesions (< 20mm).
- Lesions < 2 mm deep have an excellent prognosis, but extension beyond the dermis is associated with an increased risk of adverse outcome.
- Perineural invasion is associated with a high risk of local recurrence. It is common in lesions arising in the mid-face and lip, and is usually identified in rarer spindle cell or acantholytic variants of squamous cell carcinoma.

Malignant melanoma

Epidemiology

The incidence of melanomas has significantly increased in the last five decades. This is largely attributed to excessive sun exposure of fair skinned people. In the UK, its prevalence is 4% per annum and the incidence is 8/100,000 for men and 11/100,000 for women. It is more common in middle aged and elderly people. Between 40–70% of lesions develop in a pre-existing naevus. Although development is primarily associated with exposure to ultraviolet light, certain predisposing genetic conditions also exist. Dysplastic naevus syndrome is caused by mutations on chromosome 9. Patients with a positive phenotype and two relatives with a history of melanomas have a 100% lifetime risk of developing a lesion.

Clinical manifestation

Early diagnosis can be achieved by self screening and regular assessment by primary care physicians. Urgent referral to specialist clinic is indicated where there is:

- A new mole appearing after the onset of puberty which is changing in shape, colour or size.
- A long-standing mole which is changing in shape, colour or size.
- Any mole which has three or more colours or has lost its symmetry.

- A mole which is itching or bleeding.
- Any new persistent skin lesion especially if growing, if pigmented or vascular in appearance, and if the diagnosis is not clear.
- A new pigmented line in a nail especially where there is associated damage to the nail.
- A lesion growing under a nail.

Remember the simple assessment tool – ABCD rule.

A   Asymmetry.
B   Border – benign lesions have a symmetrical border, while malignant lesions have uneven or notched borders.
C   Colour – Usually colour is uniform in benign lesions, while variable in malignant lesions.
D   Diameter – Lesions > 6mm are more likely to be malignant, especially if other changes are also present.

Histology

There are four main subtypes of melanoma recognised by variations in their histological growth.

Superficial spreading melanoma

This is the most common type accounting for approximately 70% of all melanomas. They may develop from an existing lesion, and tumour cells continue to grow outward horizontally above the basement membrane (radial growth phase). Gradually a vertical growth phase will commence as the tumour penetrates the basement membrane, allowing the lesion to metastasise.

Nodular melanoma

This is the second most common lesion making up approximately 25% of melanomas. They often arise de novo and are more symmetric in shape and protuberant. They display more vertical growth and therefore are more aggressive than superficial spreading melanomas.

Lentigo melanoma

These account for 4% of all melanomas and demonstrate a direct dose-response relationship with sun exposure. They usually appear on exposed areas such as the face, developing over a period of time. Lentigo maligna is a pigmented lesion which is believed to be the premalignant form.

Acral lentiginous melanomas

This accounts for the remaining 1% of lesions, rarely seen in fair skinned people. This is the most common form seen in Afro-Caribbeans and Asian individuals. Lesions can be found on the palms and soles of the feet and subungual areas. Patients often present late with advanced disease.

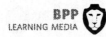

Biopsy for suspected melanoma (Adapted from NICE)

- A suspected melanoma should be photographed, then excised completely.
- The axis of excision should be orientated to facilitate possible subsequent wide local excision.
- The excision biopsy should include the whole tumour with a clinical margin of 2 mm of normal skin, and a cuff of fat.
- Diagnostic shave biopsies should not be performed (risk of incorrect diagnosis due to sampling error, inaccurate pathological staging).
- Incisional or punch biopsy is occasionally acceptable, for example in the differential diagnosis of lentigo maligna (LM) on the face or of acral melanoma.
- Prophylactic excision of naevi or of small (< 5cm diameter) congenital naevi in the absence of suspicious features is not recommended.

Staging

An adequate excision biopsy gives information regarding lymphatic or vascular invasion, presence of mitoses, ulceration, the host response and the depth and invasion. The two methods of histopathological staging are the Breslow's thickness and Clark's levels of invasion (Table 2.12). If diagnosis is confirmed, patients should go on to have baseline CT scan for staging purposes.

Tumour thickness and depth (Breslow)	
Thickness (mm)	Ten-year survival (%)
< 0.75	98
0.75-1.5	91
> 3	55
Clark's levels of invasion	
Level I – Lesions involving only the epidermis	
Level II – Invasion of the papillary dermis	
Level III – Invasion fills the papillary dermis but does not reach the reticular dermis	
Level IV – Invasion of reticular dermis	
Level V – Invasion through reticular dermis into subcutaneous tissue	

Table 2.12. Classification systems for malignant melanoma

Management

Wider excision

On confirmation of diagnosis the patient often requires a wider margin (1–3cm). Closure can be achieved in most cases otherwise flaps (pedicled/free) are necessary.

Lymph node surgery

Most metastatic spread is via the lymphatics, with approximately 70% spreading to local lymph nodes, with occult micro metastases seen in a small proportion. Options for patients in this case are:

- Elective lymph node dissection, removing all the regional nodes draining the primary melanoma site, or
- A sentinel lymph node biopsy/ultrasound surveillance

The principle of sentinel lymph node biopsy states the first node draining a lymphatic basin (sentinel node) should be able to predict the presence of metastatic spread. This technique has aided the management of melanomas in a number of ways, allowing accurate staging and identifying unpredictable patterns of lymphatic spread for certain lesions. The technique involves the injection of 1% isosulfan blue dye around the lesion for intraoperative localisation of the node. Current indications include melanomas > 1mm or lesions with ulceration or histological regression. As lesions on the trunk may have more than one sentinel node, preoperative lymphoscintigraphy with technetium labelled tracing can be used as an alternative.

Adjuvant therapy

Melanomas are rarely sensitive to chemotherapeutic drugs. *Dacarbazine* produces a complete response rate of 3–5%. Perfusion chemotherapy, such as limb perfusion with chemotherapeutic agents including *melphalan*, *cisplatin* and *Tumour Necrosis Factor-A* have shown encouraging results for local recurrence. Adjuvant therapy with interferon has also sparked interest in patients with tumour thicknesses of > 4mm, with some encouraging results. Other biological routes have also been studied, including *interleukin-2*, *monoclonal antibodies* and *vaccines*.

Preventative measures

- Physical protection: Avoidance of direct sunlight, especially for children, fair-skin individuals, those with increased number of naevi and family history of melanoma.
- Appropriate clothing.
- Sunscreens and creams.
- Avoid sunbeds and tanning salons.
- Public education.

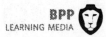

Breast pathology

Breast cancer

Epidemiology

Increasing incidence is noted, with life time risk of disease for women being 1:9. Less than 1% of breast cancer occurs in men. The UK mortality is 28 women/100,000/year, among the highest worldwide, but decreasing. Five per cent of breast cancers are hereditary, 95% sporadic; the incidence increases with age.

Risk factors

Family history, early menarche, late menopause, nulliparity, long-term use of oral contraceptive pill and hormone replacement therapy have been recognised as risk factors for breast cancer.

Histology

Breast cancer is classified into the following types:

1. Epithelial, non-invasive
   - Ductal carcinoma in situ (DCIS): This is mainly detected by breast screening and is less commonly palpable. It comprises of neoplastic epithelial proliferation within breast ducts and is limited by the basement membrane, although the process may extend into lobules. It grows within a single duct system of the breast, can vary in size and has not metastasised. Based on the cytonuclear features of the cells, DCIS is classified into low, intermediate or high cytonuclear grade. The higher the grade, the higher the risk of progression into invasive breast cancer and local recurrence after excision. It may occur alone or in association with invasive ductal carcinoma (IDC).
   - Lobular carcinoma in situ (LCIS): A monotonous proliferation of epithelial cells with expansion of the lobules. The relationship between LCIS and invasive carcinoma is not as distinct as between DCIS and IDC.
2. Epithelial, invasive
   - Ductal (85%)
   - Lobular (1%)
   - Mucinous (5%)
   - Papillary (< 5%)
   - Medullary (< 5%)
3. Mixed connective tissue and epithelial
4. Miscellaneous

Diagnostic work up

Evaluation of breast lump / screening detected abnormality is achieved by the 'Triple assessment', including:

1. **Clinical evaluation** (discussed in Chapter 7: *Clinical examinations – Breast examination*)
2. **Radiological imaging**, leading to the following potential outcomes:
   - R1: Normal
   - R2: Benign
   - R3: Indeterminate
   - R4: Abnormal probably malignant
   - R5: Malignant

The available imaging modalities include:

- Breast ultrasound, as the sole imaging modality in young patients (< 35) with a palpable abnormality, pregnancy, lactation, immobile or wheelchair bound patient, extreme tenderness/inflammation. It is also useful in the presence of implants (consider MRI as second investigation), to differentiate cystic from solid opacities, when mammography is equivocal and in evaluating suspected abscesses. Pre treatment ultrasound evaluation of the axilla should be performed for all patients being investigated for early invasive breast cancer and, if morphologically abnormal lymph nodes are identified, ultrasound-guided needle sampling should be offered (NICE, 2009) following discussion at the multidisciplinary meeting for all R4 and R5 nodes.
- Mammography for women over the age of 35 (bilateral 2 view mammogram with lateral/magnification/paddle views if necessary), and under the age of 35, with a suspicious ultrasound or where the cytological suspicion of malignancy is high.
- MRI scanning can be used:
  - If breast density or the presence of implants preclude accurate mammographic assessment.
  - If there is discrepancy regarding the extent of the disease from clinical examination, mammography and ultrasound assessment for planning treatment.
  - To assess the tumour size if breast conserving surgery is being considered for invasive lobular cancer.

3. **Cytology/Histopathology**, which can be obtained by:
   - Fine needle aspiration (FNA) cytology (if the lesion is impalpable the FNA can be performed under ultrasound or mammographic guidance).
     - C1: Inadequate
     - C2: Benign
     - C3: Cell atypia probably benign/possible malignancy
     - C4: Suspicious of malignancy
     - C5: Malignant
   - Core biopsy, under radiological guidance if the lesion is impalpable, when FNA is unhelpful or tissue diagnosis is necessary prior to initiation of further management, eg for primary medical therapy where ER (oestrogen receptor) status is required.
   - Open diagnostic biopsy, less common.

Management

This is determined by the Breast Multidisciplinary Team meeting (MDT) attended by breast surgeons, radiologists, pathologists, oncologists and breast care nurses. The treatment options to be considered in confirmed diagnosis of breast cancer are:

- Surgery followed by adjuvant chemotherapy, radiotherapy and hormonal treatment.
- Primary hormonal therapy.
- Neoadjuvant chemotherapy or hormonal treatment.
- Oncological management of metastatic disease.

Surgical treatment of breast cancer

The surgical management involves treatment for the breast disease and the axilla.

Breast surgery options include:

- Breast conserving surgery: Wide local excision.
- Total mastectomy, conventional or skin-sparing.
- Radical (Halstead) mastectomy, involving total mastectomy, axillary node clearance and excision of pectoralis muscles is now rarely done.

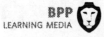

The options for surgical management of the axilla include:

- Axillary node dissection or clearance: A defined surgical block dissection to remove all the lymph node tissue in the axilla.
- Axillary node sampling (four node sampling).
- Sentinel lymph node (the first draining lymph node) biopsy (SLNB) by use of combined isotope and blue dye, isotope or blue dye alone.

NICE Guidance (Adapted from NICE, 2009): Minimal surgery, rather than lymph node clearance, should be performed to stage the axilla for patients with early invasive breast cancer and no evidence of lymph node involvement on ultrasound or a negative ultrasound-guided needle biopsy, with SLNB being the preferred technique using the dual technique with isotope and blue dye.

Adjuvant therapy

Adjuvant therapy should be considered for all patients with early invasive breast cancer after surgery, based on assessment of the prognostic and predictive factors, the potential benefits and side effects of the treatment and following discussion of these factors with the patient. Options include:

- Endocrine treatments
  - Direct treatments: tamoxifen or aromatase inhibitors (anastrozole, exemestane and letrozole) for patients with hormone receptor-positive tumours.
  - Indirect treatments such as radiation menopause, medical oophorectomy by luteinising hormone-releasing hormone agonists (LHRHa) and ovarian ablation by surgery.
- Chemotherapy
- Radiotherapy for patients with early invasive breast cancer who have had
  - Breast conserving surgery with clear margins
  - A mastectomy and are at a high risk of local recurrence
- Targeted biological agents
  The presence and overexpression of the HER2 receptor (a member of the family of human epidermal growth factor receptors) in about 15% of early stage invasive breast cancers is associated with a poor prognosis. The humanised monoclonal antibody Trastuzumab (Herceptin®) targets the extracellular domain of HER2 and is recommended as an adjuvant treatment to women with HER2-positive early invasive breast cancer following surgery, chemotherapy and radiotherapy. It is contraindicated in cardiac failure.

(See Further Reading: Adjuvant! Online – a software tool for the need and type of adjuvant therapy.)

Breast reconstruction

Breast reconstruction can be immediate or delayed. Methods used include the following:

- Tissue expanders, subsequently replaced by a permanent implant containing silicone gel or saline.
- Autologous tissue: skin and underlying muscle (myocutaneous flap) transferred with its original blood supply intact (pedicled flap) or new arterial and venous blood supply created by microsurgery (free flap).
- Pedicled myocutaneous flaps. The two commonest are the latissimus dorsi flap based on the thoracodorsal vessels and the transverse rectus abdominis based on the superior epigastric vessels (TRAM).

- Free myocutaneous flaps, such as the free TRAM flap and the deep inferior epigastric perforator (DIEP) flap.

Prognosis

Prognostic factors in invasive breast cancer include tumour type, size, grade, vascular invasion, lymph node involvement, oestrogen receptor status, HER-2 receptor status. The Nottingham Prognostic Index (below) has been used to classify patients into groups of good, intermediate and poor prognosis:

$$(NPI) = (0.2 \times \text{tumour size (cm)}) + \text{tumour grade} + \text{stage}$$

Stage 1: lymph nodes uninvolved
Stage 2: 1–3 axillary lymph nodes or one internal mammary lymph node involved
Stage 3: 4+ axillary lymph nodes or an axillary and an internal mammary lymph node involved

Classification in prognostic groups:

- Good (< 3.4)
- Intermediate (3.41–5.4)
- Poor (> 5.41)

Gynaecomastia

Gynaecomastia is a generalised enlargement of the male breast, both of ductal and stromal tissue, manifesting as a firm mobile disc of tissue. It is the commonest benign condition affecting the male breast.

Aetiology (Table 2.13)

Diagnostic work up

- History and physical examination.
- Consider investigations in adult men: Chest X-ray, electrolytes, liver function tests and assays for follicle-stimulating hormone, luteinizing hormone, human chorionic gonadotropin, thyroid-stimulating hormone, thyroxine, oestrogen, oestradiol, and testosterone levels in patients with progressive disease.
- Also, in adult men, fine needle aspiration cytology.
- Patients < 35 years old ultrasound only; if > 35 years old bilateral mammograms and ultrasound of palpable abnormality.

Management

- Reassure.
- Treatment of any underlying cause is priority.
- If drugs are involved, withdraw and review after few months.
- Medical treatment: *Danazol* as first line treatment; if no response, consider *Tamoxifen*. The medical treatment is most effective during the proliferative phase; once present for over 12 months, the gynaecomastia tends to become inactive fibroid tissue that is less likely to respond to medication.
- Surgery: Cosmetic results of surgery can be disappointing. It can be considered if gynaecomastia is painful or cosmetically embarrassing. Small areas of gynaecomastia can be excised through a peri-areolar incision. More extensive areas require either liposuction or breast reduction.

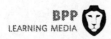

Physiological causes	
• Neonatal (60–90% of new babies) • Infantile (usually resolves by age 4) • Puberty (affects 38% of boys aged 10–16 years, with the majority resolving within 6 months) • Senile (can affect 75% of the over 50s)	
Pathological causes	
Primary testicular failure • Anorchia • Klinefelter's Syndrome • Bilateral cryptorchidism	**Endocrine tumours** • Testicular • Adrenal • Pituitary
Acquired testicular failure • Mumps • Irradiation	**Non-endocrine tumours** • Bronchial carcinoma • Lymphoma • Hypernephroma
Secondary testicular failure • Generalised hypopituitarism • Isolated gonadotrophin deficiency	**Hepatic disease** • Cirrhosis • Haemochromatosis
Drugs • Oestrogens and oestrogen agonists – digoxin, spironolactone • Hyperprolactinaemia – methyldopa, phenothiazines • Gonadotrophins • Testosterone target cell inhibitors – cimetidine, cyproterone acetate • Cannabis	

Table 2.13. Causes of gynaecomastia

Thyroid pathology

Thyroid tumours

Epidemiology

Approximately 4–7% of the population can have palpable nodules; most of them are benign dominant nodules in a nodular goitre or follicular adenomas. In contrast the incidence of thyroid cancer is low at about 4 per 100,000 population per year, accounting for 1% of all malignancies. Thyroid cancer is the commonest type of endocrine malignancy with a peak incidence at 30–50 years and a female preponderance. Although the incidence is believed to be rising, this could be attributed to earlier detection of micro-carcinomas.

Assessment of a thyroid nodule

Clinical assessment

Clinical assessment is of paramount importance (see Chapter 7: *Clinical examinations – Examination of the neck and thyroid*). Hard or fixed nodules are more suspicious for malignancy, as is recurrent laryngeal nerve palsy or dysphagia.

Laboratory evaluation

The most important laboratory test is a sensitive thyroid-stimulating hormone (TSH) assay, to screen for hypothyroidism or hyperthyroidism. In addition, obtaining serum thyroxine (T4) and triiodothyronine (T3) levels may be helpful. If there is clinical suspicion for Hashimoto thyroiditis, serum antithyroid peroxidase (anti-TPO) antibody and antithyroglobulin (anti-Tg) antibody levels need to be obtained.

Imaging

- Ultrasonography: Highly sensitive in determining the size and number of thyroid nodules, but cannot reliably distinguish a benign nodule from a malignant nodule.
- CT/ MRI: Not first line, but may be useful in the assessment of thyroid masses that are largely substernal. PET scanning with 18F-fluorodeoxyglucose might have some role in thyroid imaging in the future, particularly in the evaluation of metastatic disease.
- Thyroid scintigraphy: Not used routinely in most centres; nuclear imaging can be used to describe a nodule as hot, warm, or cold on the basis of its relative uptake of radioactive isotope. Hot nodules indicate autonomously functioning nodules, warm nodules suggest normal thyroid function, and cold nodules indicate hypofunctional or non-functional thyroid tissue. Hot nodules are rarely malignant, but 5–8% of warm or cold nodules are malignant.

Fine needle aspiration cytology (FNAC)

Fine needle aspiration cytology is a simple, safe, cheap reproducible procedure that can be performed on the patient quickly. A mean sensitivity of greater than 80% with a mean specificity of greater than 90% are reported. It has reduced the necessity for surgery for thyroid nodules by 20% to 50%, also increasing the yield of cancers from 15% to 50%. Note full assessment includes radiological and clinical findings together with the results of FNAC.

(See also Chapter 8: *Procedural skills – Fine needle aspiration cytology and biopsy*.)

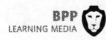

Potential outcomes of FNAC include:

- Thy 1: Not diagnostic – Insufficient material
- Thy 2: Benign lesion
- Thy 3: Follicular lesion (adenoma / carcinoma)
- Thy 4: Suspicious for malignancy
- Thy 5: Diagnostic of malignancy

The distinction between follicular adenoma and cancer can only be made on histological findings and the follicular adenoma usually requires lobectomy to confirm the diagnosis.

Benign thyroid tumours

Follicular adenoma

This benign tumour usually presents between 30–50 years of age and is 20 times more common in women than men. Most of the solitary nodules are non-functioning but can cause hyperthyroidism at times. They are usually encapsulated and of 2–4cm in size. They are white to tan or brown in colour. These lesions are clinically and cytologically indistinguishable from follicular carcinomas and therefore should be excised. Diagnosis can be made on histological examination as to whether capsular or vascular invasion is present. The distinction should be made between adenoma and carcinoma. The diagnosis of adenomas is made if there is no capsule or vascular invasion but detailed histological examination must be made to exclude the interface between tumour and normal gland. These lesions can be managed by lobectomy alone providing paraffin section histological examination does not reveal any sign of carcinoma.

Malignant thyroid tumours

Follicular carcinoma (10–15%)

Three categories of follicular lesion exist:

- Follicular lesions without vascular or capsular invasion, considered benign.
- Follicular tumours with papillary differentiation, regarded as variants of papillary cancer.
- Invasive, purely follicular carcinoma.

Follicular carcinoma is more common in women and usually presents in the fifth decade. It has a thicker capsule than an adenoma. The vascular invading tumours have a higher risk of distant metastases than only capsular invading tumours. The metastatic spread is through the vascular route particularly to lung and bone. In certain cases the distinction between benign and malignant is very difficult as signs of invasion are very subtle. Such lesions are described as minimally invasive with a 10-year survival of 70–100%. Other lesions are described as widely invasive and show obvious spread throughout the gland and beyond that seen by the naked eye. Such lesions have a 10-year survival of 25–45%. Follicular carcinomas present in different forms ranging from colloid filled follicles to more solid forms. In some cases histological changes are seen following preoperative FNAC which can pose diagnostic problems. Disruption of the capsule on passing the needle can raise the possibility of invasion if the needle track is not clearly visualised.

Management of invasive follicular carcinoma is total thyroidectomy followed by radioiodine therapy. Regional nodes should be excised by block dissection. Lifelong suppressive thyroxine therapy is also given to patients.

Oncocytic (Hurthle cells) follicular tumours

Hurthle cells are follicular cells full of mitrochondria and constitute an oncocytic variant of follicular tumours. These are single nodules usually with a deep brown cut surface. They were initially treated as malignant tumours but now go through similar assessment with any other follicular lesions. They differ from other follicular tumours as malignancy is more common with higher risk of lymph node or distant metastatic spread. In the majority of cases these tumours can be managed as benign and a lobectomy is sufficient.

Papillary carcinoma (70%)

Papillary carcinoma was originally defined on the basis of papillary architecture but now it is believed that some follicular tumours shared the same nuclear features. As such the new definition describes them as a malignant epithelial tumours showing evidence of follicular cell differentiation and characterised by specific nuclear features.

These tumours occur commonly in young adults (30–40 years) with a 4:1 predominance in women. Macroscopically they are grey-white masses with a firm texture. Most of the tumours are small at presentation (< 2cm). The classic papillary tumour consists of well formed papillary structures. Psammoma bodies (concrete calcification) are typical findings and correlate with lymph node metastases. Many papillary carcinomas comprise a mixture of papillary and follicular areas.

Surgical management includes a minimal resection of total thyroid lobectomy and isthmusectomy in cases of microcarcinoma without capsular invasion or metastatic lymph nodes. In cases of local invasion or distant metastases a total thyroidectomy with or without lymph node dissection is indicated.

Overall the prognosis is good. These tumours often metastasise to local lymph nodes however this does not seem to alter the prognosis. Poor prognostic indicators include advanced age, large tumours > 5cm and extrathyroidal extension.

Anaplastic carcinoma (3–5%)

This rare tumour is one of the most aggressive of all malignancies, with a 90% mortality within one year of diagnosis. Generally these tumours are found in older women who often present late with a fixed mass causing pressure effects or invasion of local structures (recurrent laryngeal nerve, carotid artery, oesophagus, trachea).

Biopsy (core, open) is important to distinguish between lymphoma and anaplastic carcinoma. Curative surgery is almost never feasible and certain patients may undergo debulking procedures to free the trachea or oesophagus. Some patients continue to be treated with external beam radiotherapy. The median survival is 2.5–6 months.

Poorly differentiated carcinoma

These tumours are derived from follicular cells and are indeterminate between differentiated (follicular/papillary) and undifferentiated (anaplastic) carcinoma. Incidence is higher over the age of 50 years and more are seen in women. Patients present with a large solitary mass usually > 3cm with a focus of central necrosis. Regional and distant metastatic spread is seen and the five-year survival is approximately 50%.

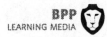

Medullary carcinoma (10%)

This is a tumour of the parafollicular C cells producing calcitonin which can be a useful tumour marker. Three specific clinical forms are recognised:

- Sporadic (75%)
- Familial associated with multiple endocrine neoplasia type 2 (MEN2).
- Familial without other signs of multiple endocrine neoplasia.

Sporadic cases are commonly seen in patients > 40 years with 25% presenting with lymph node metastases. Familial cases are often bilateral and multifocal and of younger age, while sporadic cases are solitary and unilateral. The tumours are grey and firm but rarely encapsulated. The C cells are mostly present in the middle to upper third of the gland. Familial patients show signs of C cell hyperplasia before tumour development.

Diagnosis is usually made by fine needle aspiration cytology and measurement of markers – calcitonin and carcinoembryonic antigen. The mainstay of treatment is radical surgery as the majority of patients have involved lymph nodes at surgery. A total thyroidectomy is performed with ipsilateral lymph node dissection from the thyroid cartilage to the upper mediastinum and laterally to the sternocleidomastoid muscle. In familial cases bilateral neck dissection should be performed. Postoperative follow up with sequential calcitonin levels is imperative to identify persistent or recurrent disease.

Thyroid lymphoma

The thyroid gland may be affected by lymphoma primarily or secondarily. It is important to distinguish anaplastic carcinoma from primary lymphoma. Coexisting thyroiditis can be found with over one-third of resected lymphomas found to have histological changes of Hashimoto's disease. Thyroid lymphoma is typically B cell type, and can arise from mucosa-associated lymphatic tissue. The presenting complaint is usually a rapidly expanding goitre with symptoms of compression. Surgery (thyroidectomy) is performed for histological diagnosis when FNAC is inconclusive and for some cases of disease contained to the thyroid gland. The preferred treatment is with chemotherapy and radiotherapy. When contained within the thyroid gland the five-year survival rate is 86%, while with nodal or soft tissue involvement this drops to 38%.

The NICE guidelines recommend urgent specialist referral for patients presenting with symptoms of tracheal compression (stridor) secondary to thyroid enlargement; also, for patients with thyroid swelling increasing in size, with associated cervical lymphadenopathy or unexplained hoarseness or voice changes, or if there is history of neck irradiation or family history of an endocrine tumour, particularly if the patient is very young (pre-pubertal) or 65 years and older.

Primary care physicians should request thyroid function tests and if patients have hyper- or hypothyroidism with an associated goitre, they could be referred, non-urgently, to an endocrinologist. No other investigations (ultrasonography or isotope scanning), need to be requested, as they are likely to result in unnecessary delay.

(Adapted from NICE, 2005)

Multiple Endocrine Neoplasia (MEN)

These syndromes are characterised by the presence of tumours in two or more endocrine glands. There are two major forms, type 1 (Wermer's syndrome) and type 2 (Sipple's syndrome) which are inherited by autosomal dominance.

MEN type 1

The gene for MEN 1 is located on chromosome 11 and this syndrome is characterised by tumours of the parathyroid gland, pancreatic islet cells, and anterior pituitary gland. The commonest clinical presentation is of hyperparathyroidism (adenoma) with prolactinomas the commonest pituitary lesion (others include non functioning lesions and somatotropinomas). Lesions of the pancreatic islet cells include insulinomas, gastrinomas and ViPomas. Surgical management depends on the lesions present, subtotal or total parathyroidectomy is performed for adenomas, with resection for insulinomas. Pituitary lesions can be managed by dopamine agonists (prolactinoma) or hypophysectomy and external beam radiation.

All patients should undergo lifelong screening due to the multiple and metachronous nature of the tumours. Family members should undergo genetic screening. Biochemical screening includes regular serum calcium and parathyroid hormone levels, glucose, insulin, gastrin and prolactin measurement. Cranial MRI scans should also be performed every 3–5 years after the age of 20.

MEN type 2

This syndrome can be divided into two forms.

- MEN 2a: This is characterised by medullary thyroid carcinoma associated with phaeochromocytoma and primary hyperparathyroidism.
- MEN 2b: This is characterised by medullary thyroid carcinoma and phaeochromocytoma associated with a Marfanoid habitus and mucosal neuromas.

A further group of familial patients with medullary thyroid carcinoma without other associations with MEN 2 is also recognised.

The gene for this group is RET which is a proto-oncogene located on chromosome 10. Point mutations in parts of the gene determine the severity of the syndrome. The most common presenting complaint is a thyroid nodule caused by medullary thyroid carcinoma. Management includes a total thyroidectomy and neck dissection as discussed above with prophylactic measures in high risk groups. Genetic screening for point mutations of the RET gene has 100% accuracy for identifying carriers. Other biochemical choices available are calcitonin and carcinoembryonic levels, calcium and parathyroid hormone levels and 24-hour urine metanephrines.

Hyperthyroidism

Hyperthyroidism is the consequence of excessive thyroid hormone action.

Aetiology

- Toxic diffuse goitre (Grave's disease).
- Toxic adenoma, (Plummer's disease).
- Toxic multinodular goitre
- Painful subacute thyroiditis.
- Silent thyroiditis, including lymphocytic and postpartum variations.
- Iodine-induced hyperthyroidism (for example, related to amiodarone therapy).
- Excessive pituitary, TSH or trophoblastic disease.
- Excessive ingestion of thyroid hormone.

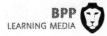

Nervousness and irritability
Palpitations and tachycardia
Heat intolerance or increased sweating
Tremor
Weight loss or gain
Alterations in appetite
Frequent bowel movements or diarrhoea
Dependent lower-extremity oedema
Sudden paralysis
Exertional intolerance and dyspnoea
Menstrual disturbance (decreased flow)
Impaired fertility
Mental disturbances
Sleep disturbances (including insomnia)
Changes in vision, photophobia, eye irritation, diplopia, or exophthalmos
Fatigue and muscle weakness
Thyroid enlargement (depending on cause)
Pretibial myxoedema (in patients with Graves' disease)

Table 2.14. Clinical manifestations of hyperthyroidism

Diagnostic work-up

As per clinical, laboratory and imaging work up for thyroid nodule.

Less commonly:

- Triiodothyronine (T3) radioimmunoassay (RIA).
- Thyroid autoantibodies, including TSH receptor antibodies (TRAb) or thyroid-stimulating immunoglobulins (TSI).
- Radioactive iodine uptake and thyroid scan with either I^{123} (preferably) or Tc^{99m}.

Management

There are three types of therapy.

- Surgical intervention: thyroidectomy.
- Antithyroid drugs.
- Radioactive iodine.

Thyroidectomy

A thyroidectomy is a commonly performed procedure for both benign and malignant conditions. Preoperatively patients should be assessed for potential nerve palsies and in cases of thyrotoxicosis managed with antithyroid medication.

Procedure

- Patient is positioned supine with a sandbag under the shoulders and a head ring.
- Make a collar incision two fingers above the clavicle / suprasternal notch.
- Divide the subcutaneous tissue and platysma carefully ensuring haemostasis.
- Raise the inferior and superior skin flaps.
- Staying within the midline, incise the deep cervical fascia onto the thyroid gland.
- Create a space between the lobe of the gland and overlying strap muscles. Division of the strap muscles may be required for large goitres.

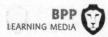

- Identify the middle thyroid vein and ligate.
- Open the plane between the posterior gland and oesophagus and other tissue to identify the recurrent laryngeal nerve.
- Identify the inferior thyroid artery following its course to where it arches, a landmark for both the nerve and superior parathyroid glands.
- Follow the recurrent laryngeal nerve to the larynx. Do not use diathermy.
- Identify the superior pole vessels and ligate protecting the external laryngeal nerve.
- Isolate the inferior thyroid vessels and ligate.
- Dissect the thyroid gland carefully off the anterior aspect of the trachea moving from one lobe to the other.
- Finally dissect the lateral thyroid ligament attachment to the lobe ensuring haemostasis and protecting the recurrent laryngeal nerve at all times.
- Lymph node dissection is recommended in certain malignancies. The central dissection consists of removal of perithyoid tissue, skeletonising the trachea and oesophagus, taking the lymphatics and upper thymus and also in certain cases the jugular nodes.
- Reapproximate the strap muscles and the platysma and close the skin.

Specific complications of thyroidectomy

- Haemorrhage.
- Recurrent laryngeal nerve injury can lead to hoarseness of the voice.
- External laryngeal nerve injury can lead to weakness and fatigue of the voice.
- Hypocalcaemia – injury to the parathyroid glands.
- Tracheomalacia can develop following removal of large goitres.

Hypothyroidism

Hypothyroidism results from undersecretion of thyroid hormone from the thyroid gland.

Aetiology

- Primary causes:
  - Chronic autoimmune thyroiditis (Hashimoto's disease) – most common cause.
  - Thyroidectomy.
  - Thyroid gland ablation with radioactive iodine, or external irradiation.
  - Biosynthetic defect in iodine organification.
  - Replacement of the thyroid gland by tumour (lymphoma).
  - Drugs, such as lithium or interferon.
- Secondary causes: pituitary and hypothalamic disease.

Fatigue	Constipation
Weight gain from fluid retention	Memory and mental impairment
Dry skin and cold intolerance	Decreased concentration
Yellow skin	Depression
Coarseness or loss of hair	Irregular or heavy menses and infertility
Hoarseness	Myalgia
Goitre	Hyperlipidaemia
Reflex delay, relaxation phase	Bradycardia and hypothermia
Ataxia	Myxoedema, fluid infiltration of tissues

Table 2.15. Clinical manifestations of hypothyroidism

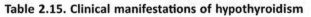

Diagnostic work up

As per hyperthyroidism, detailed above.

Management

Hormonal replacement therapy with levothyroxine is indicated, with follow-up TSH measurement. The mean replacement dosage is 1.6 µg/kg of body weight per day, which should be individualised according to age, cardiac status of the patient and the severity and duration of the hypothyroidism.

Thyroglossal cyst

This is a midline cystic neck lump arising from the thyroglossal duct (a persistent epithelial tract that represents the descent of thyroid gland between its initial area of embryological development and its final position, which normally atrophies before birth). It may be present in up to 7 % of the population.

Clinical manifestations

It can be located at any point along the thyroglossal duct, but more commonly between the isthmus of the thyroid and the hyoid bone or just above the hyoid bone (Figure 2.4). It moves up on protruding the tongue as it is attached to the foramen caecum of the tongue.

Usually it is non-tender and mobile. Infected thyroglossal cysts may manifest as tender masses with associated dysphagia, dysphonia, draining sinus, fever, or increasing neck mass. They often manifest after an upper respiratory tract infection. Airway obstruction is possible, especially with intralingual cysts.

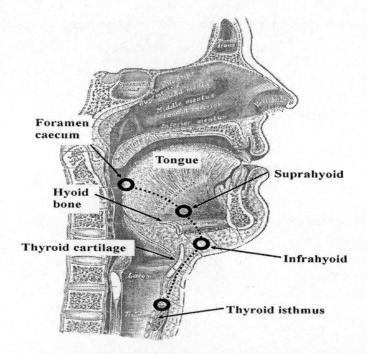

Figure 2.4. Thyroglossal tract, duct and potential locations of thyroglossal cysts
Based on Gray H (1918) Anatomy of the Human Body, 20th edition, Lea & Febiger, Philadelphia
(*This image is in the public domain because its copyright has expired. This applies worldwide.*)

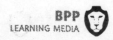

Diagnostic work up

Ultrasound and CT scanning are the radiologic tools of choice. Ultrasound can distinguish between solid and cystic components. CT scanning may reveal a well-circumscribed cystic lesion with capsular enhancement.

If a fistula present, a fistulogram may reveal the course of the tract. Thyroid scanning is suggested to rule out the possibility of the cyst containing the only functioning thyroid tissue, albeit in an ectopic site.

Management

Surgical treatment of choice for thyroglossal cysts: The Sistrunk operation; en block resection of the sinus tract and above (including the midportion of the hyoid bone). Recurrence is approximately 3–5%.

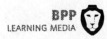

Further reading

- *Adjuvent! Online. Decision making tools for health care professionals.* Available at: www.adjuventonline.com.
- Atkin, WS, Saunders, BP. Surveillance guidelines after removal of colorectal adenomatous polyps. *Gut* 2002; 51: v6-v9.
- British Association of Day Surgery (2004) Day Case Laparoscopic Cholecystectomy. [Online] Available at: http://www.daysurgeryuk.net/bads/joomla/files/Handbooks/LaparoscopicCholecystectomy.pdf.
- Derm Atlas (2011) Dermatology Image Atlas. Available at http://dermatlas.med.jhmi.edu/.
- Gurusamy, KS, Samraj, K, Fusai, G and Davidson, BR. Early versus delayed laparoscopic cholecystectomy for biliary colic. *Cochrane Database Syst Rev* 2008; (4): CD007196.
- Hardin, DM. Acute appendicitis: review and update. *Am Fam Physician* 1999; 60: 2027-34.
- Lau, H, Lo, CY, Patil, NG, Yuen, WK. Early versus delayed-interval laparoscopic cholecystectomy for acute cholecystitis: a meta-analysis. *Surg Endosc* 2006; 20(1): 82-7.
- Marsden, JR *et al.* Revised UK guidelines for the management of cutaneous melanoma 2010. *J Plast Reconstr Aesthet Surg* 2010; 63(9): 1401–19.
- Martin, DJ, Vernon, DR, Toouli, J. Surgical versus endoscopic treatment of bile duct stones. *Cochrane Database Syst Rev* 2006; (2): CD003327.
- MBBS Medicine (Humanity First) *Inflammation* [Online]. Available at: http://Medicinembbs.blogspot.co.uk/2011/02/inflammation.html.
- NICE (2005, updated 2011) *CG27 Referral guidelines for suspected cancer.* Available at: www.nice.org.uk/nicemedia/live/10968/29814/29814.pdf.
- Purkayastha S *et al.* Laparoscopic v open surgery for diverticular disease: a meta-analysis of nonrandomized studies. *Dis Colon Rectum* 2006; 49(4): 446–63.
- Rouvelas, I, Zeng, W, Lindblad, M, Viklund, P, Ye, W, Lagergren, J. (2005) Survival after surgery for oesophageal cancer: a population-based study *Lancet Oncol* ; 6(11): 864–70.
- Sanabria, AE, Morales, CH, Villegas, MI. Laparoscopic repair for perforated peptic ulcer disease. *Cochrane Database Syst Rev* 2005; (4): CD004778.
- Scottish Intercollegiate Guidelines Network (2008) *Management of acute upper and lower gastrointestinal bleeding, a national clinical guideline.* Available at: www.sign.ac.uk/pdf/sign105.pdf.
- Stulberg, DL, Crandell, B, Fawcett, RS. Diagnosis and treatment of basal cell and squamous cell carcinomas. *Am Fam Physician* 2004; 70(8): 1481–8.
- Toorenvliet, BR, Swank, H, Schoones, JW, Hamming, JF, Bemelman, WA. Laparoscopic peritoneal lavage for perforated colonic diverticulitis: a systematic review. *Colorectal Dis* 2010; 12(9): 862–7.
- www.websurg.com/MEDIA/?noheader=1&doi=vd01en1354e.

Chapter 3
Applied surgical science

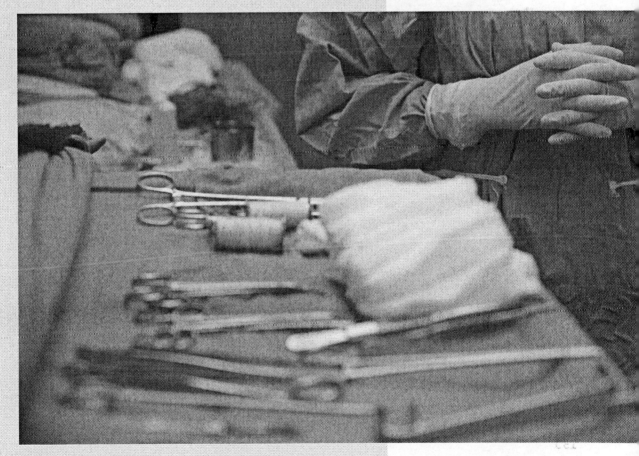

Overview

This chapter focuses on some of the essential topics concerning areas of surgical science with particular application in the intra-operative and peri-operative care of surgical patients. Good knowledge of these areas is necessary not only for the exam purposes, where they appear to be frequently tested, but also for the daily safe surgical practice on the wards, outpatient clinic setting and in theatre. Additionally, some of these aspects (such as venous thromboembolism prophylaxis, day surgery guidelines) reflect areas of clinical priority for Hospital Trusts across the country, driven by corresponding government initiatives and strict guidelines.

Day surgery

Day surgery is defined as an episode of surgery that does not include an overnight stay in hospital. There has been a substantial increase in this area of surgery over the last two decades; 15% of patients underwent day surgery in 1989 and over 80% in 2007. This increase has been facilitated by minimally invasive procedures, improved peri-operative care using specific anaesthesia with short recovery times, and purpose-built day surgery units. Guidelines have been initially produced by the Royal College of Surgeons and Department of Health in establishing a new day surgery service in hospitals. An extensive number of procedures have been recommended to be suitable for day surgery, providing other criteria are met (Table 3.1). Certain emergency procedures previously performed as inpatient ones, are now also recognised as suitable for day case surgery, thereby minimising unnecessary hospital stay and prolonged starving. Examples include incision and drainage of abscesses or repair of painful hernias.

Inguinal / umbilical hernia repair	Carpal tunnel decompression
Laparoscopic cholecystectomy	Arthroscopy
Haemorrhoidectomy	Transurethral excision of bladder tumour
Varicose vein stripping / ligation	Diagnostic laparoscopy
Excision of breast lesion	Termination of pregnancy
Tonsillectomy	Cervical dilatation / hysteroscopy

Table 3.1. Procedures suitable for day surgery

Factors suggesting suitability of procedures for day surgery

- Low risk of postoperative haemorrhage or airway problems
- Expected early commencement of oral intake
- Minimal postoperative pain
- Minimal postoperative nausea / vomiting
- No specific postoperative nursing requirements

Patient selection

Following an outpatient appointment, all patients booked for day case procedures are required to undergo and attend a pre-assessment clinic. Patient screening is performed by trained nurses with many trusts having now developed specific integrated care pathways (ICPs) for completion. The pre-assessment must include both a full medical history and, importantly, social history. Thorough preoperative assessment of patient co-morbidities and previous surgery is essential to ensure stability of chronic conditions and identify those who may need early anaesthetic review. Even patients with ASA (American Society of Anaesthesiology) grades of 3 can undergo day case procedures with the correct preoperative optimisation.

Specific patient factors and suitability for day surgery

Diabetes mellitus

It is not a contraindication for day case surgery, providing the patient has been stable on their oral hypoglycaemic treatment or low dose insulin, for at least three months. Any cardiac or renal complications must be flagged at pre-assessment together with a recent HbA1C (glycated haemoglobin) and cholesterol. Serum HbA1C level of less than 8% suggests the patient is suitable for day surgery. Preoperative starvation may also cause problems with diabetic control, so at assessment it is important to reconfirm the patient or carer's ability to monitor blood glucose

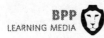

levels and recognise and treat hypoglycaemia. The main principle of peri-operative management of diabetics is to schedule the patient as early as possible on the list and return them to their diet and routine medication as soon as possible. Oral hypoglycaemics should be omitted on the day of surgery and the insulin dose halved. Glucose levels are monitored from admission throughout the operation and post-operatively with small doses of subcutaneous insulin given as necessary. Once full diet is resumed they can recommence their normal regime. Patients are advised to monitor their blood glucose for a day following discharge, warning them of the possibility of hyperglycaemia or even delayed hypoglycaemia.

Anticoagulants

Patients taking anticoagulants for previous thrombotic disease and atrial fibrillation can undergo small procedures by omitting their anticoagulant preoperatively and allowing their INR to normalise. In cases where anticoagulants cannot be stopped, such as metallic valves, patients are better managed as inpatients with the use of peri-operative heparin infusions.

Obesity

Concerns exist regarding the inclusion of patients with significantly raised body mass indexes (BMI) for day case procedures. Main issues include longer operative times, difficult anaesthesia and prolonged recovery times. Assessment aids identify those at risk or with associated conditions such as obstructive sleep apnoea. Despite this, BMI is gradually being excluded from the list of contraindications to day surgery in various policies/trust.

Age

While a higher incidence of peri-operative morbidity and mortality is associated with elderly patients, higher age is not a definite contraindication for day case procedures.

Perioperative care

Anaesthesia for day case surgery needs to be performed by an appropriately experienced anaesthetist, with a quick induction and recovery. A preferred agent for such patients is *propofol* which also has anti-emetic properties. Other common inhaled agents include *isoflurane* and *sevoflurane*. The preferred method of airway control in day surgery is via a laryngeal mask although in cases of higher aspiration risk (obesity, gastro-esophageal reflux) endotracheal intubation is more appropriate. Alternative anaesthesia can be performed via the local or regional route. Many centres now favour the repair of uncomplicated inguinal hernias under local anaesthesia. Alternatively spinal anaesthesia can be offered for certain orthopaedic and urological procedures. This has the advantages of reducing postoperative nausea and vomiting and offering a suitable alternative for those with significant comorbidities (cardiac, respiratory).

A correct balance must be achieved with analgesia postoperatively. Adequate pain relief to allow mobilisation and discharge must be provided without causing any side effects such as nausea and vomiting. First and foremost, preoperative assessment into previous pain control issues is essential and, if present, consultation with the pain team and anaesthetist may be beneficial. In cases of severe peri-operative pain control difficulties, inpatient stay may need to be considered. Preoperative analgesia is often prescribed usually in the form of NSAIDs (providing no contraindication present) with short acting opiates administered during surgery as required, with the advantage of reduced side effects. Administration of local anaesthesia to wounds or regional nerve blocks can also aid control in the first few postoperative hours. Patients should be discharged with common analgesics such as dihydrocodeine and ibuprofen.

Postoperative nausea and vomiting

Postoperative nausea and vomiting (PONV) is a common problem with a reported incidence of about 35% causing delays in discharge. Severe cases can lead to the development of aspirational pneumonia, haemorrhage and even incisional hernias. Prolonged symptoms in patients can cause hypokalaemia, metabolic alkalosis and dehydration. Contributing factors for postoperative nausea and vomiting can be divided into patient factors, surgical factors and anaesthetic factors.

Patient factors	Surgical factors	Anaesthetic factors
Age (young)	Long duration of surgery	Pre-medication
Gender (female)	Laparoscopy	Opiates
Obesity	Gynaecological procedure	Nitrous oxide
Previous PONV	Middle ear procedure	Neuromuscular blockade reversal
Motion sickness	Ophthalmic procedure	
Anxiety		
Gastroparesis		
Non smoker		

Table 3.2. Factors predisposing to PONV

Based on these risk factors, a preoperative assessment can be completed and management planned accordingly. The following recommendations are provided by the British Association of Day Surgery.

- Low risk individuals (0–1 risk factors): No prophylaxis is necessary. Administer non-opioid analgesia, minimise fluid deficit (intravenous fluids), administer short acting anaesthetic agents titrating to effect.
- Intermediate risk individuals (2–3 risk factors): Single agent prophylaxis (eg Ondansetron) with the above general measures.
- High risk individuals (> 3 risk factors): Combination prophylaxis (ondansetron and dexamethasone) with the general measures to reduce PONV.

Discharge criteria

Recovery time will always vary with the patient and procedure performed. All patients should be reviewed by the anaesthetist and surgeon postoperatively. If satisfied, the assessment of when the patient is fit for discharge can be made by the nursing staff on the unit. The following are criteria to be assessed when planning for discharge:

- Stable observations for over one hour.
- Patient orientated to time, place and person.
- Pain is controlled and adequate oral analgesia is prescribed, with instructions for discharge.
- There is minimal nausea or vomiting and patient is able to tolerate at least oral fluids.
- Patient can mobilise safely (as appropriate).
- There is no or minimal bleeding or wound discharge.
- Patient has passed urine (for certain procedures – rectal surgery, inguinal hernia repair).
- There is a responsible carer to take patient home and be available for next 24 hours.
- Clear post-operative instructions have been provided with emergency contact details.

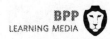

135

Venous thromboembolic disease

Deep vein thrombosis (DVT) involves the formation of a thrombus in the deep venous system, commonly within the lower limbs; however the upper limb, subclavian vein or superior vena cava, may also be involved. DVT and pulmonary embolism (PE) constitute the spectrum of venous thromboembolism (VTE) disease.

Incidence

- DVT occurs in > 20% of patients after major surgery in general and in 40% of patients having major orthopaedic surgery in particular.
- Venous thromboembolism (VTE) accounts for 25,000 deaths per year in the UK.
- Pulmonary embolism occurs in approximately 1% of all admissions, accounting for approximately 10% of hospital deaths.
- There is no difference between men and women in the incidence of VTE.

Major risk factors	Minor risk factors

Age > 60 years
Hip or knee surgery (replacement)
Major pelvic or abdominal surgery
Metastatic cancer
Hospitalisation
Lower limb fracture
Late pregnancy
Varicose veins
	Oral contraceptive, hormonal replacement therapy
	Smoking
	Obesity
	Congestive cardiac failure
	Prothrombotic disorders
	    Factor V Leiden
	    Protein C deficiency
	    Protein S deficiency
	    Antiphospholipid antibodies
	Continued travel

Table 3.3. Risk factors for DVT

Pathophysiology of DVT

Virchow's triad of prothombotic factors

1. Abnormalities of the vessel wall (vessel injury)

Tissue plasminogen activator (TPA) and plasminogen activator inhibitor-1 are normally produced by endothelial cells. TPA, prostacyclin and nitric oxide protect against the formation of a thrombus. Trauma to the endothelial wall exposes the basement membrane and disrupts this balance, thus activating the platelets. Trauma and surgery can cause thrombosis by two means; firstly the plasma activator inhibitor-1 levels are increased, reducing local fibrinolysis, and secondly the release of tissue factor secondary to trauma stimulates the clotting cascade.

2. Abnormalities of the constituents of blood (hypercoagulability)

Alterations in constituents of blood may change its viscosity and flow within the vessel predisposing to thrombosis. Also, abnormalities within the coagulation cascade or fibrinolytic system due to either inherited or acquired causes may lead to thrombosis:

- Inherited thrombophilic defects: Inherited prothrombotic causes can be identified in approximately 50% of patients presenting with DVT. These may include deficiencies of antithrombin III, protein C or protein S or even an increase in factor V Leiden (present in 5% of the population). Heterozygotes for factor V Leiden have three times the risk of DVT in comparison with the normal population, with homozygotes at 50–80 times higher risk.

- Acquired thrombophilia: Together with the risk factors listed on the previous page (Table 3.3), there are certain other conditions predisposing to thrombus formation by altering the blood, such as myeloproliferative disorders, antiphospholipid syndrome, heparin-induced thrombocytopenia, active heart or respiratory disease, inflammatory bowel disease, nephrotic syndrome and severe sepsis.

3. Changes in the dynamics of blood flow (stasis)

Both competent valves within the veins and regular contraction of the calf muscle pump are necessary for venous return. Immobility leads to stagnation of blood flow in the deep veins predisposing to thrombus formation. Stasis can also be caused by external compression on the veins resulting from a gravid uterus or pelvic tumours. Conditions reducing the haemodynamic flow rates such as congestive cardiac failure may also lead to DVT formation.

Presentation

The clinical presentation of DVT can vary from asymptomatic to extensive iliofemoral thrombosis presenting as pale, swollen painful leg. If the thrombus extends into venules and capillaries secondary arterial insufficiency can develop leading to cyanosis of the leg (and less frequently, potential by progress to *phlegmasia alba dolens, phlegmasia cerula dolens*, and venous gangrene). Differential diagnosis includes: cellulitis, torn calf muscle, ruptured Baker's cyst and haemorrhage into a calf muscle. Signs of DVT include calf pain and tenderness, pyrexia, persistent tachycardia and unilateral pitting oedema.

The diagnosis of DVT can sometimes be difficult and a high level of suspicion is necessary. The Wells criteria (Table 3.4) constitute a classification system useful for stratifying patients into groups of low, moderate and high probability.

Wells' criteria	Score
Lower limb trauma, surgery or immobilisation in plaster of Paris	+1
Bedridden for three days	+1
Tenderness along lines of femoral / popliteal veins	+1
Entire limb swollen	+1
Difference in calf circumference ≥ 3 cm	+1
Pitting oedema confined to symptomatic leg	+1
Malignancy (treatment ongoing or within previous six months, or palliative)	+1
Dilated superficial collateral veins	+1
Previous DVT, PE or thrombophilia (positive diagnostic D-dimer test)	+1
Alternative diagnosis as or more likely than DVT	−2

Table 3.4. Wells' score (Possible score: −2 to +9)

Interpretation:

Score ≥ 3: high risk (75%); score 1-2: moderate risk (17%); score <1: low risk (3%)

Investigations

- D-dimers assay: D-dimers are fibrin degradation products arising during the fibrinolytic response to thrombus formation. Their plasma levels are raised in the presence of thrombosis, but can also be raised in hospital patients with infection or malignancy and immediately postoperatively; the specificity for DVT ranges between 30–40%. DVT can be excluded in patients with low probability scores and negative D-dimer assays with a sensitivity of > 90%.
- B-mode ultrasound imaging: This inexpensive, non-invasive method is the mainstay investigation. The thrombus appears as echoic material within the vein and the vein becomes less compressible. Thrombus in deep thigh veins and popliteal veins can be diagnosed with sensitivity and specificity of 90 and 99% respectively.
- Duplex ultrasound scanning: It combines B-mode imaging with pulsed Doppler providing information about blood velocity. The 'no flow' areas show up black against the colour flow due to thrombus. This technique is ideal for detection of proximal asymptomatic DVT and is also useful in detecting isolated thrombus in calf veins, albeit with lower sensitivity. These patients with DVT of the calf are treated conservatively initially and the test is repeated in one or two weeks to exclude propagation of thrombus (20% of cases).
- MRI: It has been increasingly used to investigate iliac vein thrombosis and is particularly useful during pregnancy. It is non-invasive and a useful confirmatory test but rather expensive and not universally available.
- Contrast-enhanced CT and CT pulmonary angiography: It has replaced the isotope ventilation/ perfusion scan as a first line of investigation for PE. It can be useful for central venous occlusion and is also increasingly used in detecting peripheral venous thrombosis.
- Ascending venography: It is an invasive technique requiring venous contrast injection into veins of the dorsum of the foot. DVT can be visualised as a filling defect on high resolution film. However its use has been limited due to the invasive nature coupled with a risk of contrast reaction and extravasation.
- Impedance plethysmography: It is rarely used apart from population studies of patients with increased risk of DVT.
- Isotope-labelled fibrinogen imaging: It can demonstrate calf vein thrombosis but it is unreliable in detecting more proximal thrombosis.

Risk assessment

All patients should be risk assessed, according to the parameters listed in Table 3.5, on admission to hospital, 24 hours post admission and whenever a change in the clinical condition occurs, in order to determine optimum VTE prophylaxis regime. A reassessment after 48–72 hours of admission is also recommended.

Risk of thrombosis	Risk of bleeding
Age> 60 years	Active bleeding
Active malignancy	Acquired bleeding disorder
Dehydration	Anticoagulant treatment
Obesity (BMI>30)	Thrombocytopaenia (< 75 x 10^9/L)
Thrombophilia, history of VTE including 1st degree relative	Inherited bleeding disorder- untreated
Oral contraceptive, hormonal replacement therapy	Acute cerebrovascular event
Late pregnancy/early post-partum	Poorly controlled hypertension
Varicose veins	Severe renal/hepatic disease
Hip or knee surgery (replacement)	Lumbar puncture, epidural/spinal anaesthesia
Major pelvic or abdominal surgery	
Prolonged immobility	
Critical illness	

Table 3.5. Risk assessment for venous thromboembolism

Prophylaxis

General methods

Maintain adequate hydration, ensure early mobilisation.

Mechanical methods

Current national guidelines recommend mechanical prophylaxis for DVT on admission to hospital (thigh-length graduated compression stockings) unless contraindicated. The mechanical methods reduce 50–60% risk of DVT.

- The graduated compression stockings (Thrombo Embolus Deterrent stockings or TEDs) provide pressure compression of 18mmHg at the ankle, 14mmHg at mid calf and 8mmHg at the upper thigh, increasing the blood flow within the deep venous system by approximately 75%. Correct sizing and fitting should be ensured on admission, with review postoperatively to accommodate oedema. They should be worn until patient returns to normal day to day activity. Contraindications for use include; peripheral arterial disease/grafting, skin changes – recent graft, gangrene, friable skin, severe leg oedema secondary to cardiac failure or significant leg deformity preventing correct fit.
- Intermittent pneumatic compression: It is delivered by a boot which provides intermittent but consistent pressure to the lower legs and improves venous return and stimulates fibrinolytic activity. Foot pumps or foot impulse devices improve venous outflow and reduce stasis in immobilised patients. These devices can be used alone or in addition to compression stockings.
- Electric stimulation devices can induce passive contractions of the calf muscles, promoting limb venous blood flow.

Pharmacological prophylaxis

- Unfractionated heparin (UFH) is preferred for patients with renal failure. It accelerates the action of antithrombin together with other clotting factors (IX, X, XI. XII). The risk of DVT formation is reduced by > 50%, and the risk of pulmonary embolism by > 30%. Long term administration can lead to thrombocytopaenia.
- Low molecular weight heparin (LMWH) in addition to mechanical prophylaxis, unless contraindicated. It reduces the risk of DVT formation by > 50% and the risk of pulmonary embolism by > 60% and has lower risk of thrombocytopenia compared to unfractionated heparin.
- Fondaparinux sodium: A new pentasaccharide, a specific indirect inhibitor of activated factor Xa, administered daily subcutaneously. It reduces the risk of DVT by 48%, but it is associated with higher risk of major bleeding.

Treatment

Treatment of DVT aims to prevent propagation of clot, prevent PE and optimise resolution of thrombus.

Anticoagulation

- LMWH is the first line treatment for DVT, rather than UFH.
- Warfarin, a vitamin K antagonist, is introduced simultaneously, as it is not effective for the first 48 hours of treatment because prothrombin has a half-life of 36 hours. Low molecular weight heparin is continued until the international normalised ratio (INR), achieved by treatment with warfarin, remains in the target range for two days. Anticoagulation is continued for three to six months depending on the site and extent of the DVT. Patients with an underlying familial thrombophilia often require prolonged anticoagulant treatment for life.

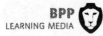

- Thrombolysis: It is reserved for PE with cardiovascular compromise and extensive iliofemoral DVT. It involves catheter-directed delivery of thrombolytic agent ie tissue plasminogen activator. It is most effective in acute thrombosis (onset less than three days) and complete or partial resolution could be achieved in approximately 80% cases. Thombolysis may carry a risk of PE without use of a vena caval filter and is associated with bleeding complications in approximately 10% of patients. Pulmonary embolism requires systemic thrombolysis, but not for peripheral thrombosis, because of the high incidence of bleeding complications.

Thrombectomy

Percutaneous mechanical and surgical thrombectomy has a limited role and is rarely used in the UK due to high morbidity and significant re-thrombosis rate.

Surgical bypass

It is rarely performed in highly specialised centres for isolated unilateral iliac vein thrombosis. The Palma bypass procedure involves use of the contralateral great saphenous vein, which is transected just above the knee, tunnelled subcutaneously and anastomosed to the ipsilateral common femoral vein in the affected leg.

Inferior vena cava (IVC) filters

Inferior vena cava filters may be temporarily or permanently placed in patients with a contraindication or significant complication related to anticoagulation, recurrent thromboembolic disease on anticoagulation, or the inability to achieve adequate anticoagulation despite patient compliance. It is contraindicated in complete IVC thrombosis or lack of access to the IVC.

Prognosis

The morbidity associated with DVT still remains high in spite of raised awareness and importance of venous thromboprophylaxis.

- Approximately 65% of patients develop chronic venous hypertension.
- 50% have post-phlebitic skin changes and 5% develop ulceration.
- 50% of patients with proximal DVT develop asymptomatic PE.
- 10% patient with symptomatic PE die with in first hour and 5% develop pulmonary hypertension.

NICE Guideline – Venous thromboembolism: reducing the risk (Adapted from NICE, 2010)

- Assess all patients for risks of thrombosis and bleeding on admission.
- Prevent dehydration in all patients.
- Encourage mobilisation as soon as possible.
- Do not regard aspirin or other anti-platelet agent as adequate prophylaxis.
- Consider inferior vena cava filters for high risk patients with contraindications to mechanical or pharmacological prophylaxis.

A comprehensive reference guide on the management of patient subgroups (medical patients, patients undergoing non-orthopaedic and orthopaedic surgery, patients sustaining major trauma or spinal injury, having lower limb plaster casts, patients in critical care units and women in pregnancy and up to six weeks post partum) is available at: http://guidance.nice.org.uk (CG92) Venous Thrombembolism – reducing the risk, NICE guideline, February 2010)

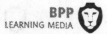

Diathermy

Introduction

Diathermy is the technique whereby the heat from electrical current is used to cut tissue and seal vessels. Such heat is generated from high frequency alternating current. It was first used in 1907 by a German physician Nagelschmidt. Knowledge of the effects, benefits and risks of diathermy requires understanding of the science and definitions behind the phenomenon.

Electricity is the flow of electrons (charge, Q) from atom to atom of an element (substance) driven by a difference in voltage (V). This flow of charge (Q) per time (t), measured in amperes, is called electric current, measured by its intensity (I). The electric current density is the quantity of current passing through tissue per unit area. The electrical resistance (R) of an element measures its opposition to the passage of current. This resistance to electron flow (impedance) generates heat. The association between the intensity of the current, the voltage driving the current through a substance (tissue) and the resistance of the tissue is described by Ohm's law:

$$I \text{ (Current)} = \text{Voltage (V)} / \text{Resistance (R)}$$

The work (heat) produced by current passing through resistance is proportionate to the electrical resistance of the element (tissue): $\mathbf{W = I^2\,R\,t}$. When passing through living tissue electricity can cause depolarisation of the cell membrane, which results in neuromuscular stimulation and myocardial fibrillation. Alternating current can pass through the body without causing such depolarisation or neuromuscular stimulation, particularly at high frequencies, generating temperatures up to 1000 ^{0}C. However, low frequency alternating current can cause neuromuscular stimulation. Muscle contractions can be seen in currents of 5–10 mA, with ventricular fibrillation at 80–100 mA. Surgical diathermy utilises current frequencies between 400 kHz–10 MHz.

Substances that allow passage of a current are called conductors, those that do not, insulators. An insulator interposed between two conductors forms a capacitor. Direct current cannot pass through a capacitor because of the insulator but high frequency alternating current can pass through insulating material. When the electrode of diathermy is in contact with the intended tissue, the energy will pass to the tissue. However in cases of energising the electrode without contact with tissue, energy can still pass through the insulation and into the surrounding tissue (capacitance coupling phenomenon). If the generator is accidently activated while the electrode is near another metal instrument this will become energised causing potential injury to the patient (direct coupling phenomenon).

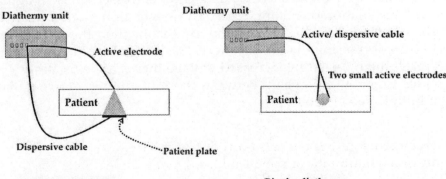

Figure 3.1. Types of diathermy

Types of diathermy
Monopolar diathermy

This involves an active electrode held by the surgeon with a small tip concentrating the current producing heat to the tissue. The return electrode plate completes the circuit spreading the current over a much wider area making it less concentrated and producing less heat. It is therefore paramount to apply the plate carefully over well vascularised areas, avoiding bony prominences and metal prostheses.

Bipolar diathermy

Bipolar diathermy involves the heating of tissue held between two small active electrodes. The patient's body is not involved in the circuit. As only small amounts of tissue can be held between the jaws of the instrument, lower voltages can be applied minimising capacitance effects. Bipolar electrosurgery does not interfere with cardiac pacemakers.

Ligasure, Gyrus

These newer feedback controlled bipolar systems have been developed in the last few years. They involve lower voltages than bipolar diathermy, but as the jaws are larger using a greater current, the feedback loop within the generator senses the tissue resistance and optimises the electrical flow.

> A Cochrane review (Nienhuijs *et al*, Rev. 2009) of 12 randomised controlled trials including 1,142 patients comparing patient tolerance of Ligasure versus conventional haemorrhoidectomy. The study reported significantly less postoperative pain in the Ligasure group in the initial few postoperative days with some trials also reporting earlier return to work.

Modes of diathermy (cutting, coagulation and blend modes)

Diathermy can be used for cutting or coagulation.

* Cutting occurs when sufficient heat is applied to tissue causing desiccation of the tissue. The alternating current generated is a continuous waveform of a few hundred volts.
* Coagulation involves a lower heating effect causing cell death by dehydration and denaturation of proteins. Bleeding is controlled by distortion of vessel walls, coagulation of plasma proteins and stimulation of clotting cascades. Coagulation mode generates output pulses on and off thousands of times per second. By this method the heat generated dissipates into the tissues decreasing the cutting effect. This form of modulation reduces the flowing current therefore necessitating increased voltage through the tissues.
* Blend modes function at voltages between those of cutting and coagulation, allowing a degree of both tissue effects.

Diathermy variables affecting the tissue impact

- Waveform: Constant (cutting) v intermittent (coagulation) v combined (blend).
- Power level.
- Electrode and tissue size: The smaller the size the higher the concentration of current.
- Time: The longer the generator is activated, the more heat will be generated and the more the thermal spread incurred.
- Manipulation of electrode: Whether the electrode is used to spark the tissue compared to continuous direct contact will determine whether coagulation or vapourisation occurs.
- Type of tissue: The level of resistance and therefore heat will vary amongst tissue types.
- Eschar: This creates increased resistance to current thereby affecting the performance of the surgical circuit.

Complications of diathermy

When using diathermy safety must be ensured by checking all equipment before use.

The following risks need to be taken into consideration during use of diathermy:

- Burns at patient plate: These injuries can occur at either open or laparoscopic surgery and are more common with monopolar diathermy. Common pitfalls are incorrect placement of plate, spirit based preparation, diathermy use on appendages or colon.
- Fire: Avoid alcohol-based skin preparations (risk of ignition from sparks from the active electrode).
- Smoke: Electrosurgical smoke has been found to contain toxic substances including carcinogens and viral particles.
- Neuromuscular stimulation: Although it is not caused by the high frequency associated with diathermy, the sparks produced may induce a Faradic effect stimulating nerves or muscle. (More common in urological procedures by stimulation of obturator nerve.)
- Pacemakers: The two risks associated with pacemakers are:
  - Interaction of high frequency current with the logic circuits of the pacemaker causing arrhythmias.
  - The use of diathermy in proximity of the pacemaker can result in the current travelling down the pacemaker wire leading to a myocardial burn.

In order to minimise these risks monopolar diathermy should be avoided in patients with pacemakers and if it needs to be used, the plate should be placed in such a location so the current does not pass near the heart.

- Laparoscopic surgery: The risks are increased due to a confined, enclosed space. Hazards include direct and capacitance coupling, described in the introduction section. Safety can be ensured by considering bipolar technique, avoiding high voltage modes and keeping the electrode in full view at all times.
- Burns from faulty insulation allowing current to travel to other non intended tissues.
- Retained heat: The tip and electrode may remain hot for some time after use so care must be taken for its position and location in relation to other structures.
- Inadvertent activation of electrodes: can be a problem with footswitches. When not being used the electrode must be placed back in the quiver.
- Flow of current from one instrument to another.

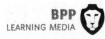

Tourniquets

A tourniquet is a constricting or compressing device used to control venous or arterial circulation to an extremity for a period of time. Pressure is applied circumferentially to the skin and underlying tissue occluding the vessels providing a bloodless operative field.

Two broad categories of tourniquets are recognised:

- Noninflatable: Composed of rubber or synthetic material.
- Inflatable (pneumatic): Composed of cuffs which can be inflated with compressed gas.

The inflatable tourniquets are the preferred method as pressure levels can be preset to control the effect exerted on the limb. Components of such pneumatic devices include an inflatable cuff, a connection tubing, a gas source, pressure display and regulator.

Indications	Contraindications

Orthopaedics
    Carpal tunnel decompression
    Fracture reduction
    Arthroscopy
    Tendon / nerve repair
Plastic / vascular surgery
    Amputation
    Resection of limb lesion
    Vascular repair
Regional intravenous anaesthesia
    Biers block
	Open fractures
	Crush injuries
	Severe circulatory compromise
	Severe hypertension

Table 3.6. Indications and contraindications for use of tourniquet

Tourniquet safety and use

Adherence to the following principles is mandatory to ensure safe use of tourniquets:

- During patient assessment, note any specific allergies, measure the patient's limb for cuff size and note the blood pressure.
- Ensure all equipment is available and not damaged.
- Calibrate the pressure equipment.
- Determine appropriate cuff pressure based on the patient's blood pressure, the cuff size, the limb circumference and the vascular status of the patient.
- Limb occlusion pressure (LOP) is the cuff pressure required to occlude the arterial flow within the limb. This can be measured by applying the cuff, identifying the arterial pulse with a Doppler and increasing the pressure until the arterial pulse stops. A safety margin of the LOP + 40–100 mmHg is recommended.
- Apply cuff over appropriate protective material.
- Monitor intraoperatively the blood pressure, tourniquet pressure and tourniquet time (recommended time < 2 hours).
- Apply dressings to the wound before deflating, deflate rapidly and check limb circulation.
- Document clearly the tourniquet use including the pressures, times, adverse events and the skin/tissue integrity at the end of the procedure.

Complications of tourniquets

Nerve injury

This is one of the most common complications from the use of tourniquets due to either mechanical stress or ischaemia of the nerve. The injury can vary from a transient neuropraxia to irreversible damage. Symptoms include the inability to sense pain, heat or cold. Tourniquet paralysis syndrome can result in the loss of motor control in the distal limb. The radial nerve is the commonest nerve injured. Such a complication can be prevented by inflating at the lowest tourniquet pressure.

Post tourniquet syndrome

This is described as profound and prolonged swelling of the limb postoperatively. Symptoms include oedema, stiffness, weakness and subjective numbness. Swelling is often caused by the return of blood to the limb together with post-ischaemic reactive hyperaemia. It is the prolonged ischaemia rather than the mechanical effect that is felt to be the cause of symptoms. The cause is usually either a prolonged tourniquet time or an inadequate pressure to prevent arterial inflow while preventing venous outflow.

Digital necrosis

This is the gangrenous destruction of a digit secondary to prolonged ischaemia. Causes include non-pneumatic devices or a prolonged tourniquet time. Risk factors include peripheral vascular disease, diabetes mellitus and Raynaud's syndrome.

Compartment syndrome

This is a rare complication of tourniquet use. The increased pressure within the myofascial compartment causes increasing pain, paraesthesia and muscle weakness with eventual absent pulses. Again, this is associated with the tourniquet ischaemia time – prolonged ischaemia time causes tissue acidosis together with increase in capillary permeability leading to compartment syndrome.

Toxic reactions

Such reactions to local anaesthetics are recognised complications of intravenous regional anaesthesia, particularly if they enter the systemic circulation. Early recognition and prompt treatment is essential to prevent serious complications such as cardiorespiratory depression and seizures leading to a coma. Causes include early or accidental deflation of the cuff.

Other complications

Tourniquet pain (dull ache together with numbness); venous thromboembolism, more common following limb surgery (the use of heparin is proposed perioperatively to prevent dislodgement of the thrombus); local tissue metabolic changes during ischaemic time (hyerkalaemia, lactic acidosis and hypercarbia), which are more significant after tourniquet time > 90 minutes; these have systemic effects once the tourniquet is deflated.

Lasers

Introduction

Lasers (light amplification by the stimulated emission of radiation) are devices for the creation of a highly directional beam of coherent electromagnetic radiation. Atoms within the lasing medium are excited by the introduction of energy. As the electrons return to their ground state a photon is emitted stimulating the emission of further photons. These are then reflected back and forth through mirrors leading to amplification.

Types

The lasing medium can be either gaseous or crystalline. The wavelength of the laser determines the absorption within the tissue. In many cases a visible guiding beam such as red helium is required.

- Carbon dioxide: This form of laser has a wavelength of 10.6μm and is rapidly absorbed by the water within tissue. Its uses generally surround the vaporisation of the tissue surface. Applications include the removal of benign and premalignant cervical and vaginal lesions.
- NdYAG: The neodymium, yttrium, aluminium garnet laser possesses a wavelength of 1.06μm with a greater depth of penetration. The uses include coagulation of tissue. Its applications include the vaporisation and debulking of oesophageal carcinomas (although now greatly replaced by the insertion of stents) together with the control of gastrointestinal haemorrhage. Success has also been reported in the management of low grade transitional cell carcinomas of the bladder.
- Argon: The argon laser light is blue/green with a principal wavelength of between 0.49–0.51 μm. Applications include the management of retinopathy and to reduce intraocular pressure in open angle glaucoma.

Risks and safety

Risks exist for both the patient and operator, therefore organised safety measures must be in place. Risks to the patients include the burning of tissue and perforation of a viscus with overly deep treatment. Operators can be accidently exposed to the laser, which can cause corneal burns or cataract formation, therefore the use of eye protection is imperative.

All departments using laser equipment must have an assigned laser protection adviser responsible for local protocols and a laser safety officer holding the laser key. Adequate training must be provided for all health professionals involved in the use of lasers with an up-to-date log kept of all training together with a nominated list of users. Laser equipment should be kept locked in a specific area with a key held by the safety officer. Other protective features include eye protection, foot pedals, emergency shut off devices and laser plume extractors.

Principles of laparoscopic surgery

One of the greatest developments in surgical practice over the last three decades surrounds minimally invasive surgery. Laparoscopic surgery is a technique by which procedures can be performed through small incisions in the abdominal cavity. Carbon dioxide is used to insufflate the peritoneum and instruments are introduced through ports placed through the small incisions. The instruments are manipulated using video camera guidance. Since the first laparoscopic appendicectomy (Semm, 1981) and the first laparoscopic cholecystectomy (Mouret, 1987) the list of laparoscopic procedures now performed continues to increase with more and more operations performed as day case or emergency (Table 3.7).

Diagnostic/staging laparoscopy	Aortic aneurysm repair
Cholecystectomy / Choledochoscopy	Obesity surgery – band / bypass
Appendicectomy	Oesophagogastric surgery
Hernia repair	Oophorectomy / Ovarian cystectomy / Tubal surgery
Splenectomy	Nephrectomy
Pancreatic resection	Colorectal resection

Table 3.7. Examples of current applications of laparoscopic surgery

There has been extensive research assessing the surgical, functional and oncological outcomes of patients undergoing laparoscopic procedures in comparison to open surgery. After overcoming the early issues related to training and surgeons' learning curves, the advantages and limitations of the laparoscopic approach have been established (Table 3.8).

Advantages	Limitations
Magnified view, better definition	Loss of tactile feedback
Reduction in wound size and pain	Remote vision
Reduction in wound complications	Reduced depth perception
Shorter hospital stay	Requires good hand-eye co-ordination
Early return to function	Motion limitation
Reduced postoperative ileus	Difficult to control bleeding
Facilitates Enhanced Recovery	Training issues
Cost effective	Increased procedure time (learning curve)

Table 3.8. Advantages and limitations of laparscopic surgery

While the indications for laparoscopic surgery continue to grow exponentially with the help of further technological developments, certain factors are still regarded as contraindications to such surgery; such examples of these are listed in Table 3.9.

Absolute	Relative
Irreversible coagulopathy	Peritonitis (Hinchey III / IV)
Severe cardiac dysfunction	Severe COPD
Haemorrhagic shock	Pregnancy
	Inability to tolerate general anaesthesia
	Bowel obstruction + massive distension

Table 3.9. Contraindications to laparoscopic surgery

Preparation

All patients should undergo a thorough preoperative assessment reviewing their pathology, comorbidities, fitness for anaesthesia (daycase / inpatient) and previous surgical history.

A note should be made of any previous surgical scars and any body deformities such as kyphosis. Following this the patient's informed consent should be obtained for the procedure including reference to conversion to open method and alternative treatment options. Patients should be warned about the possibility of postoperative shoulder tip pain and surgical emphysema. A full risk assessment and appropriate prophylaxis for venous thromboembolism should be undertaken as described already.

Routine equipment

Laparoscopic stack

This is a mobile cart with locking brakes. The stack can consist of the monitor, the insufflator together with space for other equipment. It can be placed anywhere in the theatre according to the procedure and surgeon's preference. With more hospitals developing dedicated laparoscopic theatres monitors are now fixed to the walls and ceiling on flexible arms.

Light cable and source

These can be either fibre optic or liquid crystal gel cables providing high quality optical transmission, although they can be very fragile. The light source consists of a lamp which can be either quartz halogen (300–400 hours), xenon (1,000 hours) or metal halide (100 hours) lamp.

Telescope

These can vary from 6 to 18 rod lens systems with a diameter of 1.5–15mm. Commonly used telescopes are those with viewing angle of 0° or 30°, although up to 120° are recognised.

Camera and monitor

The newer high definition cameras and monitors provide exceptional detail on widescreen monitors allowing a natural panoramic view. The high definition systems require increased illumination usually in the form of xenon light sources.

Insufflator

The carbon dioxide insufflator allows controlled pressure insufflation of the peritoneal cavity. The required pressure and flow can be set at the desired level, which is automatically maintained when the pressure changes.

Other instruments

Other instruments include trocars, cannulae and laparoscopic tools such as graspers, dissectors, scissors, diathermy electrodes (hook) and suction / irrigation systems.

Technique for safe establishment of pneumoperitoneum

Various methods have been employed to create the pneumoperitoneum for laparoscopic surgery and their use largely reflects surgeons' preferences, habits and experience. The method recommended as the safest involves open access to the peritoneal cavity and insertion of port under direct vision (open Hassan method) and is described below.

- In an anaesthetised and appropriately draped patient make an initial 1.5–2 cm incision either vertically or transversely infraumbilically.
- Continue dissection deepening the incision down to the linea alba (white fibres).
- Incise the linea alba allowing the peritoneum to be grasped separately and incised.

- Open the peritoneum under vision between two small clips.
- Insert a finger to ensure you have entered the peritoneal cavity, and assess for adhesions.
- Insert two stay sutures on either side of the linea alba and attach a clip to the end.
- Insert the trocar carefully (5 or 10mm). This may be a blunt Hassan trocar or other type.
- If the port has an inflatable balloon beneath the peritoneum, inflate this carefully.
- Tie the stay sutures (fix with clip) around the port to secure position.
- Ensure that port moves comfortably.
- Look with the camera to ensure you are in the peritoneal cavity.
- Attach the gas lead, check the pressure and insufflate the abdomen.
- Reintroduce the camera to check for any injuries.
- Perform a full laparoscopy to plan further port placement.
- Adjust the view to focus on the anterior abdominal wall (look for superficial vessels, particularly the inferior epigastric vessels) and insert further ports under direct vision.
- Ensure ports are placed in the correct positions to allow triangulation around the area(s) of focus and the correct distance for the fulcrum.
- At the end of the procedure ensure there has been no inadvertent injury or bleeding.
- All ports should be removed under direct vision confirming haemostasis and no herniation.
- Carefully remove the laparoscope under vision and expel the residual gas gently.
- Inject local anaesthetic to the surrounding tissues and fascia.
- Close the fascia with absorbable suture (using J needle) and subcuticular suture for the skin.

Physiological changes during laparoscopic surgery

The working space available intra-abdominally during laparoscopic surgery depends on a number of factors including: the anatomical size of abdominal structures (eg distended bowel, abundant abdominal fat, organomegaly, aneurysms, tumours); relaxation of the patient's abdominal musculature; and the intra-abdominal pressure created by insufflation of carbon dioxide (commonly 10–15mmHg). Higher pressures for prolonged periods of time can have several adverse effects on the body. The physiological responses to laparoscopic procedures mainly derive from the raised intra-abdominal pressure, the absorption of carbon dioxide in the circulation and the effects of patient positioning (such as Trendelenburg, reverse Trendelenburg position or rotational tilt along the longitudinal axis).

Cardiovascular response

Increased intra-abdominal pressure is the commonest reason for cardiovascular instability during a laparoscopic procedure together with patient position, pre-existing disease and vagal stimulation. Often a biphasic change in the cardiac output is seen. With low intra-abdominal pressures (5–10mmHg) an increase in venous return and cardiac output is seen due to upward mechanical pressure. As the intra-abdominal pressure increases, the compressive effects on the arterial vasculature lead to increase in afterload, systemic / pulmonary vascular resistance (raised intrathoracic pressure) and mean arterial pressure; on the other hand there is a reduction in venous return (narrowing of sub diaphragmatic vena cava) and cardiac output. In patients with significant pre-existing cardiac disease this increase in the systemic vascular resistance and myocardial oxygen requirement can lead to an acute coronary event. In a small number of cases (0.5%) the insufflation with carbon dioxide and creation of pneumoperitoneum can cause bradycardia and asystole, believed to be secondary to pressure on the vagus nerve. Given these potential changes, it is imperative for patients with cardiac disease to be thoroughly assessed preoperatively and the anaesthetists should be prepared for all possibilities.

Respiratory response

Carbon dioxide is the preferred gas for laparoscopic procedures as it is soluble and non-combustible. A rise in the intra-abdominal pressure causes a cephalad displacement of the diaphragm; this results in reduction of the lung volumes (vital capacity and functional residual capacity) and the pulmonary compliance and increases the resistance within the airways. Patients with significant respiratory disease such as chronic obstructive pulmonary disease (COPD) or morbid obesity are at risk of pulmonary decompensation and may require positive end-expiratory pressure to maintain adequate gaseous exchange. These responses can be worsened by certain positions as mentioned above (Trendelenburg). Furthermore, reports have been made of increased intra-abdominal pressure resulting in displacement of the carina in a cephalad direction, which could ultimately result in an end- bronchial intubation despite an original endotracheal intubation; signs include increase in the airway pressure with associated reduction in oxygenation. Together with the responses to the mechanical pressure, the absorption of carbon dioxide can also have significant consequences including hypercapnia and respiratory acidosis. While this excess carbon dioxide can be eliminated by increased ventilation, those with pre-existing disease are unable to eliminate as efficiently which may result in dangerous PCO_2 levels.

Renal response

Increase in intra-abdominal pressure is commonly associated with reduced renal blood flow causing oliguria. This is often reversible and should not be overtreated. The compressive effects also affect the renal parenchyma and a reduction in the glomerular filtration rate (GFR) can be seen with higher pressures. At pressures of 15mmHg the urinary output can decrease by 64% with a 21% decrease in GFR. Hormonal changes are also recorded, with increased levels of renin, aldosterone, endothelin and antidiuretic hormone causing systemic vasoconstriction and fluid retention. Such levels often reduce to normal baseline postoperatively causing a mild diuresis.

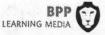

Preoperative assessment

The preoperative assessment aims to enhance patient safety, inform them of surgical risks and improve their care by optimising the surgical plan. The performed investigations aim to ascertain the function of other organ systems which may not be related to the surgical diagnosis but will have an effect on the perioperative course of the patient. In order to avoid unnecessary investigations and prevent duplication, specialised tests are agreed upon at multidisciplinary meetings or via agreed upon protocols. The outcome of such important investigations may delay or alter the surgical management of a patient, or determine referral to another specialty for further optimisation or even to a specialised department for alternative treatment.

Risk stratification scoring systems

The ASA classification system (Tables 3.10 and 3.11)

The determination of need for certain investigations is based on the functional status of the patient, in accordance with the ASA (American Society of Anaesthesiologists) grade, together with the general status of the patient and proposed procedure. Various grading and scoring systems are in place to aid predict morbidity and mortality of patients, aiming to flag up those high risk patients who may warrant a period of stay on the critical care department.

Grade	Features (mortality %)
I	Normal healthy patient (0.05%)
II	Patient with mild systemic disease and no functional limitation (0.4%)
III	Patient with severe systemic disease with functional limitation (4.5%)
IV	Patient with incapacitating systemic disease that is a constant threat to life (25%)
V	Moribund patient who is unlikely to survive 24 hours (50%)
E	Emergency case

Table 3.10. The ASA Grading classification system

	ASA II	ASA III
Cardiovascular disease		
Angina	Occasional GTN spray use (2–3 times/month)	Regular GTN spray use (2–3 times/week) or unstable angina
Hypertension	Stable with single anti-hypertensive	Not well controlled, multiple anti-hypertensives
Diabetes mellitus	Well controlled, no complications	Not well controlled, diabetic complications
Respiratory disease		
COPD	Wheeze, well controlled with inhalers	Breathless on minimal exertion
Asthma	Well controlled on inhalers, not limiting lifestyle	Poorly controlled, limiting lifestyle, taking steroids
Renal disease		
Renal impairment	Creatinine 100–200 µmol/l	Creatinine >200 µmol/l, requiring dialysis

Table 3.11. Characteristics of comorbidities according to ASA grade.

The POSSUM (Physiologic and Operative Severity Score for the enUmeration of Mortality and Morbidity) score

This is a scoring system developed in a general surgical environment in 1991. It is based on 12 physiological/biochemical variables together with six operative variables to predict mortality risk and inform patients accordingly (Table 3.12). Over the last few years specific colorectal, vascular and other specialty adaptations have been developed. Due to the overprediction of mortality in low risk patients a modified version P-POSSUM (Portsmouth-POSSUM) was devised in 1998.

Physiological parameters	Operative parameters
Age	Operation type (minor, major etc)
Cardiac (evidence of failure)	Number of procedures
Respiratory (dyspnoea)	Operative blood loss (mls)
ECG (arrhythmias)	Peritoneal contamination
Systolic blood pressure	Malignancy status (benign, metastatic)
Pulse	Mode of surgery (elective, emergency)
Haemoglobin	
White cell count	
Urea	
Sodium	
Potassium	
Glasgow Coma Scale	

Table 3.12. The POSSUM parameters

Clinical assessment

The history and examination must be thoroughly completed to ensure safety for both the patient and team, with emphasis on the following:

- The diagnosis and investigations to date should be revisited, including all histological analysis. Any specific pending investigations must be flagged up immediately.
- The planned procedure should be reconfirmed with any new information arising from recent investigations. Any specific risks associated with the procedure should be noted (eg high risk of DVT or anticipated blood loss) and any anaesthetic concerns must be discussed as soon as possible.
- A thorough assessment of the patient's comorbidities must be made in order to identify any necessary preoperative investigations that will aid patient optimisation. Patients' medications should be reviewed to allow appropriate modifications perioperatively (warfarin, oral hypoglycaemic drugs, antiplatelet therapy etc). Any specific concerns regarding the recovery and rehabilitation should be identified as early as possible to inform all relevant members of the team (critical care / physiotherapy).
- Postoperative recovery needs to be discussed with the patient, detailing the possibilities for stomas, drains, lines or catheters, particularly if patients are treated within an Enhanced Recovery Programme. Any known care that will be required following discharge should be discussed allowing time for organisation (eg dressing change).

Investigations

Blood tests

- Full blood count: This is recommended for adult women and men over the age of 60 years to look for occult anaemia. In cases of complex surgery or comorbidity (cardiovascular or respiratory) a full blood count is indicated. A blood count should also be performed in all patients with chronic inflammatory conditions.
- Renal function and electrolytes: This should be performed on all patients over the age of 60 and those with comorbidities such as diabetes mellitus, hypertension or those taking drugs which can affect the renal function and electrolytes (diuretics, steroid therapy).
- Liver function test: Indicated in patients with known liver disease or suggestive of on examination. Similarly liver function tests are useful in patients with specific surgical diagnoses such as gallstone disease or undergoing major gastrointestinal disease.
- Clotting profile: This should be performed in all patients taking anticoagulants, known coagulopathies or liver dysfunction or patients who are critically ill (sepsis). This is not generally required in healthy patients undergoing low risk procedures.
- Glucose: A random glucose test can be performed on patients over the age of 40 years undergoing moderate procedures. It can also be used as an indicator of glycaemic control in known diabetics together with a simple urine test. In known diabetics it is also useful to include a recent glycated haemoglobin result in preoperative planning as this is a good indicator of glycaemic control over the preceding few months.
- Group and save / cross matching: A group and save should be performed for any moderately complex surgery where a transfusion may be necessary although unlikely. In cases where transfusion is likely a cross match should be performed depending on the preoperative haemoglobin concentration, the planned procedure and anticipated blood loss.
- Endocrine function tests: In cases of thyroid surgery a full thyroid hormone profile should be performed. In circumstances where the patient is receiving treatment for thyroid disease a profile should be performed if there have been any recent changes to the treatment or previous tests have raised concerns. In cases of other more complex endocrine disease specific investigations may be required in consultation with their endocrinologist.
- Sickle cell test: Testing should be performed for patients whose origins are within specific malarial areas in Africa, West Indies and the Mediterranean. The Sickledex test is the most commonly used analysing the haemoglobin solubility. It is unable to distinguish between sickle cell trait and disease. The test needs only to be performed once.
- Arterial blood gas: This test can be useful in specific circumstances such as prior to lung resection or in cases of poor preoperative oxygen saturations (<90%). A preoperative hypoxaemia is associated with a higher risk of complications and in such cases it can be useful to differentiate between type I and II respiratory failure and aid plan postoperative recovery.
- B-type natriuretic peptide (BNP): This test can be used for the diagnosis of cardiac failure. Levels can be elevated in a number of cardiac conditions such as valvular disease or rhythm abnormalities. It is also regarded as a useful predictor of outcomes for certain cardiac procedures.

Urine tests

- Urine dipstick analysis: This can be used to search for protein, blood, ketones and glucose together with pH levels within the urine. It can be used to look for renal tract disease in specific conditions; otherwise rarely helps preoperative assessment.
- Pregnancy test: Elective surgery for benign disease should ideally not be undertaken during pregnancy. After obtaining informed consent a pregnancy test should be performed in female patients of reproductive age.

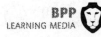

Bedside tests

- ECG: This can provide information regarding both the structure and function of the heart. It is indicated in all patients with cardiovascular disease including hypertension and in cases of abnormalities identified on clinical examination. Some institutions recommend performing routine ECGs on patients above the age of 40 years (age may vary with institution). In cases of arrhythmias which may be intermittent, 24 hour monitoring may be planned preoperatively.
- Spirometry: Lung volume and capacity testing can be useful preoperatively in lung resection surgery to predict outcome. The main parameters used include forced expiratory volume in 1 second (FEV_1), forced vital capacity (FVC), vital capacity (VC) and functional residual capacity (FRC). Spirometry can also be used together with measuring the diffusing capacity of the lung for carbon dioxide (DLCO).
- Peak expiratory flow rate: This test can provide an approximation of the level of airway obstruction, if present. The investigation is however dependent on patient understanding and compliance. It is a simple test that can be used for asthmatics and certain patients with chronic obstructive pulmonary disease (COPD) to identify any necessary preoperative optimisation (change of inhalers, steroids).

Radiology

- Chest X-ray: Preoperative chest X-ray is not necessary in most cases. Indication for preoperative X-rays in accordance with guidelines from the Royal College of Radiologists are: a recent change or deterioration in cardiorespiratory function; surgery involving the cardiorespiratory system; suspected or proven malignancy; suspected or proven tuberculosis (if no recent imaging), and the elderly (> 80 years).
- Flexion / extension cervical spine X-rays: These are often performed in patients with significant spinal disease limiting their neck movement (rheumatoid arthritis, ankylosing spondylitis, severe osteoarthritis) in preparation for the anaesthesia.
- CT / MRI / PET scans: Such complex imaging techniques are rarely used for preoperative assessment, however, they are important in confirming, staging the disease (cancer) and procedure planning, and are therefore organised by the relevant MDT meetings.

Other investigations

- Echocardiography: Transthoracic, non-invasive test easily performed in the outpatient / bedside setting. Echocardiograms should be performed preoperatively in cases of known cardiorespiratory disease or cardiac murmur or in patients where a definite murmur is identified on examination, even in asymptomatic patients. Echocardiography can also be performed under stress (exercise or dobutamine) conditions to evaluate the patient's physiological reserve.
- Cardiopulmonary exercise testing (CPEX): This combined evaluation with exercise (treadmill / bicycle) measures cardiac function via aerobic activity and respiratory function by dynamic flow volume loops and ventilation-perfusion measurements. This testing has been used to predict cardiovascular risk following major vascular and gastrointestinal surgery.
- Polysomnography: Sleep studies involve continuous monitoring of oxygen saturation during sleep to identify any periods of desaturation (sleep apnoea). Obstructive sleep apnoea can be found in patients with significant obesity or tonsillar enlargement. Such overnight desaturation can be managed by the use of positive pressure ventilation (CPAP) and these patients are often managed postoperatively in the critical care unit. Indications for polysomnography include BMI > 43 kg/m^2, significant snoring or daytime somnolence.

- MRSA screening: Guidelines developed by the Department of Health recommend preoperative screening should be considered in all surgical patients where infection could have a significant impact. Also included should be patients with previous MRSA colonisation, recent hospitalisation or those residing in homes (nursing, residential). Screening involves swabbing common areas – nose, groin and head.

Management of specific conditions

Hypertension

Patients should be continued on regular medication with a regular monitoring chart commenced. An ECG together with a chest X-ray should be performed. In cases of poor control ie a persistent diastolic > 110 mmHg or a persistent systolic > 180 mmHg elective surgery should be reconsidered. Patients can be referred to their GP for optimisation.

Severe angina

Significant angina should be managed with beta blockers and nitrates as per cardiology advice. Patients with severe angina should be referred to their cardiologist and GP for optimisation before proceeding to elective surgery. In emergency cases multidisciplinary input is necessary.

Diabetes

Patients should undergo a complete preoperative assessment and be listed ideally early on the operating list. Those having minor procedures can omit their medication on the morning of surgery while those with poor control or undergoing a major procedure will need an insulin sliding scale.

Organising the operating list

Several patient or procedure related factors can affect the order of the list and all members of the team need to be clearly informed.

Patients for early slots in the list

- Latex allergy: Preferably place first in the list. All latex products must be removed and purged from the theatre some hours in advance.
- Paediatric cases: Ideally planned for early slots to reduce starvation time and anxiety.
- Diabetic cases: The aim is to minimise the period of starvation and return to normal diet and diabetic regime as early as possible.
- Adult day cases: Aim for earlier slots to maximise recovery time and allow safe discharge.

Patients for later slots in the list

- In patients with planned overnight stay – with no specific requirements.
- Contaminated infected cases (anal surgery, abscesses, gangrenous limbs), in order to prevent infection for subsequent cases.
- Patients with transmissible infections (MRSA, blood borne viruses): Remove all non essential equipment from theatre and replace recyclable items with disposable ones. A thorough high clean of the theatre should be performed before the theatre is used any further.

Further reading

- British Association of Day Surgery (2011) Available at: www.bads.co.uk.
- Department of Health (2011) *Day surgery: operational guide*. Available at: http://webarchive.nationalarchives.gov.uk/+/www.dh.gov.uk/en/Publicationsandstatistics/Publications/PublicationsPolicyAndGuidance/Dh_4005487?IdcService=GET_FILE&dID=17206&Rendition=Web.
- Department of Health (2011) *MRSA Screening – Operational guidance*. Available at: www.dh.gov.uk/Publications and Statistics/Letters and circulars/Dear Colleague letters/DH_086687.
- NICE (2003) *CG3 Prooperative tests: The use of routine preoperative tests for elective surgery*. Available at: guidance.nice.org.uk/cg3/guidance/pdf/English.
- NICE (2010) CG92 *Venous thromboembolism – reducing the risk*. Available at: http://publications.nice.org.uk/venous-thromboembolism-reducing-the-risk-cg92.
- Royal College of Surgeons of Edinburgh. *Diathermy*. Intercollegiate Basic Surgical Skills Course. Available at: www.medkaau.com/bssc/index.html.
- Verma, R, Altadi, R, Jackson, I, *et al.* Day case and short stay surgery: 2, *Anaesthesia* 2011: 66: 417–434.
- WeBSurg (2011) *World Electronic Book of Surgery*. Available at: www.websurg.com.

Chapter 4
Critical care

Overview

The contents of this chapter refer to critical surgical disease. The basic physiology and relevant clinical applications are detailed around major system organs. Reference is made to monitoring systems and advanced therapeutic modalities employed to maintain patient homeostasis in the critical care setting. In these stations, the candidate's knowledge of pathophysiology of surgical disease is examined and basic understanding of the science behind critical care monitoring and interventions is required. Candidates need to be prepared here as well to draw graphs (eg oxygen dissociation curve) and equations on the exam day, and be familiar with normal values of important vital parameters (eg arterial blood gases).

Care of critically ill surgical patients

Critical illness can develop either gradually over a period of time or suddenly. Once multi-organ failure develops necessitating support on the intensive care unit, mortality can reach as high as 50%. Early detection and prompt treatment is therefore the aim in optimising the patient's outcome. The *National Confidential Enquiry into Patient Outcome and Death* (NCEPOD) report (2005) identified that two-thirds of patients transferred to intensive care units (ICU) more than 24 hours after hospital admission, exhibited physiological instability for more than 12 hours before ICU admission. It was deemed that up to 41% of ICU admissions were potentially avoidable.

Levels of care in the hospital setting

There is a continuing spectrum of care from the surgical ward to through the high dependency unit and to the intensive care unit. Each unit provides specific aspects of care to the patients, with increasing nursing ratios, monitoring and support. Certain accepted general principles exist for admissions to the high dependency and intensive care units.

- Admission **to a high-dependency unit (HDU)** aims to establish a single-organ support (not invasive ventilation) or close monitoring of an unstable patient (hourly) regarding:
  - Oxygenation: respiratory rate, oxygen saturation, arterial blood gases.
  - Cardiac function: pulse, blood pressure, central venous pressure.
  - Renal function: urine output.
- **ICU admission** is indicated for multi-organ mechanical support:
  - Respiratory: mechanical ventilation, non-invasive ventilation.
  - Renal: continuous haemofiltration, intermittent haemodialysis.
  - Cardiac: advanced cardiac output monitoring, inotropic support.
  - Neurological: intracranial pressure monitoring.

Escalation of monitoring and treatment is necessary for patients at risk (such as emergency patients, elderly patients with multiple comorbidities, patients with massive blood transfusion, re-bleeding and established shock) and patients at risk circumstances (such as when there has been a delay in diagnosis, incomplete assessment or failure to act on abnormal findings).

Surgical patients requiring critical care include those newly admitted, patients acutely deteriorating on the ward or those already on the high dependency / intensive care units requiring repeat assessment. Their assessment requires a systematic approach using basic clinical skills that have also been summarised into the concept of Care of Critically Ill Surgical Patients Course (CCrISP) by the Royal College of Surgeons of England (Anderson 2003). This is presented briefly in the sections that follow.

Immediate management

This process allows identification and treatment of life threatening conditions.

A – Airway

Look for central cyanosis, seesaw respiration, use of accessory muscles or reduced consciousness. Listen for abnormal sounds such as snoring, stridor or grunting. Feel for airflow with respiration.

In cases of airway obstruction, immediate resuscitation with airway manoeuvres and the administration of high flow oxygen (12–15L/min via reservoir bag) are necessary. Remember to gain help from the anaesthetist early. Securing an airway may require the following manoeuvres, in order of severity: jaw thrust and chin lift, oral Guedel airway, nasopharyngeal airway, endotracheal tube or surgical airway (cricothyroidotomy).

B – Breathing

Look for central cyanosis, respiratory rate, depth of respiration, jugular venous pressure and the use of accessory muscles. Listen for noisy breathing and the ability of the patient to complete full sentences. Auscultate the chest for breath and heart sounds. Feel for the position of the trachea, and bilateral chest movements with respiration. Look out for life threatening conditions including open pneumothorax, tension pneumothorax, flail chest, massive haemothorax and cardiac tamponade.

C – Circulation

In surgical patients, hypovolaemia must always be considered in cases of haemodynamic instability; in particular haemorrhage must be excluded primarily (unless there are obvious signs of cardiac shock–raised jugular venous pressure). Signs suggestive of compromised circulation include pallor, collapsed veins, and obvious external haemorrhage via drain output or from wounds. Concealed haemorrhage must also be considered including bleeding into the thoracic or abdominal cavities and from pelvic / lower limb fractures. Remember to assess perfusion rather than blood pressure initially as this may be normal in the early stages of circulatory dysfunction.

Insert large bore cannulae and send blood for routine investigations together with cross matching. Administer an initial fluid challenge of 10ml/kg of warmed crystalloid in the normotensive patient or 20ml/kg in the hypotensive patient. In cases of known cardiac failure a bolus of 5ml/kg should be administered unless pulmonary oedema is suspected.

These patients can be categorised into three groups:

- Obvious severe circulatory disturbance (exsanguination) in need of emergency intervention.
- Unstable patient requiring aggressive resuscitation and reassessment while investigations continue. A transient response to resuscitation may be seen, however definitive treatment is still required.
- Patient requires minor resuscitation, responding well and remaining stable on further reassessment.

Reassessment is paramount in all patients to identify those who are clearly not responding well to resuscitation and remain unstable, therefore in need of urgent definitive treatment. In cases of bleeding early organisation of cross matched blood must be made to avoid repeated administration of crystalloids. Similarly those patients who will need surgical intervention to stop bleeding should be flagged up with the relevant teams immediately.

D – Dysfunction of the central nervous system

A brief immediate assessment of the neurological status of the patient can be performed using the AVPU system:

A Alert
V Responds to verbal stimulus
P Only responds to pain
U Unresponsive to all stimuli

Reduced levels of consciousness may be seen in cases of trauma, however other causes such as hypoxia, hypercapnia, shock, drugs or hypoglycaemia must also be considered.

E – Exposure

For a full assessment and resuscitation to be performed it is essential to expose the patient adequately, preserving their dignity at all times. Note patients may require some form of warming.

Should the patient's condition deteriorate at any stage during the resuscitation, it is essential to recommence full assessment starting with the A – airway.

By the end of this stage the patient should be receiving full resuscitation and hopefully showing signs of response. All relevant members of the team and other departments should have already been called and basic procedures and investigations performed (chest X ray, ECG, urinary catheter, blood tests and arterial blood gas). If the patient is unstable then plans should already be in place for definitive treatment.

Full patient assessment

Once the patient is stabilised a full examination and review of documentation and results is necessary to diagnose the change in condition and plan for further management.

Chart review

This should include a review of the observation charts at the foot of the bed for ward patients or the specific charts for patients on the higher dependency or intensive care units. All aspects relating to respiration and circulation together with input / output charts should be reviewed carefully identifying any trends together with absolute values. Fluid balance review should also include the previous few days to determine any positive or negative balance. Pay particular attention to outputs from drains, nasogastric tubes, and hourly urine outputs to estimate renal perfusion. The patient's drug chart should be carefully reviewed looking for any new medications commenced or drugs that may have been omitted.

History and systematic examination

Review of the patient's case notes should be made and further information can be gathered from other medical and nursing staff. In certain cases the patient's family may need to be contacted to ascertain more details. A full thorough clinical examination should then be performed. Ensure full exposure and all wounds, stomas, drains sites etc should also be examined. Repeat examination is essential in such patients allowing early identification and treatment of developing infective or other complications.

Available results

All available investigations should now be reviewed including blood tests, microbiology results and radiological investigations. After completion of such reviews and examination, it must be decided whether the patient is stable or unstable.

Stable patient

Patients that are deemed stable with normal observations and not requiring more than routine fluid management can be monitored with a daily plan in place. This should include:

- Investigations – blood / radiological
- Fluid balance
- Nutrition – oral intake, supplementation

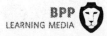

163

- Physiotherapy
- Medications including patient's regular drugs and appropriate analgesia
- Venous thromboprophylaxis in accordance with risk assessment

Unstable patient

In certain cases the patient will not show signs of progression and therefore cannot be left with a daily plan. Senior support should be sought early. In each case it is essential to question whether resuscitation is required before commencing investigations or whether this can be continued simultaneously, which further investigations are required, and whether the patient requires a higher level of care.

Investigations may be necessary to help diagnose deterioration and plan further treatment. They can range from simple to more complex tests. Routine investigations will have already been sent by this stage. In the case of specific radiological investigations the safety of the patient must be considered first. Radiology departments, particularly out of hours, have limited staffing support with minimal equipment for resuscitation; therefore a visit should be planned appropriately. In some cases it may be beneficial to transfer the patient to a higher level of support before visiting the radiology department. Remember at all times to keep reassessing the patient for response to treatment and signs of deterioration. Keep documentation up to date at all opportunities, and seek support from seniors and other specialties early.

Definitive treatment

The aim is to commence definitive treatment as soon as possible. This treatment may include medical, surgical or even radiological options. The ideal location for such treatment should be considered before commencing. Once definitive treatment is commenced, a repeat full assessment should be made to ensure the appropriate clinical response to treatment.

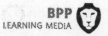

Respiratory physiology and critical care topics

The respiratory system is responsible for gaseous exchange between the circulatory system and the atmosphere. Oxygen from the atmosphere is taken in with inhalation via the upper airways (the nasal cavity, pharynx and larynx) through the lower airways (trachea, primary bronchi and bronchial tree) and into the small bronchioles and alveoli (spongy air-filled sacs surrounded by capillaries) within the lung tissue. The capillary and alveolar walls are very thin, allowing rapid exchange of gases by passive diffusion along concentration gradients.

Carbon dioxide (CO_2) moves into the alveolus as the concentration is much lower in the alveolus than in the blood, and oxygen (O_2) moves out of the alveolus as the continuous flow of blood through the capillaries prevents saturation of the blood with O_2.

Factors that influence the transmission of oxygen from the alveoli to the capillaries

- Right to left shunt (blood passes through the lungs with no contact with air).
- Diffusion defects (eg in cases where the thickness of the alveolar wall increases – such as in pulmonary fibrosis, chronically, or pulmonary oedema).
- Cardiac output changes.
- Ventilation/perfusion mismatch.
  This is a spectrum of conditions; on one end alveoli are ventilated but not perfused (pure dead space ventilation) and on the other end alveoli are perfused but not ventilated (pure shunt).

After diffusing through the alveolar membrane into the capillary blood, apart from a small fraction that dissolves in the blood, oxygen is carried by haemoglobin, via which it is delivered to the cells.

The amount of oxygen carried in the bloodstream and delivered to the tissues (DO_2) is determined by the oxygen carrying capacity, the serum haemoglobin level (Hgb), the percentage of this haemoglobin saturated with oxygen (SaO_2), the amount of oxygen dissolved ($0.003 \times PaO_2$), and the cardiac output (Q), according to the following equation:

$$DO_2 = [1.39 \times Hgb \times SaO_2 + (0.003 \times PaO_2)] \times Q$$

In turn, oxygen delivery to the tissues would be also affected by factors that influence the variables of the above equation:

- The cardiac output (Q) is determined by changes in preload, afterload and heart contractility.
- The haemoglobin concentration (Hgb) is determined by production, destruction and loss.
- The SaO_2 (the saturation of haemoglobin at arterial level with oxygen) is determined by the oxygen saturation (dissociation) curve, which equates PaO_2 (arterial oxygen tension) against SaO_2 (see Figure 4.1).

The oxygen dissociation curve describes the non-linear tendency for oxygen to bind to haemoglobin. Be prepared to draw the curve and discuss factors affecting it (right and left shift).

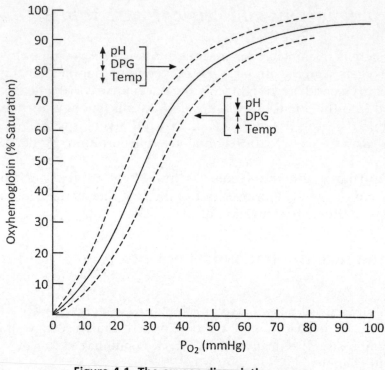

Figure 4.1. The oxygen dissociation curve
Based on Bascroft J and Roberts F.
The dissociation curve of haemoglobin. J Physiol. 1909 August 26; 39(2): 143-148.

Factors affecting the dissociation of oxygen

The position of this curve may shift rightwards (lower saturation for given PaO_2) or leftwards (higher saturation for a given PaO_2) secondary to changes in temperature, pH, and organic phosphates.

*   Temperature: Increasing the temperature denatures the bond between oxygen and haemoglobin, which increases the amount of oxygen and haemoglobin and decreases the concentration of oxyhaemoglobin (oxygenated haemoglobin). The dissociation curve shifts to the right.
*   pH: A decrease in pH (increase in acidity) by addition of carbon dioxide or other acids causes a right shift.
*   Organic phosphates: 2, 3-Diphosphoglycerated (DPG) is the primary organic phosphate in mammals. DPG binds to haemoglobin which rearranges the haemoglobin decreasing the affinity of oxygen for haemoglobin (right shift).

Lung volumes and capacities

Lung volumes and capacities refer to the volume of air associated with different phases of the respiratory cycle (capacities are the summation of volumes). These are depicted in Figure 4.2.

*   Tidal Volume (TV): Volume inspired or expired with each normal breath (Adults - 500ml).
*   Inspiratory Reserve Volume (IRV): Maximum volume that can be inspired over the inspiration of a tidal volume/normal breath. Used during exercise / exertion.
*   Expiratory Reserve Volume (ERV): Maximal volume that can be expired after the expiration of a tidal volume / normal breath.
*   Residual Volume (RV): Volume that remains in the lungs after a maximal expiration. It cannot be measured by spirometry.
*   Inspiratory Capacity (IC): Volume of maximal inspiration: IRV + TV

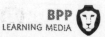

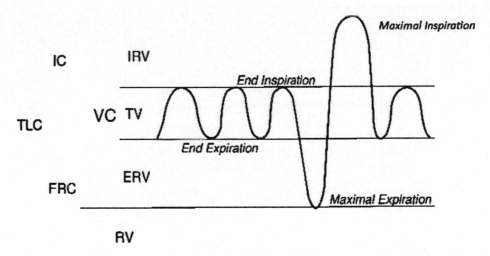

Figure 4.2. Physiological lung volumes and capacities during the respiratory cycle
Based on Whitfield AGW et al. Br. J. Soc. Med. 1950 Jul; 4(3): 113-136.

- Functional Residual Capacity (FRC): Volume of gas remaining in lung after normal expiration, cannot be measured by spirometry because it includes residual volume: ERV + RV
- Vital Capacity (VC): Volume of maximal inspiration and expiration:

$$IRV + TV + ERV = IC + ERV$$

- Total Lung Capacity (TLC): The volume of the lung after maximal inspiration. The sum of all four lung volumes cannot be measured by spirometry because it includes residual volume: IRV + TV + ERV + RV = IC + FRC
- Dead Space: Volume of the respiratory apparatus that does not participate in gas exchange, approximately 300ml in normal lungs.
  - Anatomic Dead Space: Volume of the conducting airways, approximately 150ml.
  - Physiologic Dead Space: The volume of the lung that does not participate in gas exchange. In normal lungs, is equal to the anatomic dead space (150ml), but may be greater in lung disease.
- Forced Expiratory Volume in 1 Second (FEV1): The volume of air that can be expired in one second after a maximal inspiration. It is normally 80% of the forced vital capacity, expressed as FEV1 / FVC.
  - In restrictive lung disease both FEV1 and FVC decrease, thus the ratio remains greater than or equal to 0.8.
  - In obstructive lung disease, FEV1 is reduced more than the FVC, thus the FEV1 / FVC ratio is less than 0.8.

Acute Lung Injury and Acute Respiratory Distress Syndrome

Definitions

Hypoxaemic respiratory failure with bilateral pulmonary infiltrates on chest X-ray and Pulmonary Capillary Wedge Pressure < 18mmHg is defined as

- Acute Lung Injury (ALI) if PaO_2/FiO_2 <300 or as
- Acute Respiratory Distress Syndrome (ARDS) if PaO_2/FiO_2 <200
  (FiO_2: fraction of inspired oxygen)

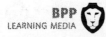

Sepsis	Fat embolism
Pneumonia	Massive blood transfusion
Major trauma	Air embolism
Pulmonary aspiration	Eclampsia
Burns	Poisoning
Inhalation of toxic fumes	Radiation

Table 4.1. Aetiology of ALI and ARDS

Epidemiology

The incidence of ARDS is reported to vary between 58/100,000 person years (USA) and 16/100,000 person years (Scotland) with sinister mortality, reported between 36–44%.

Pathophysiology

Two phases are recognised in ALI / ARDS:

- An acute phase, characterised by widespread destruction of the capillary endothelium, extravasation of protein-rich fluid and interstitial oedema with extensive release of cytokines and migration of neutrophils; the alveolar basement membrane is also damaged, and fluid seeps into the airspaces, stiffening the lungs and causing ventilation/perfusion mismatch.
- A later reparative phase, characterised by fibroproliferation, and organisation of lung tissue. If resolution does not occur, disordered collagen deposition occurs leading to extensive lung scarring.

Differential diagnosis of ARDS

- Acute cardiogenic pulmonary oedema
- Other causes of flash pulmonary oedema:
    - Renal artery stenosis
    - High altitude
    - Drugs (e.g., naloxone)
    - Head injury
- Lymphangitis carcinomatosa
- Pulmonary veno-occlusive diseases
- Pulmonary vasculitis
- Acute presentation of idiopathic interstitial lung diseases
- Acute hypersensitivity pneumonitis
- Acute eosinophilic pneumonia

Diagnostic work up

- Imaging: Chest X-ray, CT chest
- Bronchoalveolar lavage
- Haemodynamic monitoring and assessment

Treatment

The management of patients with ALI / ARDS starts with initiation of supportive measures to all systems (airway, breathing, circulation, also see CCrISP guidelines), empirical antimicrobial therapy, and treatment of underlying disease, if identified.

Low tidal volume – This lung protective strategy protects the lungs from over distension and prevents the release of inflammatory mediators. The ARDSnet multicentre RCT reported a 22% lower mortality group in the lower tidal volume group.
Moderate PEEP – Used to prevent lung injury and improve oxygenation. Lower doses are generally preferred to minimise cardiovascular compromise and risk of pulmonary oedema. A recent meta-analysis has recommended using higher levels of PEEP for severe hypoxaemia.
Prone positioning – This has been found to significantly improve oxygenation (up to 65%). Safety is paramount to minimise displacement of tubes, drains etc. Randomised controlled trials using prone positioning for shorter periods of time have not reported an improvement in survival.
High frequency oscillation – This lung protective mode of ventilation includes low positive pressure together with high respiratory rates. It prevents ventilator-assisted lung injury. A lower 30 day mortality rate was reported in a small randomised controlled trial in comparison with conventional ventilation.
Extracorporeal membrane oxygenation (ECMO) – Can be used for profound refractory hypoxaemia. No significant advantage has been identified although its role in combination therapy is under investigation. Major bleeding is the potential complication.
Low dose steroids – Certain studies have identified improved oxygenation and survival with steroid therapy. However it is recognised that therapy should not be commenced 2 weeks after the onset of ARDS due to the increased risk of infection and mortality.
Haemodynamic management – Studies have reported the benefit of conservative fluid management maintaining a low central venous pressure. This reduces the pressure in the pulmonary microvasculature thereby preventing the development of pulmonary oedema.
Inhaled nitric oxide/prostacyclin –Both treatments cause pulmonary vasodilation, reducing pulmonary hypertension and improving gaseous exchange.
Antibiotics – These should be administered in cases of infective causes after obtaining the appropriate cultures.
Nutrition – Enteral nutrition should be commenced after 48–72 hours of mechanical ventilation. A low carbohydrate, high fat formula containing anti-inflammatory and vasodilating agents such as eicosapentaenoic and linoleic acids is recommended.

Table 4.2. Current strategies in the management of ALI/ARDS

The management needs to be escalated to the critical care setting where the cornerstone of treatment is to keep the $PaO_2 > 60mmHg$ (8KPa), without causing injury to the lungs with excessive O_2 or barotrauma. Several strategies are recommended for the management of ALI/ARDS, which are summarised in Table 4.2.

Invasive Mechanical Ventilation (IMV)

The main goal in invasive mechanical ventilation is to replace the normal functions of the lungs and ventilatory pump in patients with as little disruption of their homeostasis and as few complications as possible.

Physiological objectives of IMV

*   To improve alveolar ventilation and arterial oxygenation
*   To increase the end-inspiratory lung inflation
*   To increase the end-expiratory lung volume (functional residual capacity) and
*   To reduce the work of breathing and unload the ventilatory muscles.

Clinical objectives of IMV

Invasive mechanical ventilation is used, aiming to:

- Reverse acute respiratory acidosis.
- Reverse hypoxaemia.
- Relieve respiratory distress and patient discomfort while the primary disease process resolves or improves.
- Prevent or reverse atelectasis.
- Reverse ventilatory muscle fatigue and unload the ventilatory muscles.
- Permit sedation and / or neuromuscular blockade.
- Decrease systemic or myocardial oxygen consumption in certain settings (eg severe ARDS; cardiogenic shock).
- Reduce intracranial pressure, by means of controlled hyperventilation, as in acute closed head injury.
- Stabilise the chest wall, as in chest wall resection or massive flail chest.

Clinical indications for invasive mechanical ventilation

Conditions leading to respiratory failure requiring IMV include (list non-exhaustive):

- Apnoea and impending respiratory arrest.
- Exacerbation of chronic obstructive pulmonary disease.
- Acute severe asthma.
- Neuromuscular disease.
- Acute hypoxaemic respiratory failure.
- Heart failure and cardiogenic shock.
- Acute brain injury.

Contraindications to Invasive Mechanical Ventilation

Intubation and mechanical ventilations should not be used in the following circumstances:

- No indication for ventilatory support exists.
- Non-invasive ventilation is indicated in preference to invasive mechanical ventilation.
- Intubation and mechanical ventilation are contrary to the patient's expressed wishes.
- Life-support interventions, including mechanical ventilation, would constitute medically futile therapy.

Impaired cardiac function	Impaired mucociliary clearance
Increased intracranial pressure	Mucosal injury
Gastric distension	Alteration of mouth flora
Respiratory alkalosis	Lower airway colonisation
Renal and hepatic dysfunction	Increased work of breathing
Clinical Barotrauma	Loss of ability to speak
(ventilator-related extra-alveolar air)	Tracheal stenosis (late)
Complications of Intubation, Tracheostomy	Ventilator-Associated Pneumonia
(Tissue injury; haemorrhage)	Agitation and respiratory distress developing during
Increased airway secretions	mechanical ventilation
Loss of endogenous humidification system	

Table 4.3. Complications of Invasive Mechanical Ventilation

Acute pancreatitis

Epidemiology

Acute pancreatitis is a common disease presenting to the emergency general surgical team. The annual incidence is between 5 and 80 per 100,000 population, with about 80% of patients having mild disease. Approximately 10% of all cases develop infected pancreatic necrosis with mortality rates reaching 40%. One-half of patients who die with severe pancreatitis do so within the first week of admission to hospital due to organ failure.

Aetiology

- Gallstones and alcohol are common causes (80%). Gallstones < 5mm in size are more likely to cause pancreatitis than larger stones. Approximately < 5% of patients with gallstones present with acute pancreatitis.
- Other causes include structural lesions, surgical trauma (ERCP) viral infections (HIV, mumps), medications (ACE inhibitors, azathioprine, steroids), hypercalcaemia or autoimmune disease.
- Idiopathic group have no identifiable cause found after clinical assessment, biochemistry, CT and ultrasound. Causes include microlithiasis or sludge, chronic pancreatitis, and pancreas divisum.

Pathophysiology

The main pancreatic enzyme is trypsin, activating itself and other proenzymes (see also Chapter 1: *Anatomy – the pancreas*). The injury to the acinar cells in pancreatitis leads to an acute inflammatory response within the gland stimulating further cytokine production. This, together with other mediators stimulates a systemic inflammatory response syndrome causing organ dysfunction within hours. While gallstones can stimulate the onset of pancreatitis, impaction does not cause disease progression.

Local changes can be:

- Phlegmonous (80% of cases): The secretion of pancreatic enzymes is disrupted causing activation of enzymes such as amylase, lipase. This leads to disruption of the acini and oedema. Gradually the oedema and inflammation will create a phlegmon. Persistence of fluid collections within the phlegmon leads to the development of pseudocysts.
- Haemorrhagic (15% of cases): Disruption of peripancreatic veins due to inflammation can cause bleeding. Retroperitoneal haemorrhage can manifest itself as Grey Turner's (flank) and Cullen's (periumbilical) signs.
- Necrotising (5% of cases): Severe inflammation causes significant vascular disruption developing pancreatic ischaemia and tissue necrosis. Other neighbouring organs may become involved and the tissue may become infected.

Clinical manifestations

- 95% cases present with acute moderate to severe pain in upper abdomen radiating to the back. The pain may have a sudden onset and will intensify to a constant ache.
- Nausea and vomiting are often associated symptoms (70%).
- Initial observations include a pyrexia (75%) and tachycardia (65%).
- Abdominal examination reveals epigastric / central tenderness with guarding and sometimes distension.
- Jaundice is seen in a proportion of cases (28%).

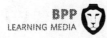

- Other signs may be related to systemic organ effects of pancreatitis; dyspnoea, tachypnoea, haemodynamic instability.
- Retroperitoneal haemorrhage is rarer and non specific and occurs late (48 hours).
- Diagnostic Specificity of serum amylase is 95% with sensitivity around 60%. A value of more than three times the upper normal limit is classed as diagnostic.
- Serum lipase remains elevated more than a week with specificity at four times normal of 95% and sensitivity 55–100%. Both can be measured in the urine.
- Features suggestive of gallstone aetiology include female gender, age > 50 years, amylase > 4000 IU/L, raised bilirubin, alanine aminotransferase or alkaline phosphatase.
- A raised serum alanine aminotransferase of > 150IU/L has a positive predictive value of 95%.
- Ultrasonography is 95% sensitive in identifying gallstones although views can be difficult in the presence of an ileus.
- Early CT scanning is useful in cases of diagnostic uncertainty to exclude alternative diagnoses (mesenteric ischaemia).

Definitions of complications

- Acute pancreatitis is termed severe if organ dysfunction or local complications are present. Prognostically, this includes a Glasgow or Ranson score of ≥ 3, APACHE II score of > 8 or a CRP of > 150mg/dl in the first 48 hours of admission (see Table 4.4).
- Pancreatic necrosis is a histological or radiological diagnosis. It can be diagnosed using contrast enhanced CT or gadolinium enhanced MRI scanning. Features include non perfused / necrotic parenchyma, perinecrotic fluid collection and haemorrhagic foci.
- Acute fluid collections refer to the peripancreatic fluid seen within the first four weeks of diagnosis. This collection lacks a defined wall.
- Post acute pseudocyst is caused by disruption of the pancreatic duct stimulating an inflammatory response and fibrous capsule formation. This can only be diagnosed after four weeks.
- Pancreatic abscesses are formed when necrosis is followed by liquefaction and infection.
- Organised pancreatic necrosis (necroma) describes the final product of liquefaction of necrosis seen at 1–3 months stage. It can also be referred to as a pseudocyst with debris.

Initial management

- Aggressive fluid resuscitation to maintain satisfactory urine output. Strict hourly fluid balance monitoring.
- Analgesia: paracetamol with NSAIDs and opiates in severe cases. PCA is required in certain circumstances.
- Supplemental oxygen.
- Venous thromboembolism prophylaxis.
- Regular monitoring of blood tests especially electrolytes.
- Regular respiratory and cardiovascular measurements.
- Nutrition support should be included, either orally in mild cases within a few days or via supplementation (nasogastric, parenteral). Early enteral feeding is preferred to protect the gastrointestinal mucosal barrier and limit bacterial translocation.
- The benefit from use of antibiotics has not been completely defined. Overuse has been found in necrosis to cause superinfection with Candida. Some studies have demonstrated benefit from use of carbapenems in severe necrotic pancreatitis. If used, the duration of treatment should not exceed 14 days without evidence of infected necrosis.
- Organ compromised patients to be monitored in ICU or HDU.
- Early discussion with specialist unit in cases of necrosis > 50%, infected necrosis or multiple organ failure.

Glasgow criteria	Ranson criteria
Age > 55 years WCC > 15 × 10⁹/L Blood glucose > 10 nmol/L Lactate dehydrogenase > 600 IU/L or Aspartate transaminase > 200 IU/L Albumin < 32 g/L Calcium < 2 mmol/L Urea > 16 mmol/L PaO₂ < 8KPa	Age > 55 years WCC > 16 × 10⁹/L Blood glucose > 11.1 nmol/L Lactate dehydrogenase > 350 IU/L Aspartate transaminase > 250 IU/L Calcium < 2 mmol/L* Urea > 1.8 mmol/L rise* Base deficit > 4 mmol/L* Arterial PO₂ < 60 mmHg* Hct fall by > 10%* Estimated fluid sequestration of > 6lt* * During initial 48 hours

Table 4.4. Scoring systems for acute pancreatitis
Glasgow/Ranson score > 3 indicates severe pancreatitis and consideration for HDU/ITU

Disease severity stratification

A simple test available is the C-reactive protein at 48 hours from admission. A CRP < 150mg/l has a negative predictive value of 90% for necrosis, but a value > 150mg/l only has a positive predictive value of 40%. The Glasgow and Ranson criteria are presented in Table 4.4.

Role of ERCP

The clearance of bile duct in severe acute pancreatitis was not advocated during the open surgical era due to higher mortality than conventional management.

The evidence on the role of ERCP with early endoscopic sphincterotomy has been conflicting:

- The Cochrane meta-analysis of three trials (Ayub *et al*, 2004) indicated that patients with predicted severe acute pancreatitis benefited from early ERCP with reduction in complication rate. There was no documented mortality reduction in predicted mild or severe disease.
- Early ERCP may be of more benefit in cholangitis or obstructive jaundice (Petrov *et al*, 2008).

Further management

- A majority of patients with mild disease recover within five days.
- As the recurrence of symptoms is reported between 32–61% of cases if a cholecystectomy is not performed during the initial admission, those with cholecystolithiasis would benefit from an urgent cholecystectomy (± cholangiography).
- In cases where the aetiological factor is not obvious, a CT or MRI scan should be performed to exclude any structural lesions. ERCP can also be performed to identify ampullary lesions, while endoscopic ultrasound has the benefit of diagnosing early stage alcohol induced chronic pancreatitis.
- Severe acute pancreatitis progresses to SIRS (systemic inflammatory response syndrome) and MODS (multi-organ dysfunction syndrome). Early organ failure within the first week is usually respiratory and transient in > 40% of patients. Persistent organ failure (> 48 hours) is associated with 35% mortality. Intensive care support and follow up imaging is essential.
- CT scanning using the Balthazar's index scores the appearance of the pancreas and degree of necrosis, thereby predicting mortality. Secondary infection and necrosis should be considered if improvement or stability in weeks 2–4 is not apparent.

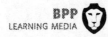

- Fine needle aspiration under image guidance to confirm infection before intervention is recommended. The complication rate of this procedure is low and sensitivity and specificity is 90%. Acute fluid collections consisting of enzyme rich fluid commonly develop in the periphery of the gland within 48 hours. Patients are rarely symptomatic and drainage is not recommended.

- Surgical intervention for acute pancreatitis should be reserved for infected necrosis. Surgical intervention for necrosis within the first two weeks is associated with high mortality and should be avoided; delay to the third or fourth week to minimise intra-operative haemorrhage is recommended. In certain cases of sterile necrosis who fail to thrive, surgery is performed. Surgical options available for infected pancreatic necrosis include necrosectomy with lavage, or newer techniques involving interventional radiology and minimally invasive surgery. In certain specific cases of infected necrosis without organ failure success has been achieved with prolonged treatment with antibiotics only.

- Haemorrhage can occur in cases of early necrosectomy or de novo. The bleeding ranges from slow and intermittent to sudden which is often fatal. Arterial bleeding can occur from pseudoaneurysms of the left gastric, splenic or gastroduodenal arteries. Embolisation is the preferred method of management. Venous bleeding is uncommon in comparison and can be more difficult to manage, requiring emergency surgery in certain cases.

Guidelines on the management of acute pancreatitis (UK Working Party, 2005)

- The diagnosis should be confirmed within 48 hours of admission to hospital with the aetiology confirmed in ≥80%.
- Severity scoring should be performed on admission and patients with severe acute pancreatitis should be aimed to be treated on a high dependency unit or intensive therapy unit with full monitoring.
- In cases of gallstone aetiology with a predicted or actual severe acute pancreatitis an urgent ERCP should be planned ideally within 72 hours from the onset of symptoms. This is also recommended for cases of cholangitis, jaundice or a dilated common bile duct.
- Patients with acute pancreatitis of gallstone aetiology should undergo a definitive procedure for their gallstones either during the same admission or within two weeks.
- In cases of necrosis with signs of sepsis or significant necrosis (>30%), image guided fine needle aspiration should be performed to obtain material for culture. Cases of infected necrosis should be considered for debridement.

Chronic pancreatitis

Definition

Chronic pancreatitis refers to continuous inflammatory process within the gland that can cause irreversible changes (fibrosis) which can lead to both endocrine and exocrine insufficiency.

Epidemiology and risk factors

The incidence described is 5 cases per 100,000 population in Europe, with higher prevalence in males. The commonest aetiological agent for chronic pancreatitis is alcohol, accounting for over 70% of cases. Idiopathic makes up the majority of the remaining causes with rarer cases such as pancreas divisum, pancreatic tumours or hereditary pancreatitis accounting for the rest.

 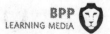

Pathology

Various proposals have been made regarding the pathways leading to parenchymal destruction. One theory is based upon the toxic effects of alcohol together with malnutrition, while another describes the fibrosis as a sequel of repeated episodes of acute pancreatitis and necrosis.

Clinical manifestations and differential diagnosis

The commonest presenting symptom is abdominal pain which can be deep and boring, radiating into the back. Patients often require significant amounts of analgesia including opiates to control the pain. Gradually over years pancreatic insufficiency develops causing steatorrhoea and endocrine complications such as diabetes. The differential diagnosis includes pancreatic or other upper gastrointestinal tumour, peptic ulcer disease and gallstone disease.

Investigations

- Blood tests, including routine haematology and biochemistry. Both serum amylase and lipase are often not helpful even during acute episodes due to little functioning parenchyma. Liver function tests should be performed and may be deranged in cases of alcoholic pancreatitis or biliary obstruction. Similarly a clotting profile should be performed.
- Radiological: A plain abdominal X-ray can sometimes identify pancreatic calcification. Ultrasound can be used to assess the pancreatic duct and identify pancreatic stones, or pseudocysts. CT scanning is the preferred method allowing full assessment of the size, shape and texture of the gland together with the pancreatic duct and biliary tree. Local involvement of vascular or gastrointestinal structures can also be identified. MRCP (magnetic resonance cholangiopancreatography) can offer a useful, detailed examination of the pancreatic duct with the addition of *secretin* stimulation quantifying exocrine function. One of the most sensitive investigations for diagnosing early changes in chronic pancreatitis is endoscopic ultrasound (EUS); it can help exclude pancreatic cancer (fine needle aspiration cytology) and identify small ductal changes.

Complications of chronic pancreatitis

- Pain: This is probably the most significant symptom suffered by patients, often requiring long term opiates. Acute exacerbations can require hospital admission necessitating strong opiates, bowel rest and nutritional support. Some positive results have been reported with procedures such as coeliac axis blocks or thoracoscopic splanchnicectomy, although repeat procedures are often required.
- Pancreatic insufficiency:
  - Endocrine insufficiency takes a progressive course often requiring insulin. With minimal glucagon levels, patients are more prone to hypoglycaemia. Strict control should be aimed for particularly in alcoholic patients with nutritional insufficiency, to minimise complications.
  - Exocrine insufficiency leads to various deficiencies and can be managed by pancreatic enzyme supplements. Supplements should be taken with meals and a proton pump inhibitor.
- Pseudocysts: Peripancreatic fluid collections can be seen in chronic pancreatitis which can become infected or cause other local effects such as biliary or duodenal obstruction or pain. Drainage of the pseudocysts can be performed either percutaneously or by creating a cystogastrostomy or cystojejunostomy by either laparoscopic or open surgery.
- Biliary obstruction: This occurs either due to the pseudocysts or pancreatic parenchymal fibrosis. Management involves ERCP and introduction of a biliary stent. In certain cases

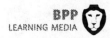

a more long term solution is required in the form of a choledochoduodenostomy / choledochojejunostomy.

- Haemorrhage: This can be caused by erosion of the splenic artery causing a pseudoaneurysm or in alcoholic cases variceal bleeding. Management includes angiography and embolisation and endoscopic management.
- Portal hypertension: This is seen either secondary to alcoholic liver cirrhosis or thrombosis of the splenic vein.
- Pancreatic cancer: The risk of cancer is increased by five to ten fold in cases of chronic pancreatitis.

Management of chronic pancreatitis

The common management principles are based on supportive therapy, including pain management, nutritional support with pancreatic enzyme supplementation, and psychological support. Surgical procedures can be offered for cases of persistent pain and a dilated pancreatic duct. Procedures include lateral pancreaticojejunostomy with or without resection of the pancreatic head. In cases of disease only in the tail of the gland, a distal pancreatectomy can be offered. Unfortunately total pancreatectomy may not relieve pain in some individuals, due to damage of the autonomic pathways, together with the patient developing brittle diabetes. Overall, the five-year survival in chronic pancreatitis is approximately 70%.

Renal physiology and critical care

The functions of the kidney

- The kidney regulates fluid and electrolyte balance by filtration, secretion and re-absorption.
- It also acts as an endocrine organ, activating **erythropoietin** (for production of red blood cells) and **vitamin D** (which regulates calcium metabolism). It also produces **renin** which affects various aspects of water and electrolyte homeostasis.

Glomerular filtration

The renal blood flow is 25% of cardiac output. Approximately 1% of the filtered load is excreted as urine. The rate at which fluid is filtered by the glomerulus is the glomerular filtration rate (GFR). The major determinants of GFR are:

- Renal blood flow and renal perfusion pressure.
- The hydrostatic pressure difference between the tubule and the capillaries.
- The surface area available for ultra-filtration.

Oliguria and causes of low urine output post-operatively

(See Chapter 8 – Procedural skills)

How to minimise the risk of peri-operative renal injury

- Avoid nephrotoxins if pre-existing renal injuries are present.
- Prevent rhabdomyolysis by aggressively fluid loading patients at risk (trauma patients, those with compartment syndromes and those undergoing limb revascularisation).
- Identify patients at risk: patients undergoing cardiac surgery, major vascular surgery.
- Maintain adequate preoperative and intraoperative hydration.
- Maintain renal perfusion pressure (watch for anaesthetic drugs with vasodilatory effects).
- Pharmacologic interventions.

	GFR criteria	Urine output criteria
Risk	Increased Creatinine × 1.5 or Decrease GFR > 25%	UO <0.5ml/kg/hr × 6 h
Injury	Increased Creatinine × 2 or Decrease GFR > 50%	UO <0.5ml/kg/hr × 12 h
Failure	Increased Creatinine × 3 or Decrease GFR > 75%	UO <0.5ml/kg/hr × 24 h or Anuria × 12 h
Loss	Persistent ARF (complete loss of renal function) > 4 weeks)	
End-stage renal disease	Persistent ARF > 3 months	

Table 4.5. RIFLE classification to determine the extent of acute kidney injury

Renal replacement therapy

Renal replacement therapy is required to prevent endogenous poisoning or fluid overload. The most common clinical indications for renal replacement therapy are fluid overload, hyperkalaemia, metabolic acidosis and uraemia.

Indications for renal replacement therapy

- Oliguria (urine output < 200mL/12h)
- Anuria / extreme oliguria (urine output < 50mL/12h)
- Hyperkalaemia ([K] > 6.5 mEq/L)
- Severe acidemia (pH < 7.1)
- Azotemia ([urea] > 30mg/dL)
- Clinically significant organ (especially pulmonary) oedema
- Uraemic encephalopathy
- Uraemic pericarditis
- Uraemic neuropathy / myopathy
- Severe dysnatremia ([Na] < 115 or > 160 mEq/L)
- Hyperthermia
- Drug overdose with dialyzable toxin

Modes of renal replacement therapy

- Intermittent haemodialysis (IHD): The most efficient mode, as large amounts of fluid can be removed and electrolyte abnormalities can be rapidly corrected; not suitable in unstable patients (risk of severe hypotension).
- Peritoneal dialysis (PD): Simple and cost effective; disadvantages include poor solute clearance, poor uraemic control, risk of peritoneal infection, mechanical obstruction of pulmonary and cardiovascular performance.
- Continuous renal replacement therapy (CRRT): is an effective preferred method for critically ill patients. It can be utilised in cases of haemodynamic instability, fluid overload and catabolic states. It enhances recovery from acute renal failure whilst maintaining electrolyte and acid base balance. CRRT has been shown effective to remove some of the inflammatory mediators in multi organ dysfunction syndrome. Indications for continuous renal replacement therapy include renal causes such acute renal failure with either haemodynamic instability or sepsis, or non renal causes such as SIRS, acidosis or crush syndrome (traumatic rhabdomyolysis).
  - Advantages
    - Low rate of fluid removal allows a steady state fluid equilibrium for haemodynamically unstable patients.
    - CRRT allows electrolyte (potassium, phosphate) and acid-base balance and removal of fluid (ARDS).
    - CRRT can lower intracranial tension.
    - Mediators of inflammation can be removed, aiding treatment of sepsis.
  - Disadvantages
    - Anticoagulation is required.
    - Expensive therapy
    - Hypothermia
    - Thrombosis and air embolism can complicate the treatment.

Interpretation of arterial blood gases

Acid base physiology

The pH is defined as the power of hydrogen (**p** denotes for power and **H** Hydrogen) as described by Soran Sorensen in 1909 and expresses the measure of activity of dissolved hydrogen [H⁺] ions in a solution:

$$pH = -\log^{10} [H^+],$$

with [H⁺]: the concentration of hydrogen ions

Even a small change in the pH is indicative of a large change in the H⁺ ion concentration in the contrary direction. A change in pH of 0.3 approximately doubles or halves the [H⁺]. A change in pH of 1 reflects 10 fold changes in [H⁺] (Table 4.6).

pH	[H⁺] nmol/l
6.0	1,000
7.0	100
8.0	10
9.0	1

Table 4.6. Association between pH and [H⁺]

The pH values range within 0–14, with water having a pH of 7.0 at 25°C. A balance in the acid-base status is necessary for the correct functioning of reactions within the body, as significant imbalance causes enzyme deactivation. Blood pH is normally maintained at 7.35–7.45. Approximately 60mmol/l of H⁺ ions are produced in 24 hours through metabolism in the form of organic acids (amino acids), which are oxidised to form carbon dioxide and water or inorganic acids (such as hydrochloric acid) excreted by the renal system.

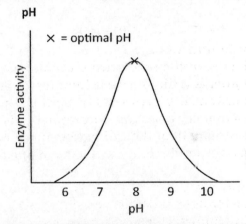

Figure 4.3. Effect of pH on enzyme activity
Based on Sorensen SPL. Biochem. 2. 21,131 (1909); 22,352 (1909)

Respiratory acid

Carbonic acid (H_2CO_3) is the respiratory acid; carbon dioxide (CO_2), although not an acid itself, has the potential to create an equivalent amount of carbonic acid. Carbon dioxide is produced from various oxidative processes involving carbohydrates and fatty acids. It is excreted via the respiratory system, a process which needs to be rapid and efficient.

Given a resting adult has an oxygen consumption of 250ml/minute and a carbon dioxide production of 200ml/minute (respiratory quotient – 0.8), the total daily carbon dioxide production equals to approximately 13,000mmol/day. An increase in activity will increase the oxygen consumption; thereby the daily carbon dioxide production also increases depending on the metabolic activity.

Metabolic acid

This refers to the non-volatile acids produced by the body (incomplete metabolism of carbohydrates, fats and proteins) and are therefore known as fixed acids. Apart from carbonic acid the remaining acids within the body are mainly fixed acids. The total production of H⁺ in form of metabolic acid is about 70–100mmol per day in an adult, which is excreted by the kidney.

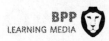

This total excludes the lactate produced by the body, because most of the produced lactate is metabolised and not excreted. In order to maintain balance the quantity of acid excreted per day should equal the quantity produced per day. The carbonic acid is excreted via the lungs and the fixed acids via the kidneys.

The response of the body to alterations in the acid-base balance in order to maintain homeostasis within the body are by three mechanisms: buffering, respiratory responses (alteration in partial pressure of carbon dioxide) and metabolic (renal) responses (alteration of bicarbonate excretion).

Buffers

Buffers are solutions which have the ability to minimise changes in the pH when acids or bases are added. Typically this will consist of a weak acid solution (HA) and a salt of the acid:

$$HA \leftrightarrow H^+ + A^-,$$

where A^- is any anion (eg chloride) and HA is an undissociated acid (eg organophosphate).

The addition of a strong acid, such as hydrochloric acid, to this solution shifts the equation to the left. The H^+ ions are 'used up' in the formation of undissociated acid. The salt provides a reservoir of A^- to replenish $[A^-]$ when A^- is removed by reaction with H^+. On the contrary when a base is added, the H^+ ions react with the OH- ions and form water (H_2O). The pKa is the logarithm to base 10 of **Ka**, the acid dissociation constant, and is equivalent to the pH at which 50% of the substance is ionised. Generally, the closer the pKa of the buffer is to the pH of the solution the more efficient the buffering system.

Within the blood system, bicarbonate (HCO_3^-) is the most important buffer system, accounting for approximately 80% of extracellular buffering. H^+ ions combine with HCO_3^- and are then removed from the body in the form of CO_2 and H_2O:

$$CO_2 + H_2O \leftrightarrow H_2CO_3 \leftrightarrow H^+ + HCO_3^-$$

Despite the pKa of bicarbonate being much lower (6.1) than the pH of blood, it is still an efficient system due to the large quantity available and thanks to the independent ability of the respiratory and renal systems to alter the levels of carbon dioxide and bicarbonate. An increase in H^+ ions in the blood creates an increase in H_2CO_3, causing a rise in CO_2 (as they are in equilibrium), which is excreted via the lungs. The Henderson-Hasselbalch equation (below) describes the association between the serum concentration of HCO_3^-, the partial pressure of CO_2 and blood pH:

$$pH = 6.1 + \log_{10} [HCO_3^-] / [H_2CO_3] = 6.1 + \log_{10} [HCO_3^-] / 0.03 \times PCO_2$$

Oxygen

As discussed already (see the earlier section *Respiratory physiology and critical care topics*), two forms of oxygen exist within the blood; dissolved in plasma or combined with haemoglobin. The partial pressure of oxygen (kPa) determines the quantity dissolved. For each 1 kPa, 0.027ml oxygen is dissolved per 100ml blood. Therefore, each 100ml of normal arterial blood contains about 0.3ml dissolved oxygen.

Haemoglobin is composed of an iron porphyrin compound (haem) joined to a globin protein made of four polypeptide chains, each able to combine reversibly with oxygen to form oxyhaemoglobin. Therefore, each haemoglobin molecule can bind four molecules of oxygen. Each binding of an oxygen molecule stimulates a conformational change in the haemoglobin increasing the affinity for oxygen. Such a change aids the loading and unloading of oxygen in various tissues and explains the nature of the oxygen dissociation curve (see the section *Respiratory physiology*). Every 100ml of normal arterial blood with a [Hb] of 15 g/dl contains approximately 20ml of oxygen of which only 1.5% is dissolved in plasma. The oxygen saturation of haemoglobin defines the percentage of available binding sites that have combined with oxygen. Arterial blood has an oxygen saturation of approximately 97% (corresponding to a PaO_2 of 13.5 kPa).

Alveolar gas equation

The alveolar gas equation is

$$PAO_2 = PiO_2 - PaCO_2/RQ, \text{ with}$$

PAO_2 = Partial Alveolar oxygen pressure
$PaCO_2$ = Arterial partial carbon dioxide pressure
PiO_2 = partial pressure of inspired oxygen (PiO_2) = barometric pressure × FiO_2
RQ (respiratory quotient) = the ratio of the amount of CO_2 produced for each molecule of O_2 used in metabolism, typically equals 0.8.

This equation helps calculate the expected alveolar partial oxygen pressure (PAO_2) for a given fraction of inspired oxygen (FiO_2) and from that, the 'A-a gradient'.

As the oxygen in the blood passes through the alveoli in the lungs, it is completely taken up making the arterial and alveolar partial pressures the same. The actual difference between the two values (actual PaO_2 and expected PAO_2) is known as 'A-a gradient' and it is increased when more deoxygenated blood is leaving the left ventricle due to a pathological process.

Effect of PiO_2

Hypoxia can develop with changes in altitude, due to reduction in the PiO_2. Hypoxia stimulates an increase in ventilation reducing $PaCO_2$ resulting in respiratory alkalosis, fatigue and cerebral oedema – altitude sickness. The bicarbonate leaves the cerebrospinal fluid normalising its pH and then is excreted via the kidneys. Once the blood pH is normal again the ventilation also returns to normal. Contrarily an increase in pressure below sea level increases the PiO_2 forcing more uptake into the arterial blood.

Carbon dioxide

Carbon dioxide (CO_2) is carried in the blood in three forms: as carbamino compounds, as bicarbonate, and as dissolved in the blood. CO_2 is much more soluble than oxygen. In arterial blood, about 90% is in the form of bicarbonate ions, with the rest split between carbamino compounds and dissolved. In the venous blood only 60% of CO_2 is found in bicarbonate ions and 30% as carbamino compounds.

Bohr effect

This describes the effect of carbon dioxide on the release of oxygen to tissues. The combination of carbon dioxide and water forms carbonic acid (under the influence of carbonic anhydrase) which dissociates into hydrogen and bicarbonate ions. The increase in hydrogen ions causes acidosis

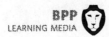

181

encouraging the release of oxygen from haemoglobin (right shift, see oxygen dissociation curve section). In the lungs where carbon dioxide is excreted, alkalosis encourages uptake of oxygen.

Haldane effect

This describes the increased ability of blood to carry carbon dioxide when the haemoglobin is in a deoxygenated state. Deoxygenated haemoglobin is over three times more effective at forming carbamino compounds than oxyhaemoglobin. Both these effects result in carbon dioxide loading at the tissue level and the unloading of oxygen.

Blood gas analysis

Blood gas analysers measure the pH, PaO_2 and $PaCO_2$ in the blood. Modern equipment consists of automated systems requiring minimal intervention. The pH electrode compares the potential difference between a known solution and the unknown sample solution at 37°C. The $PaCO_2$ is measured by allowing the carbon dioxide to undergo a chemical reaction producing hydrogen ions which creates a measurable difference in the potential difference. Similarly the PaO_2 is estimated by measuring electrical currents generated by reactions of the polarographic electrode.

Anion gap

Under normal conditions a state of electroneutrality exists with the major cations and anions in balance. The anion gap is an artificial disparity between the concentrations of the major plasma cations and anions routinely measured – normally sodium, potassium, chloride, and bicarbonate and is defined by the equation below:

$$\text{Anion gap} = ([Na^+] + [K^+] - ([Cl^-] + [HCO_3^-])$$

The normal range is 8–18mmol/l and 11mmol/l is commonly due to albumin.

- A reduced anion gap is caused by hypoalbuminaemia or even increased concentrations of minor cations such as calcium or magnesium.
- An increased anion gap acidosis is due to dehydration and processes that increase the concentrations of minor anions, lactate, ketones and renal acids, or even drug therapy such as penicillin and salicylates.
- Metabolic acidosis without an increased anion gap is commonly associated with an increase in plasma chloride concentration caused by gastrointestinal loss.

Base excess / deficit

Base excess or deficit refers to the amount of base required to restore 1 litre of blood to normal pH (assuming CO_2 is normal) at 37°C. If there is a deficit of base, metabolic acidosis develops, thus base has to be added; excess base leads to alkalosis which requires removal of the base to normalise the pH. In cases of a raised CO_2 the excess base may be compensatory.

Lactate

This is the end product of anaerobic glycolysis with normal range between 0.6–2.0 mmol/l. An increase in anaerobic metabolism increases the lactate concentration causing acidosis. Shock and sepsis can cause extremely high levels of lactate implying poor tissue perfusion and cellular hypoxia.

Compensation

Compensation is the active process whereby independent mechanisms of the body (respiratory ventilation, kidney function) tend to resist to changes in the acid-base balance that cannot be addressed by the buffering systems alone.

The compensation for abnormalities in acid–base balance is either metabolic or respiratory. For cases of primary metabolic disturbance (such as diabetic ketoacidosis) the compensation is respiratory, by the way of increase of the minute ventilation to eliminate the CO_2, and vice versa; primary respiratory abnormality (such as CO_2 retention in COPD) tends to be compensated by retention of HCO_3^- from the kidneys.

There are three main terms used in reference to compensation:

* Uncompensated: Acid base disturbance, where no successful correction of pH is achieved.
* Partial compensation: where some attempt is made to correct pH but pH stays outside the normal range.
* Fully compensated: where complete pH correction is made to normalise the pH.

In general, the body can never over-compensate an acid-base abnormality.

Interpretation of arterial blood gas

As PO_2, pH and PCO_2 are the only measured variables, it is good practice to look at these first, before reviewing the derived variables.

1. Look at PO_2
    * Is there hypoxia?
    * What FiO_2 is the patient receiving?
    * Calculate the A-a gradient.
    * Leave oxygen on.
2. Look at pH
    * Is it normal? A normal pH may be seen with a fully compensated acid base disturbance. If this is due to respiratory compensation, the patient may be hyperventilating to maintain a normal pH and will need regular review as they may develop exhaustion.
    * Is it high? There is alkalosis.
    * Is it low? There is acidosis.
3. Look at PCO_2
    * Together with the pH this will determine if the primary disturbance is respiratory in origin.
    * If the pH is low and the PCO_2 is elevated, there is a respiratory acidosis.
4. Assess metabolic component
    * Evaluate the $[HCO_3^-]$, compare it with normal.
    * Calculate the anion gap.
5. Is there any compensation?

Also see Figure 4.4 for diagnostic algorithm of acid-base imbalance.

Normal range for ABG analysis

* pH: 7.35–7.45
* H^+: 35–45 nmol/litre
* PO_2: 10.3–13.3 kPa (80–100 mmHg)
* PCO_2: 4.7–6.0 kPa (35–45 mmHg)

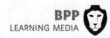

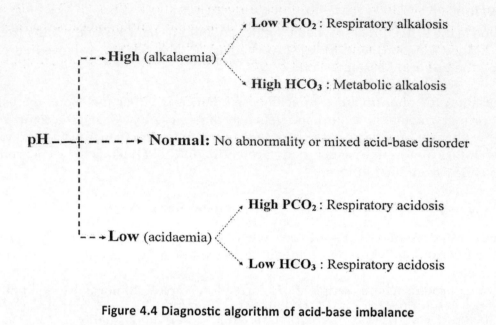

Low PCO$_2$: Respiratory alkalosis

High (alkalaemia)

High HCO$_3$: Metabolic alkalosis

pH — — — — — → Normal: No abnormality or mixed acid-base disorder

High PCO$_2$: Respiratory acidosis

Low (acidaemia)

Low HCO$_3$: Respiratory acidosis

Figure 4.4 Diagnostic algorithm of acid-base imbalance

- Bicarbonate: 22–26 mmol/litre
- Base excess: -2- +2

Abnormalities of acid-base balance

There are four basic types of primary acid-base disturbance which may exist alone or as a mixed presentation. In some cases the disturbance may be acute and in others chronic with compensation and a normal pH.

1. Respiratory acidosis: A rise in PCO$_2$, caused by hypoventilation or ventilation/perfusion inadequacy. This increases the PCO$_2$/ HCO$^-_3$ ratio and depresses the pH. Persistent cases lead to renal compensation conserving bicarbonate.

    Signs and symptoms include headache, confusion, dyspnoea, cyanosis, normal cardiac output (deteriorates if severe).

    Causes include central nervous system depression due to head injury or drugs, impaired respiratory muscles due to neuromuscular disorder, and pulmonary disorders such as atelectasis or pneumonia, hypoventilation due to chest wall injury.

2. Respiratory alkalosis: A decrease in PCO$_2$ leads to a decrease in PCO$_2$/ HCO$^-_3$ ratio and elevates the pH due to hyperventilation. Renal compensation occurs by increasing the amount of HCO$^-_3$ excretion thus returning the ratio back to normal.

    Signs and symptoms include confusion, cardiac arrhythmias, ischaemic ECG changes, peri-oral and extremity numbness, tetania.

    Causes include anxiety, pain, respiratory stimulants, increased metabolic demands such as fever, sepsis, pregnancy.

3. Metabolic acidosis: A primary fall in the HCO$^-_3$ leading to an increase in the PCO$_2$/ HCO$^-_3$ ratio thereby depressing the pH. The reduction in bicarbonate may be due to the accumulation of acid within the blood as seen in diabetics (ketones) or by tissue hypoxia producing lactic acid. The respiratory compensation increases the minute ventilation reducing the PCO$_2$ increasing the ratio and normalising the pH.

    Signs and symptoms include hyperventilation, dyspnoea, reduced cardiac output and blood pressure, increased metabolic demands, insulin resistance.

    Causes include renal failure, diabetic ketoacidosis, anaerobic metabolism, starvation, salicylate intoxication.

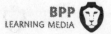

4. Metabolic alkalosis: Increased bicarbonate decreases the PCO_2 / HCO^-_3 ratio and with that decreases the pH. Subsequent reduction in alveolar ventilation causes a rise in PCO_2, increase respiratory compensation, although this may be small.

    Signs and symptoms include lethargy, arrhythmias, hypoventilation, hypokalaemia, hypocalcaemia, muscle cramps.

    Causes include vomiting, diuretic therapy and hyperaldostonism.

Burns

Burns affect approximately 1% of the population in the UK per year, with approximately 10% requiring admission to hospital. Management of burns includes treating of a range of injuries and diseases, from minor injuries to devastating thermal trauma affecting every organ system. Care can continue for many years, with many undergoing reconstructive procedures, necessitating a multidisciplinary approach. Burns are more prevalent in young children and the elderly.

Aetiology

Most burns occur at home, commonly in the kitchen, with the aetiology varying somewhat with different age groups.

Thermal burns

Wet injuries such as scalds are common in children and the elderly due to spillage of hot liquids. They usually cause superficial partial thickness burns. Adults are more likely to suffer from flame burns due to ignition of volatile substances. Patients usually suffer from deep partial or full thickness burns and in some cases with associated inhalation injuries. Contact burns are caused by prolonged contact with hot objects which are also associated with deep partial or full thickness burns. The extent of the burn depends on the length of time of contact with the object.

Chemical burns

These are usually caused by industrial accidents. Basic / alkaline substances cause deeper burns than acidic substances as they cause liquefactive necrosis instead of coagulative necrosis. Chemical burns also usually cause deep partial or full thickness burns.

Electrical burns

These amount to about 5% of all burns hospital admissions. The degree of injury is dependent on the amount of heat generated ($0.24 \times$ voltage^2 $\times$ resistance). Household low voltage electricity can cause deep burns at entry and exit points, causing cardiac arrhythmias. In comparison, high voltage burns can be either flash burns where a patient is in the arc of current, or a true electrocution.

Pathophysiology

The tissue injury sustained by a burn stimulates an inflammatory response which causes local and systemic effects.

*   Local: Disruption of the capillaries causes loss of protein-rich fluid into the interstitial space causing oedema.
*   Systemic: Systemic inflammatory response syndrome (SIRS) can be seen in significant (> 25% body surface area) cases. This has multiple potentially life threatening consequences, such as hypovolaemia due to increased capillary permeability, increased basal metabolic rate, global hypoperfusion (cardiac, renal), bacterial translocation leading to sepsis, acute lung injury causing acute respiratory distress syndrome (ARDS) and immunosuppression.

Assessment of burns

The initial assessment requires a structured and methodological approach to resuscitate and identify injuries; management and treatment may be prioritised and delivered comprehensively. The Advanced Trauma Life Support™ (ATLS™) guidelines provide a universally applicable and co-ordinated approach to injury.

Primary injury is the immediate damage caused by the burn. The aim should be to minimise the extent of injury by various methods:

- Removal of heat source (thermal injury) including clothing
- Rapid cooling of burn area (approximately 20 minutes for thermal burns). Cooling should be with tepid water (15°C) to reduce pain and minimise oedema. Ice cold water should be avoided as it causes vasoconstriction and excessive cooling which can lead to burn progression and hypothermia.
- Chemical injury is often ongoing therefore it requires prompt and copious irrigation, guided by pH testing.
- Burns should be covered with cling film (loosely to avoid constriction). This allows protection of the burn with the opportunity for easy inspection.

Secondary injury includes the sequelae resulting from the primary injury. The extent of this injury depends upon the management of the team to improve tissue survival and minimise morbidities and refers to: heat loss; fluid shifts and electrolyte disturbances; massive inflammatory response (endogenous / exogenous toxins); secondary infection; oedema of tissue and coagulopathy.

Jackson's burn model

Jackson's model describes three areas within a burn wound (Figure 4.5):

- Zone of coagulation, centrally, representing the irreversibly damaged tissue as a result of the primary injury.
- Zone of stasis, surrounding the zone of coagulation, consists of less damaged tissue with impaired vascular supply, considerable inflammation, but with potential to recover in certain circumstances.
- Zone of hyperaemia, with marked vasodilation and increased blood flow.

These zones are dynamic and are influenced by local and systemic factors, such as infection, disrupted blood flow and excessive oedema that can alter the extent of each zone.

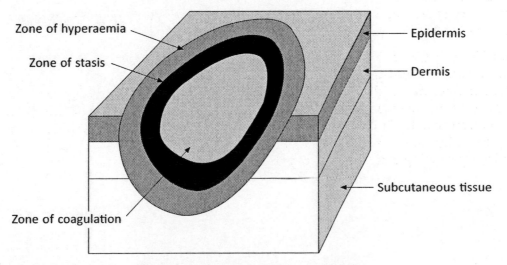

Figure 4.5. Jackson's burn wound model

Injury severity

The severity of the injury depends upon numerous factors including the extent, depth of the burn and whether there is an associated inhalational injury. Different tools exist for the estimation of the total burn surface area. When making such an assessment two factors should be considered. First, the anatomical position of the burns and second, the overall patient's condition including comorbidities. Note that burns are dynamic injuries, with damage continuing for 24–48 hours after the initial insult due to oedema, coagulation and pressure. Regular evaluation is therefore necessary to plan management and further procedures (debridement).

Assessment of burn area

Various tools have been developed to assess the total burn surface area (TBSA). Ideally if possible the burns should be cleaned and blisters de-roofed before assessed.

The Wallace 'rule of nines'

This tool (Figure 4.6) is quick and easy to use as an initial estimate for medium and large burns. In children with small burns this can be inaccurate. The body is divided into areas of 9% and calculations are made based on this. Erythema should not be included when calculating the total burns surface area.

Other methods, such as the Lund and Browder chart, are utilised; these take into consideration the variation of body shape with age, giving an accurate assessment (more important in children).

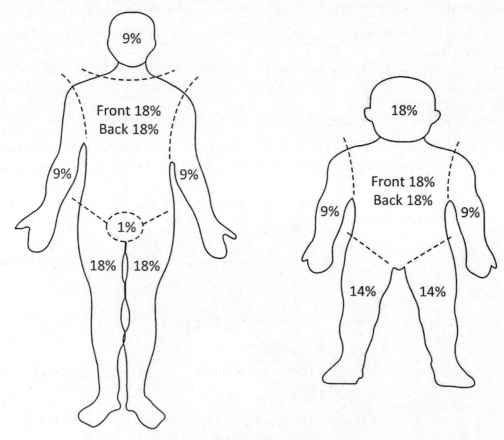

Figure 4.6. The Wallace 'rule of nines'

Burn classification depending on depth assessment (Figure 4.7)

Depth assessment of burns provides an estimation of the local blood supply and tissue elasticity from which one can determine the healing time and management options of the injury (see also Table 4.7).

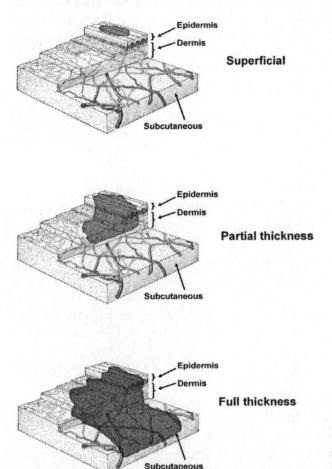

Figure 4.7. Burn classification based on depth of damaged tissue
Based on Gray H (1918), Gray's Anatomy, 20th edition, Lea & Febiger, Philidelphia.
(*This image is in the public domain because its copyright has expired. This applies worldwide.*)

- Superficial burns just cause erythema involving the epidermis only. Healing time is minimal without scarring. Examples include sunburns and minor scalds during accidents within the kitchen. Topical ointments can be used for soothing.
- Partial thickness burns involve the dermis and can be classified into superficial and deep. They often blister and are painful. Examples include flash flame burns. Healing can occur slowly over a period of weeks with some cases requiring surgical intervention.
- Full thickness burns involve the entire thickness of skin thereby preventing re-epithelialisation. They are often leathery in appearance and insensate. Deeper tissue involvement can also be seen carrying the associated risks of rhabdomyolysis, compartment syndrome and hyperkalaemia. Debridement and grafting are often required for such injuries, with recovery taking from months to years.

Management

The initial assessment of a burns injury should follow guidelines set out for all trauma patients via the Advanced Trauma and Life Support (ATLS) course. A slight modification is made to the primary survey. It is important not to be distracted by the burn initially to ensure a logical thorough assessment without missing any associated injuries.

Type	Depth	Healing time	Appearance	Blanching	Blisters	Sensation	Surgery
Superficial	Epidermis	Days	Pink, dry without blisters	Yes	No	Painful	No
Superficial dermal (partial thickness)	Papillary dermis	1–2 weeks	Moist / wet, pink	Yes	Yes	Painful	No
Deep dermal (partial thickness)	Reticular dermis	> 4 weeks	Dry, red, thick blisters	No	Yes	Reduced sensation	In certain cases
Full thickness	Whole thickness	> 4 weeks	White, dry, leathery	No	No	Insensate	Yes

Table 4.7. Classification of burns according to depth, clinical features and management

Primary survey

1. Airway and cervical spine control: The assessment of whether the airway is compromised or at risk of compromise is principal. An inhalation injury can cause oedema over the course of hours leading to occlusion. Direct inspection of the oropharynx is essential with a low threshold for intubation. Inhalational injuries are serious complications significantly increasing the severity and required resuscitation. A high index of suspicion should be maintained (Table 4.8). They are grossly classified into upper airway (supraglottic - usually thermal, causing significant rapid oedema); and lower airway (subglottic - often from chemical and particulate inhalation, causing narrowing and excessive mucus and exudate production, atelectasis, bronchospasm, oedema, leading to pneumonia and ARDS).

Signs	Indications
History of flames in enclosed space	Erythema or oedema of oropharynx on direct inspection
Deep partial or full thickness burns to the face (peri-oral)	
Singed nasal hair	Change in voice – hoarseness
Carbonaceous sputum	Stridor, tachypnoea
Hoarse voice	
Stridor / dyspnoea	
Reduced level of consciousness	

Table 4.8. Signs of inhalational injury and indications for intubation.

Management of inhalational injuries include: intubation and ventilation, prompt therapeutic bronchoscopy – to remove plugs, chest physiotherapy, nebulised heparin and salbutamol therapy.

2. Breathing: All patients should receive 100% oxygen through a humidified non re-breathing mask on presentation to hospital. Deep dermal partial thickness or full thickness burns to the chest can limit expansion and respiration, requiring escharotomies in some cases. Treatment of pneumothorax if present in blast injuries to the chest. Carbon monoxide binds to deoxyhaemoglobin with a 40 times affinity to that of oxygen causing both intra and extra cellular hypoxia. Arterial blood gas analysis is required to identify the carbon monoxide levels together with metabolic acidosis. If the carboxyhaemoglobin levels reach 25–30%, intubation is recommended. Concentrations of > 60% are considered fatal. Treatment is by 100% oxygen to displace the carbon monoxide.

3. Circulation: Two large bore cannulas should be inserted through normal tissue and all bloods including a group and save and clotting screen taken and sent for analysis. Ensure to check the peripheral circulation carefully as full thickness burns can have a tourniquet effect once the oedema develops.

    Fluid resuscitation: Burn injuries can result in significant fluid changes due to fluid evaporation, capillary leak and exudation of systemic inflammatory response. The primary aim in fluid management should be to restore the appropriate circulating volume and ensure adequate tissue perfusion. A urinary catheter is compulsory for all patients suffering from > 20% total body surface area burns to monitor urine output (providing not involved in the injury).

    The Parkland formula is used to guide fluid administration:

    Resuscitation fluid volume / first 24 hours = 3-4 × TBSA (%) × body weight (kg)
    - Half of this volume is given over the first 8 hours after injury.
    - The second half is given over the remaining 16 hours.

As a rule, intravenous fluid resuscitation is required for children (aged < 12 years) with a ≥ 10% TBSA injury, and in individuals (aged ≥ 12 years) with a ≥ 15% TBSA injury. Children also require provision of maintenance fluid, in addition to calculated resuscitation fluids according to the following rule:

– 100 ml/kg/24 hours for the first 10 kg body weight
– 50 ml/kg/24 hours for the next 10 kg body weight
– 20 ml/kg /24 hours for each kg body weight over 20 kg

Thromboprophylaxis should be administered to all patients unless contraindicated.

4. Disability: A full assessment of responsiveness using the Glasgow coma scale should be performed. A reduced level of consciousness could be indicative of hypoxia or hypovolaemia.

5. Exposure: A full patient assessment should be performed including the back to calculate the total body involvement – depth and surface area. Pay close attention to the body temperature and cover the patient as soon as possible.

6. Temperature: Significant burn injuries can affect the thermoregulatory function of the skin leading to local hyperaemia thereby increasing the skin surface. Heat is therefore lost through convection, radiation and evaporation with a breach in the epithelial surface. The dermal receptors sense the hyperaemia and the patient feels hot seeking cooling despite a falling temperature. This could ultimately lead to hypothermia. A warm environment should be created for the patient.

Nutrition in burns

Burn injuries create a marked hypermetabolic states, more so than many other injuries. Early intervention to improve this will impact all aspects of recovery. Ambient temperatures should be increased to eliminate shivering and evaporative loss of heat. Major burns patients should have a nasogastric tube inserted to decompress the stomach and commence early enteral nutrition, thereby maintaining gastrointestinal function and homeostasis and preventing bacterial translocation. Proton pump inhibitor cover should also be given to prevent stress ulcer formation. High calorific diets should be planned with carbohydrate and protein dominance, with early input from the dietician. Supplementation of vitamins and trace elements will most probably also be required.

Infection

Rapid colonisation takes place of the burn site and together with the altered metabolic state the patient is at high risk for infection. Topical products can be used to reduce the colonisation with bacteria, with antibiotics reserved for invasive infections. Similarly patients with open wounds from burns should receive tetanus immunisation.

Dressings

Significant burns often require specialist input for dressings. The preferred choice of dressings is cling film which reduces the evaporative losses and allows visualisation of the injury for inspection. Caution should be placed for circumferential application causing oedema. Thorough documentation of assessment and procedures performed is essential for such wounds with regular irrigation and debridement as required. Burns units commonly use Flamazine (silver sulphadiazine) dressings which contains an antibacterial cream which can penetrate the eschar. In cases of transfer to specialist burns units, the appropriate dressings should be discussed.

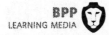

Escharotomy

For circumferential deep partial thickness or full thickness burns on a limb or involving the chest, escharotomy should be performed. This procedure involves incising the burn eschar and not the underlying fascia. For limb injuries the incision should be placed on the medial aspect avoiding any neighbouring structures, and for the chest wall longitudinal incisions along the midaxillary lines and joined with a subcostal incision allowing a mobile sternum. It is best to discuss such procedures with a specialist unit.

Systemic	Local
Hypovolaemia, shock	Eschar affecting chest expansion / peripheral circulation
Hypothermia	Infection
Electrolyte imbalance – hyperkalaemia, hypomagnesaemia	Scarring
Renal impairment – acute tubular necrosis due to haemoglobinuria, myoglobinuria	Contractures
Respiratory compromise – pneumonia, ARDS Curling's ulcers (stress) Rhabdomyolysis	
Ileus	

Table 4.9. Complications of burns

Referral to a specialist burns unit

Guidelines have been developed by the British Burns Association for referrals to specialist burns units. The proposal is to refer the patient to an appropriate burns care centre based on complexity of the injury rather than surface area.

- All complex burns need referral to a specialist burns centre (six hours)
- Complex burn cases include:
  - Extremes of age (< 5 years and > 60 years).
  - Deep partial or full thickness injury to difficult sites (face, hands, perineum, feet, flexural surfaces, neck, axilla).
  - Inhalation injury (excluding poisoning by isolated carbon monoxide).
  - Large areas (paediatric > 5% TBSA, adult > 10% TBSA).
  - Specific mechanisms (chemicals, ionizing radiation, high-pressure steam, high-tension electricity and hydrofluoric acid).
  - Significant comorbidities (cardiorespiratory limitation).
  - Burns in a multiply injured patient (head injury, multiple fractures).
  - Suspicion of non-accidental injury.
- Non-complex are considered those with:
  - Size of skin injury for children (up to 16 years) – 2–5% TBSA if dermal or smaller if full thickness.
  - Size of skin injury in adults 5–10% TBSA if dermal or smaller injury if full thickness.

Non-accidental burns in children

It is believed that between 3–10% of paediatric burns are non-accidental. Suspicions should be raised early with involvement of the paediatric team for full assessment.

Suspicions should be raised in the following situations

- Child brought into hospital by an unrelated adult.
- Unexplained delay in seeking medical attention.
- History of injury inconsistent with developmental capacity of the child.
- History of injury inconsistent with injury.
- Historical accounts of injury vary over time.
- Prior history of injury or accidents to child or siblings.
- Scalds with clear-cut immersion lines.
- Scalds with no splash marks.
- Scalds involving specific sites – perineum, genitalia and buttocks.
- Mirror-image injury of extremities.
- Other signs of physical abuse (eg bruises, fractures).

In such situations the assessment should include an examination for other signs of abuse, photographs of the injuries, an assessment of the parent-child interaction, further information from the general practitioner and individual interviews of the family members involved.

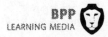

Sepsis

Sepsis is a clinical condition defined by the presence of both infection and inflammation. It is associated with significant morbidity and the mortality is reported up to 60% worldwide. A central role in the manifestations of sepsis is played by Systemic Inflammatory Response Syndrome (SIRS), which in surgical patients requires early recognition and prompt management to prevent its progression to multi-organ failure.

Systemic Inflammatory Response Syndrome (SIRS)

The definition of SIRS requires the presence of two of the following criteria:

- Body temperature < 36°C or > 38°C
- Heart rate > 90/minute
- Respiratory rate > 20 breaths/minute or PCO_2 < 4.3 kPa (32mmHg)
- WBC < 4 or >12 × 10^9/l or the presence of > 10% immature neutrophils

SIRS is caused by inflammatory, ischaemic or traumatic insult to the body. In normal circumstances the immune and neuroendocrine systems control the response removing the source, however in certain situations where such local control fails sepsis can develop (see also Chapter 2: *Surgical pathology – Acute inflammation*).

Classification of sepsis

- The term sepsis is reserved to describe the presence of SIRS together with proven or suspected infection.
- Severe sepsis occurs when it is complicated by organ dysfunction or tissue hypoperfusion. Many patients with severe sepsis develop signs of pulmonary complications (ranging from acute lung injury to acute respiratory distress syndrome) and circulatory dysfunction (tissue hypoperfusion and lactic acidosis) and in almost a half of cases renal impairment.
- Septic shock indicates the presence of hypotension refractory to fluid resuscitation.
- Multi organ dysfunction syndrome (MODS) is defined as failure of two or more organs which require intervention in order to maintain homeostasis.

Aetiology

The majority of cases of sepsis are caused by infections such as pneumonia, urinary tract, soft tissue or intestinal infections. In 90% of cases such infections are due to either Gram positive (Streptococcus, Staphylococcus) or Gram negative bacteria (E. coli, Klebsiella or Pseudomonas). The remainder of infections are caused by fungi (Candida) and viruses. In over one-third of cases a causative organism is not identified.

Pathogenesis

The pathogenesis of the sepsis involves various pathways triggered by components of the immune system, already described in the Chapter 2: *Surgical pathology – Acute inflammation*. Briefly,

- Pro-inflammatory cytokines such as tumour necrosis factor, interleukin – 6 and interleukin – 1 are elevated in sepsis; they further stimulate other mediators (interleukin-8, complement, histamine, kinins) which contribute to organ dysfunction, pyrexia and hypermetabolism. At the same time, other cytokines such as interleukin 10 inhibit the release of those pro-inflammatory cytokines from macrophages and lymphocytes, thereby antagonising systemic inflammation.

- Neutrophils migrate from the pulmonary vasculature and enter the infected tissue, where with the release of free radicals and proteolytic enzymes can induce directly a tissue insult; if this occurs in the lung parenchyma a decrease in lung compliance is noted, followed by complications of Acute Lung Injury and ARDS.
- Coagulopathy: The combination of activation of the coagulation system and inhibition of fibrinolytic pathway can lead to fibrin deposition in the microvasculature impairing oxygenation. Both thrombocytopaenia and coagulation disorders can be seen in severe sepsis.

Pathophysiology

- Fluid loss due to leaky capillary endothelium leads to intravascular hypovolaemia and arterio-venous shunting.
- Such abnormalities lead to reduction in stroke volume and ultimately cardiac output with further myocardial depression caused by circulating cytokines. There is biventricular failure, reduced ejection fraction and myocardial ischaemia.
- Despite adequate fluid resuscitation the blood pressure often needs to be supported by vasoconstrictors to ensure adequate tissue delivery of oxygen.
- During the early stages of sepsis a high volume of circulating acute phase proteins is found, believed to exert a protective effect.
- An increase in the release of stress hormones such as catecholamines, vasopressin, ACTH and growth hormone is seen together with insulin resistance and hyperglycaemia.

Management – Surviving Sepsis Campaign

In 2002 a combined survey was conducted by the European Society of Critical Care Medicine and Society of Critical Care Medicine of 1,050 physicians to assess their views on sepsis, focusing on definitions, diagnosis and management. About 86% of responses agreed that symptoms of sepsis can be misattributed to other conditions with 89% of physicians eagerly awaiting a breakthrough in management of sepsis.

This led to the initiative of the Surviving Sepsis Campaign aiming to improve the diagnosis and management of patients with sepsis and ultimately reduce the associated mortality by 25% in five years.

Initial resuscitation (first six hours)

- Begin resuscitation immediately in patients with hypotension or elevated serum lactate >4 mmol/L; do not delay pending ICU admission.
- Resuscitation goals include:
  - CVP 8–12 mmHg
  - Mean arterial pressure -65 mmHg
  - Urine output 0.5ml/kg/hr
  - Central venous (superior vena cava) oxygen saturation -70% or mixed venous -65%

1. Give high flow oxygen (15L) via non-rebreathe bag.
2. Take blood cultures (ideally 2 sets) and consider source control.
3. Give intravenous antibiotics according to local protocol.
4. Commence intravenous fluid resuscitation with Hartmann's solution or equivalent.
5. Check haemoglobin and lactate.
6. Monitor actively hourly urine output (consider catheterisation).

Table 4.10. The Sepsis Six tasks to be completed within the first hour of recognition of sepsis

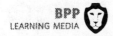

- Obtain appropriate cultures before starting antibiotics, provided this does not significantly delay antimicrobial administration. Obtain two or more blood cultures and culture all other sites as clinically indicated. Use imaging studies to confirm and sample any source of infection.
  - Begin intravenous antibiotics as early as possible and always within the first hour of recognising severe sepsis and septic shock.
  - Broad-spectrum: one or more agents active against likely bacterial/fungal pathogens and with good penetration into presumed source.
  - Reassess antimicrobial regime daily to optimise efficacy, prevent resistance, avoid toxicity, and minimise costs.
  - Consider combination therapy in Pseudomonas infections and neutropenic patients.
  - Limit duration of therapy to 7–10 days; longer if response is slow or there are non drainable foci of infection or immunologic deficiencies.
  - Stop antimicrobial therapy if cause is found to be noninfectious.
- Source identification and control
  - A specific anatomic site of infection should be established within the first six hours of presentation.
  - Evaluate patient for a focus of infection amenable to source control measures (eg abscess drainage, tissue debridement).
  - Implement source control measures as soon as possible following successful initial resuscitation (exception: infected pancreatic necrosis, where surgical intervention is best delayed).
  - Choose source control measure with maximum efficacy and minimal physiologic upset.
  - Remove intravascular access devices if potentially infected.

Further management
Source control

This describes all the measures taken to control the focus of infection and modify factors related to the environment that promotes microbial growth or impairs the host defences. A thorough clinical assessment involving all systems is required to identify the source and in some cases the use of radiology is required to confirm presence and plan the appropriate procedure for control. Techniques employed for control include:

- Drainage of abscess
- Administration of antibiotics
- Removal of devices
- Debridement of necrotic tissue
- Definitive surgery
- Damage control surgery

Cardiovascular support

Sepsis adversely affects the cardiovascular system; prompt identification and management of cardiovascular disturbances is necessary. Adequate fluid volume status monitoring is essential to optimise oxygen delivery to tissues. Together with the traditional methods of invasive monitoring, newer techniques such as the oesophageal Doppler have reported benefits in assessing fluid status.

Vasoactive drugs

These are indicated when the blood pressure is not stabilised with sufficient fluid resuscitation.

- **Adrenaline**: A potent alpha-1 and beta (high affinity) agonist which augments the cardiac rate and contractility thereby increasing the cardiac output and blood pressure. Drawbacks of its use include an increase in myocardial oxygen demand, an increase in serum lactate (possibly due to poor perfusion to tissue), and adverse effects on splanchnic blood flow. Adverse effects include cardiac arrhythmias.
- **Nor-adrenaline**: This is mainly an alpha agonist used to maintain systemic vascular resistance when it remains inappropriately low. By its action on alpha 1 receptors, contraction of the smooth muscle causes vasoconstriction, thereby improving organ perfusion. Nor-adrenaline reduces serum lactate levels and is also as effective as dopamine in improving renal perfusion in an adequately resuscitated state. Adverse effects also include arrhythmias.
- **Dobutamine**: This potent beta-1 agonist also increases myocardial contractility and with it the stroke volume and cardiac output. It also possesses a vasodilatory effect aiding reduce the mean arterial pressure in cases of cardiogenic shock. In septic shock dobutamine aids improve cardiac performance and splanchnic perfusion; it can be administered with nor-adrenaline and its adverse effects include hypotension.
- **Dopamine**: This has predominantly beta adrenergic effects in low to moderate doses with alpha adrenergic effects such as vasoconstriction seen with higher doses. Its effect as a chronotrope is seen with all doses. Other proposed effects include vasodilation of renal, mesenteric and coronary vessels, theoretically increasing the urinary output and protecting the kidneys. The concept of the renal protective dose remains controversial.

Respiratory support

Patients with severe sepsis requiring admission to the intensive care unit will most probably require some form of respiratory support via mechanical ventilation. Urgent endotracheal intubation should be performed in cases of impaired ventilation and oxygenation (hypoxia and hypercapnia), to control the upper airway or protect the lower airway. The decision to initiate mechanical ventilation should be based on clinical situation and should not be delayed. In cases of non-invasive ventilation this can be administered using tightly fitting masks in the form of continuous positive airway pressure (CPAP); this method helps reduce the work of breathing, recruit alveoli and reduce cardiac afterload. (See also the section on *Invasive Mechanical Ventilation* in this chapter.)

Renal support

Approximately 40% of critically ill patients develop some form of renal impairment. Renal failure is regarded as an important independent risk factor for mortality. In a majority of cases it is reversible, however between 8–16% of patients may require long-term renal replacement therapy. (For further information see the section in this Chapter *Renal physiology and critical care*.)

Gastrointestinal support and nutrition

- Prevention of villous atrophy of gastrointestinal mucosa and bacterial translocation involves correction of splanchnic blood flow and appropriate enteral nutrition.
- Nutrition should be considered as a part of the daily plan.
- Septic patients are catabolic and dehydrated and their caloric requirements increase significantly.
- The enteral route should be considered whenever possible (nasogastric feeding). Occasionally prokinetics such as metoclopramide or erythromycin are also given.

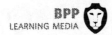

- Where enteral feeding is not possible parenteral feed is utilised with monitoring for risks such as line related sepsis and volume overload.
- Limited evidence exists reporting the benefits of immune modulating feeds (combining glutamine, omega-3 fatty acids) particularly in those undergoing surgery.

Activated protein C

- Activated protein C possesses anticoagulant, anti-inflammatory and fibrinolytic properties.
- Together with the standard therapy, activated protein C can be used in cases of severe sepsis (APACHE score > 25) and organ failure.
- The PROWESS study showed 6.1% absolute reduction in 28 – day mortality using recombinant human activated protein C in patients with severe sepsis.

Additional therapy for sepsis

- In septic shock intravenous hydrocortisone should be administered (200–300 mg/day for seven days).
- Peptic (stress) ulcer prophylaxis.
- Venous thromboembolism prophylaxis.
- Glycaemic control – tight monitoring of blood glucose has been shown to reduce both morbidity and mortality.
- Infection control measures when handling lines, devices and hand washing to prevent cross infection (particular risk of drug resistant pathogens).
- Regular physiotherapy for chest and limbs to prevent muscle atrophy.
- Multidisciplinary input from microbiologists, pharmacists, nutritionists and physiotherapists.
- Control of sleep deprivation and delirium.
- Intravenous immunoglobulin G can be administered in cases of toxic shock due to Group A haemolytic streptococcus infection.
- Psychological support.

Multi Organ Dysfunction Syndrome (MODS)

MODS was initially described after massive blood loss from a ruptured abdominal aortic aneurysm; now a group of disorders are recognised as causes – sepsis, pre-eclampsia, trauma and pancreatitis. Once the cascade commences it generally follows a predictable course irrespective of the aetiology.

- Initial changes are seen in the cardiovascular system with signs such as tachycardia, hypotension and arrhythmias. Myocardial depression is a late event. Management depends on optimisation of intravascular volume and vasoactive drugs.
- Respiratory involvement includes local injury within the alveoli and increased microvascular permeability leading to alveolar oedema. The respiratory insult can progress to ARDS (see the section on *Respiratory physiology* earlier in this chapter).
- This hypoxaemia further leads to renal, gastrointestinal and central nervous system dysfunction necessitating renal replacement therapy and other support.

Management centres on early identification and aggressive support of failing organs together with source control. Prognosis is directly related to the number of failing organs.

Temperature regulation in the surgical patient

The body maintains a strict balance of the core temperature to ensure optimum function of cells and their enzyme reactions. Normal temperature is 37°C (±0.5°C) with an element of diurnal variation. In women there is also a monthly variation associated with ovulation.

Physiology

A uniform temperature is maintained by temperature-sensitive neurons found in the great veins, abdominal viscera, spinal cord and hypothalamus, which ensure control despite fluctuating environmental temperatures. Various pathways under neural and hormonal control are integrated in the pre-optic anterior hypothalamus. Here a set point of acceptable core temperature is assigned and any deviation by ± 0.2°C initiates reflexes to either gain or lose heat.

Two separate compartments are recognised in the body:

- Core compartment (66% of body mass): Little variation in temperature occurs here. This component includes the main organs.
- Peripheral compartment (34% of body mass): Here the temperature varies widely from 36-28°C allowing thermal energy to be absorbed and released.

In infant and neonates the peripheral compartment is extremely small which can cause accelerated heat loss due to an increased temperature gradient between the skin surface and the environment.

Physiological mechanisms for temperature regulation

Heat production is a result of essential cellular functions at rest constituting the basal metabolic rate. Physical activity generates approximately 90% of the heat during strenuous activity. Heat can be exchanged with the environment by a number of methods:

- Radiation: This is the exchange of heat with nearby objects not in direct contact such as theatre lights, metal equipment. Radiation is responsible for approximately 40% of heat loss in anaesthetised patients.
- Convection: This is the exchange of heat with the environmental air, accounting for approximately 30% of heat loss. Continuous air movement as seen in theatres increases the heat loss by convection.
- Conduction: This accounts for a small amount of heat loss. It refers to the exchange of heat by direct contact with another object such as the operating table.
- Evaporation: This accounts for 25–30% of heat loss and refers to the energy required to break down the bonds within liquids and convert them to gas. A significant amount of heat is lost during laparotomies due to the evaporation of water from the exposed bowel.

Mechanisms to preserve heat

- Vasoconstriction: An initial sympathetic response acts on the adrenoceptors of blood vessels supplying the skin causing vasoconstriction thereby reducing the radiation and convective heat loss. The cooler tissue and fat surrounding the core provide insulation. A difference of up to 6°C can be tolerated between hands and core organs without damage to tissues.
- Piloerection: Stimulation of the alpha adrenoceptors on the erector pilae muscle can cause the hairs on the skin to stand to trap warm air.
- Increase in both voluntary and involuntary muscle activity: Increased activity generates heat, a response not possible in the anaesthetised state.

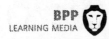

- Shivering, an activity controlled by the hypothalamus, can double heat production and increase metabolic activity. Non-shivering thermogenesis is more important in children. It involves the stimulation of beta adrenergic receptors in brown fat in children (nape of neck) stimulating lipid oxidation by the mitochondria generating heat.
- Counter-current exchange: It is a mechanism by which heat is transferred from the warmer arterial blood to the colder venous blood. By this method the heat loss in digits and the scrotum (counter-current cooling to 32°C) can be maintained.

Mechanisms to decrease heat

Opposing sympathetic response causes vasodilation of the blood vessels to the skin allowing loss of heat by convection and radiation. The sympathetic cholinergic fibres stimulate the sweat glands to produce sweat which can be easily evaporated aiding heat loss. Approximately up to 2 litres of sweat can be produced per hour. Other behavioural responses are also stimulated such as a reduction in physical activity and locating to a cooler area.

Hormonal regulation of temperature

- Thyroid hormones: The thyroid gland plays an important role in regulation of body temperature. Thyroid hormones can act directly on ion channels in cells to increase expression of specific uncoupling proteins which ultimately generates heat. Thyrotropin releasing hormone is released by the hypothalamus in response to the cold. This sets off a cascade to increase the production of thyroxine and triiodothyronine.
- Catecholamines: Cold environments stimulate the production of catecholamines. Noradrenaline acts upon the beta 3 adrenoceptors on brown fat to increase lipolysis causing generation of heat.
- Melatonin: A circadian variation in core body temperature is seen at rest (0.5°C to 0.7°C). The temperature falls during the night. Melatonin, produced by the pineal gland is believed to be associated with such diurnal variation.
- Progesterone: This thermogenic hormone is associated with the changes in core body temperature seen with the menstrual cycle and during pregnancy.

Pyrexia

Pyrexia is a regulated rise in the body temperature in response to an insult (such as infection, inflammation, or trauma). It is defined as core temperature of > 38°C and it is regulated by a new set-point being created in the hypothalamus. This explains why the above mechanisms of preserving heat are activated until the new temperature is reached. Pyrexia is an immune response resulting from stimulation by cytokines produced by macrophages and monocytes. These cytokines (interleukin-1, -8, interferon, tumour necrosis factor) act upon the hypothalamus stimulating the release of prostaglandins. Thus drugs inhibiting cyclo-oxygenase (paracetamol) have antipyretic effects. The duration and magnitude of the pyrexia is determined by the interaction between the pyrogen and antipyretic cytokines. Injuries or cerebrovascular insults near the preoptic hypothalamus can disrupt the protective mechanisms resulting in pyrexias not responding to traditional treatment.

Hyperthermia

Hyperthermia is the elevation of the core body temperature above the normal diurnal set-point of 36°C to 37.5°C due to failure of thermoregulation. This differs from pyrexia which is stimulated by a cytokine rise and regulated at the hypothalamus. With rises in the core temperature the hypothalamus stimulates sweating and peripheral vasodilatation. Up to a relative humidity of 75% evaporation is the main mechanism to lose heat. If the environmental temperature exceeds the skin temperature, the mechanisms of heat loss are not efficient. The three commonest causes of severe hyperthermia include:

- Heat stroke, from exposure to environmental temperature of >40°C causing a rise in core temperature and neurological disruption. This can occur either in individuals with underlying conditions that impair their thermoregulation or prevent their removal from the hot environment. Examples include cardiovascular disease, anhidrosis or extremes of age. An exertional form can also be seen in healthy young individuals following strenuous exercise in high ambient temperatures. Complications include renal failure, disseminated intravascular coagulation, sepsis due to bacterial translocation, ARDS, seizures and non cardiogenic pulmonary oedema. Treatment involves cooling the individual with tepid water and fans.

- Neuroleptic malignant syndrome: This is a rare condition precipitated by antipsychotic drugs and their antidopaminergic action blocking the hypothalamic receptors. The condition is characterised by hyperthermia, muscle rigidity and extra-pyramidal dysfunction. Dopamine agonists such as bromocriptine can have beneficial effects.

- Malignant hyperthermia: This is a life-threatening pharmacogenetic disorder which occurs when a susceptible person is exposed to specific trigger factors. Classical malignant hyperthermia is characterised by hypermetabolism, muscle rigidity and muscle injury. Its reported incidence in the general population is between 1:10,000 and 1:15,000. Susceptibility to malignant hyperthermia is inherited as autosomal dominant with variable penetrance. In 50–70% of affected families there are links to the ryanodine receptor gene (RYR1) on chromosome 19. Exposure to trigger factors (succinylcholine and halothane) leads to an uncontrollable release of calcium from the sarcoplasmic reticulum of skeletal muscle. Onset is usually within one hour of administration of the anaesthesia.

The clinical presentation is a direct consequence of the loss of skeletal muscle calcium homeostasis. Initial signs may be an unexplained CO_2 production and tachycardia. The blood pressure becomes unstable and the temperature begins to rise at a rate of 1°C every five minutes. Muscle rigidity (initially masseter) becomes more generalised and rhabdomyolysis, arrhythmias and disseminated intravascular coagulation may develop.

Management involves firstly discontinuing the inhalation agents and suxamethonium. The patient should be hyperventilated with 100% oxygen. If possible the surgery should be stopped. Dantrolene (2–3mg/kg) should be administered until the tachycardia, pyrexia and carbon dioxide production start to normalise. Active cooling should also be performed including gastric and bladder lavage if necessary. Any effects of the malignant hyperthermia such as electrolyte imbalance (hyperkalaemia), arrhythmia and disseminated intravascular coagulation will also need attention.

Perioperative hypothermia

Under anaesthesia hypothermia is defined as a core temperature less than 36°C. The effects of hypothermia are proportional to the change in body temperature. Care must be taken to prevent its development.
Aetiological factors for perioperative hypothermia include:

- Abolished behavioural responses (shivering).
- Increased heat loss through radiation in the operating theatre.
- Increased heat loss through evaporation from body surfaces and open cavities.
- Cooling effect of cold anaesthetic gases.

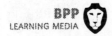

- Hypothalamic function altered by anaesthetic agents decreasing heat production.
- Reduced metabolic heat production.
- Reduced muscle activity.

With the induction of anaesthesia hypothermia develops in three stages:

- Redistribution: This represents the largest drop in core temperature. Heat is redistributed from the core to the periphery with vasodilation.
- Linear phase: Commences at the start of surgery when exposed to cleaning solutions and cool air flow. During this stage heat loss will exceed that produced.
- Plateau phase: At a certain threshold the thermoregulatory mechanisms tend to increase peripheral vasoconstriction. The reduced peripheral heat loss balances the heat produced by the core creating a plateau.

Hypothermia

Hypothermia is defined as a body temperature below 35°C. The thermoregulatory mechanisms remain intact. A reduction can be seen in platelet adhesion which may affect the coagulation status of the patient. With progressively lower temperatures a variety of physiological impairment can be seen:

- Cardiovascular – decreased cardiac output (anaesthetised), arrhythmias, vasoconstriction, ECG – increased PR interval, wide QRS complex.
- Respiratory – increased pulmonary vascular resistance and V/Q mismatch, decreased ventilator drive. Increased gas solubility.
- Renal – decreased renal blood flow and glomerular filtration rate, cold diuresis.
- Haematological – reduced platelet function and coagulation, increased fibrinolysis, increased haematocrit, left shift of oxygen dissociation curve.
- Metabolic – reduced basal metabolic rate, metabolic acidosis, insulin resistance, hyperglycaemia.
- Gastrointestinal / hepatic – reduced gut motility.
- Neurological – reduced cerebral blood flow, impaired conscious state leading to coma.

Therapeutic hypothermia

Hypothermia has a protective effect on the brain by reducing the metabolic rate and therefore oxygen requirements. By this principle hypoxic injuries take longer to develop. Therefore certain procedures can use the advantage of a controlled hypothermia. In both cardiac and neurosurgery hypothermia allows a reduced metabolic rate without damage despite a decreased perfusion.

The following NICE Guidelines (adapted from NICE, April 2008) provide recommendations to prevent, diagnose early and minimise the effect of inadvertent perioperative hypothermia:

- **Perioperative care**: Advise patient regarding keeping warm before the procedure and warn them regarding the temperature in hospital advising them to bring additional clothing and inform nursing staff if feeling cold.

- **Preoperative period**: Risk assessment is necessary for inadvertent hypothermia.
  - High ASA grade
  - Preoperative temperature < 36.0°C
  - Major / intermediate surgery
  - Combined anaesthesia (general/regional)

- **Intraoperative period**
  - Measure patient's temperature before induction and every 30 minutes until end of surgery
  - Ensure temperature is 36.0°C or above before commencing induction of anaesthesia
  - Intraoperative warming should be planned for all cases lasting more than 30 minutes

- **Postoperative period**
  - Measure the patient's temperature on admission to recovery and every 15 minutes
  - Do not transfer the patient to the ward unless the temperature is 36.0°C or above. If below commence active warming.

Cardiovascular physiology and shock

Haemodynamics

The cardiovascular system is made up of three key elements: the pump (heart), tubing (vessels) and a fluid (blood). Under normal conditions these elements interact with each other, and if one element malfunctions, the others compensate to maintain the system homeostasis.

In any closed tubing system the flow of fluid between two parts is proportional to the pressure difference between these two points (ΔP) and inversely proportional to the resistance of the system. In the systemic circulation, the blood flow equals the cardiac output (CO), the pressure difference equals the mean arterial pressure (MAP) minus the central venous pressure (CVP) and the resistance is the total peripheral vascular resistance (TPR). Their relations are defined by the following equation:

$$CO = (MAP-CVP) / TPR$$

or, rearranged,

$$MAP = (CO \times TPR) + CVP$$

It is extracted from the above that the mean blood pressure increases if the cardiac output or total peripheral resistance increase.

Peripheral resistance

Three factors determine the resistance to flow within a vessel: the vessel diameter (radius), length, and frictional forces or viscosity of the blood as described by Poiseuille's Law:

Resistance = 8nL/ πr^4 (1)
(with **r** = vessel radius, **L** = vessel length, **n** = blood viscosity).

The vessel radius is the most important physiologically, as it changes by contraction and relaxation of the smooth muscle in the vessel wall (vascular tone); small changes in the vessel diameter lead to large changes in its resistance. On the contrary, vessel length does not change significantly in vivo, and therefore remains a constant, and viscosity also stays within a normal range, unless the haematocrit or temperature changes significantly.

As blood flow equals to the ratio of the pressure gradient (ΔP) between these points divided by the resistance to flow (**Flow = ΔP/Resistance,**) and combining with Poiseuille's equation (1) it is concluded that **(Flow) = ΔP πr^4 / 8nL.** In other words, the blood flow is proportional to the fourth power of vessel radius.

Blood vessels are mainly arranged in parallel with each other, as are the vascular beds within the organs. Therefore the total resistance in the system is calculated as parallel vessels, with three important consequences:

* The total resistance is less than if they were arranged in series.
* The total resistance is lower than the individual resistance of an artery.
* Very little change is seen in the total resistance with changes in the resistance of a small proportion of such parallel vessels.

The venous system vessels have diameters ranging from 50–200μm with low resistance. They are known as *capacitance vessels* as they contain approximately 70% of the total circulating blood volume. Constriction of these veins increases the venous pressure and return, thereby affecting the cardiac output. In comparison, the arterial system vessels demonstrate a change in resistance, but with very small differences in the mean pressure between the aorta and peripheral arteries. However, the largest drop occurs at the level of the muscular arterioles (diameter 10–100μm) which are known as *resistance vessels*. These vessels are innervated by the sympathetic nervous system and respond to changes in nervous and hormonal activity by constricting or dilating, thus affecting the arterial blood pressure.

Types of flow

The blood flow to an organ can be increased in two ways, either by increasing the pressure gradient or by reducing the resistance of the arterioles within the system. Three forms of blood flow are recognised within blood vessels.

Laminar flow

This is the normal condition for blood flow within most of the circulation. It is characterised by concentric laminae of blood moving in parallel along the length of the vessel. The highest velocity is found in the centre of the vessel with the lowest along the wall due to cohesive forces (friction). The flow profile once developed is parabolic. Sliding of the laminae past each other helps direct the red blood cells preferentially in the direction of flow and towards the central axis also known as axial streaming. A thin plasma layer is created beside the vessel wall which aids flow through resistance vessels. Disruption of this flow causes turbulence increasing energy losses.

Turbulent flow

Under conditions of high flow, eg in the ascending aorta, disruption of the laminar flow can occur causing turbulent flow. The fluid layers disperse becoming chaotic which results in the dissipation of energy. Triggers for turbulent flow are branch points in large arteries, diseased, stenotic vessels and valves and a low fluid viscosity. A greater amount of energy is required to drive the blood flow during turbulence as there is a greater loss due to friction. Therefore turbulence increases the perfusion pressure required for a given flow. Once the velocity of flow reaches a certain point the flow laminae split apart creating turbulence. Sounds can also be heard due to turbulence (murmurs). The *Fahraeus-Lindqvist* effect refers to the change in viscosity of blood with changes in the diameter of the vessel. In smaller vessels the apparent viscosity decreases.

Bolus flow

As the diameter of red blood cells is less than the average capillary size, the cells deform in order to enter the vessels. The red cells move as a bolus of uniform velocity with plasma between them eliminating the friction that occurs with laminar flow.

Cardiac Output (CO)

Cardiac output (CO) is the volume of blood pumped through the heart every minute. It is a product of the stroke volume and heart rate (CO = SV × HR). The resting cardiac output in the average adult is 5l/minute, rising to up to 35l/minute in exercise states. The cardiac output can be corrected for body surface area giving the *cardiac index* that ranges normally between 2.5 and 4.2l/min/m^2.

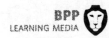

The cardiac output is a dynamic volume, responding to changes in the environment and is split between the organs as follows: heart 5%, kidneys 22%, liver 25%, muscle 20%, brain 14% and remaining body 14%. The cardiac output is pivotal in maintaining the arterial blood pressure: Blood pressure (BP) = Cardiac output (CO) × Systemic vascular resistance (SVR) or

$$BP = SV \times HR \times SVR$$

Stroke volume

The three parameters determining the stroke volume (SV) are; the *preload* (degree of filling of the ventricle), the myocardial *contractility* and the *afterload* (resistance against the ventricle).

Preload

The more the heart muscle fibre is stretched before stimulated to contract, the greater will be the overall force of contraction. This theory is referred to as Frank-Starling's law, it is an intrinsic property of cardiac myocytes and refers to passive stretching of the ventricular walls before systole. During diastole blood returns to the ventricle causing stretching. It is the end diastolic pressure / volume (preload) that determines the force of contraction and therefore the stroke volume, providing the myocardial contractility and afterload remain stable. However, beyond a specific point the contractility fails and failure develops (Figure 4.8). Factors affecting preload include overall blood volume, the phase of respiration (intrathoracic pressure) and valvular regurgitation.

Contractility

This refers to the intrinsic ability of cardiac muscle to contract and remains independent of the degree of preload and afterload. Release of nor-adrenaline and adrenaline, stimulated by the sympathetic nervous system, have a positive inotropic effect on the heart by increasing intracellular calcium ions. Acidosis, hypoxia and certain anaesthetic agents exert negative inotropic effect on the myocardium (Figure 4.9).

Afterload

At the completion of diastole the ventricle begins to contract; the afterload relates to the force against which the ventricle must contract in order to eject the blood. In healthy states the afterload is determined by the vascular tone of the arteries, which is under control of the

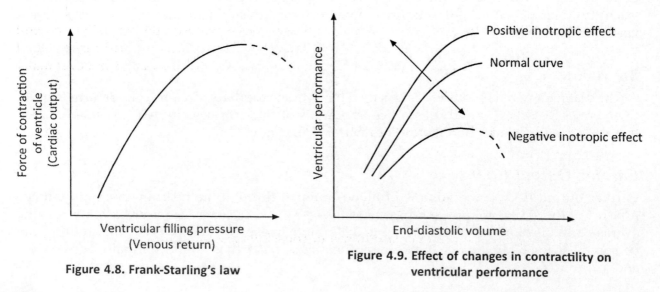

Figure 4.8. Frank-Starling's law

Figure 4.9. Effect of changes in contractility on ventricular performance

sympathetic nervous system, and varies between the left and right sides of the heart; the left ventricular afterload equals approximately the systemic vascular resistance and the right side the pulmonary vascular resistance. Other factors affecting afterload include aortic stiffness, valvular regurgitation, metabolic rate and preload.

Autonomic control of cardiovascular haemodynamics

The arterial blood pressure and end-organ perfusion is under local control by various autonomic reflexes. Afferent fibres transmit information to the *nucleus tractus solitarius* in the brainstem. From here modulation of the vagal and pre-sympathetic activity occurs. The main involved reflexes include the baroreceptor, cardiopulmonary and chemoreceptor reflexes.

Baroreceptor reflex

Baroreceptors are stretch receptors located in the walls of the carotid sinus, subclavian arteries, carotid arteries and aortic arch. They monitor changes in the vessel wall stretch caused by changes in the arterial blood pressure. The nucleus of tractus solitarius is the central projection for the chemo and baroreceptors. The baroreceptors play an important role in the short term management of arterial pressure responding to changes in cardiac output, arterial pressure and peripheral resistance. Longer term control is the responsibility of the renal system.

Cardiopulmonary reflexes

Various intrinsic cardiovascular reflexes stem from the heart and lungs. Vagal fibres mediating these reflexes reduce the heart rate and vascular tone. The *Bainbridge reflex* (atrial reflex) stimulated by receptors in the veno-atrial junctions is a positive feedback mechanism where a rise in right atrial pressure causes a sympathetically mediated tachycardia together with reduction in the secretion of anti-diuretic hormone, renin and cortisol.

Chemoreceptor reflexes

These receptors are located in the aortic and carotid bodies. They are sensitive to hypoxia, hypercapnia and acidosis. Stimulation of the receptors results in increased pulmonary ventilation and blood pressure via sympathetic peripheral vasoconstriction and splanchnic venoconstriction together with an indirect tachycardia by stimulating lung inflation.

Shock

Shock is defined as acute circulatory failure leading to inadequate tissue perfusion and end organ injury. It is associated with an attempt to maintain homeostasis by prioritising blood flow to the vital organs (brain and heart), resulting in cellular hypoxia, damage and eventually multi-organ failure.

Clinical signs of decreased tissue perfusion

- Cool peripheries, clammy skin.
- Poor peripheral venous filling.
- Tachypnoea.
- Prolonged capillary refill time (> 2 s).
- Reduced urine output.
- Restlessness / agitation or decreased level of consciousness.
- Metabolic / lactic acidosis.

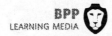

There are four main categories of shock (see Table 4.11), although many investigators believe in a fifth category of 'cellular or cytotoxic shock', where mitochondria are unable to utilise the oxygen delivered.

Hypovolaemic	Cardiogenic	Vasodilatory	Obstructive
Blood loss Saline loss Burns Dehydration	Myocardial infarction Cardiac failure Valvular heart disease Arrhythmia	Sepsis Neurogenic Anaphylactic Adrenal crisis	Pulmonary embolus Cardiac tamponade Tension pneumothorax Abdominal Compartment Syndromes

Table 4.11. Types of shock and examples of causes (non exhaustive)

Hypovolaemic shock

Hypovolaemic shock is an example of a low output shock associated with a reduced venous return and reduced cardiac output. Causes include:

- Haemorrhage – effects vary according to severity, duration and patient factors (see Table 4.12).
- Vomiting / diarrhoea – loss of significant quantities of fluid (electrolytes) or even by high output fistulae.
- Burns – leads to direct loss of fluid and sequestration.
- Renal disease – loss of significant quantity of fluid can be seen in endocrine emergencies – diabetic, addisonian crisis.
- Iatrogenic – administration of mechanical bowel preparation or inadequate fluid administration.

Pathophysiologic response to hypovolaemic shock

- Cardiovascular response: Increased sympathetic outflow causes increase in the heart rate and contractility, vasoconstriction, and increase in the cardiac output. Blood is also redistributed to the main organs and away from the skin and muscles.
- Renal response: The stimulation of *renin* secretion from the juxtaglomerular apparatus initiates the cascade leading to *angiotensin II* production which acts as a powerful vasoconstrictor of arterioles together with *aldosterone* release which stimulates sodium and water reabsorption.

	Class I	Class II	Class III	Class IV
Blood loss (ml)	Up to 750	750–1500	1500–2000	> 2,000
Blood loss (% blood volume)	Up to 15%	15–30%	30–40%	> 40%
Pulse rate	< 100	> 100	> 120	> 140
Blood pressure	Normal	Normal	Decreased	Decreased
Pulse pressure (mm Hg)	Normal or increased	Decreased	Decreased	Decreased
Respiratory rate	14–20	20–30	30–40	> 35
Urine output	> 30	20–30	5–15	Negligible
CNS/mental status	Slightly anxious	Mildly anxious	Anxious confused	Confused lethargic

Table 4.12. Classification of haemorrhagic shock

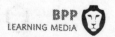

- Haemotological response: Clotting cascade and platelets are stimulated. Any damage to vessel walls stimulates fibrin deposition and clot stabilisation.
- Neuroendocrine response: This is detected by the cardiopulmonary stretch receptors, arterial baroreceptors and arterial chemoreceptors (discussed above). Increased sympathetic outflow and raised levels of vasoactive hormones (including adrenaline, noradrenaline, vasopressin and angiotensin II) cause tachycardia and vasoconstriction in the cutaneous, splanchnic, renal and skeletal circulations. The total peripheral resistance and, consequently, blood pressure is increased. Reflex venoconstriction also improves venous return to some extent.
- The neuroendocrine system responds to haemorrhagic shock by causing an increase in circulating antidiuretic hormone (ADH) from the posterior pituitary gland in response to a decrease in BP (as detected by baroreceptors) and a decrease in the sodium concentration (as detected by osmoreceptors). ADH indirectly leads to an increased reabsorption of water and salt (NaCl) by the distal tubule, the collecting ducts, and the loop of Henle.

Cardiogenic shock

Cardiogenic shock is defined as sustained hypotension (a systolic BP of < 90mmHg for greater than 30 minutes) with inadequate tissue perfusion in spite of adequate left ventricular filling pressure (a cardiac index of <2.2L/min/m^2 in the presence of a pulmonary capillary wedge pressure of > 15mmHg). This is manifested with organ dysfunction such as oliguria, confusion, cool extremities and lactic acidosis.

Aetiology

- Acute myocardial infarction
  - Pump failure (large infarction, smaller infarction with pre-existing disease, right ventricular failure)
  - Mechanical complications (papillary muscle rupture, ventricular septal defect, cardiac rupture, tamponade)
- Other conditions
  - Septic shock with myocardial depression
  - End-stage cardiomyopathy
  - Myocarditis
  - Drugs – eg beta-blocker overdose
  - Aortic dissection with acute aortic regurgitation
  - Myocardial contusion
  - Left ventricular outflow tract obstruction

Pathophysiology of cardiogenic shock

Once a critical ischaemic ventricular mass is affected, then there is pump failure and reduction in cardiac output. This in turn leads to reduced coronary perfusion, lactic acidosis from reduced tissue perfusion and an increase in the left ventricular end-diastolic volume. These factors all contribute to worsening afterload and contractility. The compensatory mechanisms of increased heart rate and increased contractility can further contribute to a worsening myocardial oxygen demand and ischaemia.

Low-resistance / distributive or vasodilatory shock

In low-resistance shock, the vascular capacity is increased and the blood volume does not adequately fill the circulatory system, thus a 'relative hypovolaemia' is noted. In this category the following types are included:

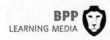

Neurogenic shock

This is characterised by a sudden loss of vasomotor tone throughout the body with massive vasodilation. The increased vascular capacity reduces the systemic filling pressure leading to reduced venous return to the heart. Causes include deep general anaesthesia (depression of the central vasomotor centres), spinal anaesthesia or spinal cord trauma (blockage of the sympathetic outflow from the spinal cord).

Anaphylactic shock

The mast cell degranulation and the release of histamine and other histamine-like substances cause both venodilatation and arteriolar dilatation. Arterial blood pressure falls and increased vascular permeability causes the rapid loss of protein and fluids into the interstitium. This type of shock is similar to septic shock.

Septic shock

Septic shock causes profound vasodilation and loss of fluid into tissues; these conditions are often complicated by a relative hypovolaemia. Clinically it can manifest with warm peripheries as a result of vasodilation, which is in contrast to hypovolaemic shock. In the early stages, the patient may not show any signs of circulatory collapse and the cardiac output may actually be increased as a result of systemic inflammatory response / sepsis. Despite a normal blood pressure, cellular perfusion may still be inadequate for the increased metabolic demands of the tissue. As the infection becomes more severe, the loss of fluid into the tissues combined with impaired cardiac function results in depressed cardiac output, which the patient may eventually be unable to compensate.

Obstructive shock

Obstructive shock is seen where there is a mechanical impairment of blood flow. This can be the result of either impaired venous return to the heart (tension pneumothorax or excessive positive pressure ventilation in intubated patients) and / or reduced arterial outflow from the heart (pericardial tamponade or abdominal compartment syndrome). It is characterised by reduced cardiac output, hypotension, tachycardia and a raised central venous pressure (a reflection of transmitted pressure rather than increased cardiac filling).

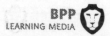

Principles of fracture healing

A fracture is defined as the structural failure of bone and depends on several factors, such as the load, rate and direction of loading, and the properties of the bone itself.

Factors affecting bone fractures

- Extrinsic factors: Forces such as tension, compression, rotation or shearing cause the bone to fail. Specific patterns of failure can be seen according to both mechanical characteristics of the bone together with the direction of the load applied (eg twisting forces cause spiral fractures).
- Intrinsic factors: These factors are related to the biomechanical features of bone. Components of bone include an outer strong brittle cortical layer made up of compact Haversian systems, and an inner cancellous layer where the Haversian systems are less organised. The proportion of cortical and cancellous bone will affect the degree of fracture.

Factors affecting bone healing

- Blood supply to the bone.
- Quantity of force involved in the fracture site.
- Condition of the surrounding soft tissue.

Fracture classification

Fractures can be classified based on:

- Cause (traumatic, stress, pathological).
- Fracture pattern (transverse, spiral, compression, oblique).
- Degree of displacement (displaced or undisplaced).
- Section of the bone is fractured (intra-articular, metaphysis, diaphysis).
- Whether the skin is intact (closed fracture) or damaged (open fracture) allowing the underlying soft tissue to communicate with the fracture and haematoma.

Fracture healing

Fracture healing depends on the biomechanical stability of the fracture together with the method of fixation employed.

- Rigid internal fixation or anatomical reduction creates absolute stability allowing primary healing of the fracture.
- In other cases, if left alone, healing takes place secondarily involving *callus* formation.

Secondary bone healing

Fracture healing may be considered as a series of phases that overlap and occur sequentially.

Initial haematoma

Injury results in tearing of the periosteum and disruption of the Haversian systems. Bone has a good blood supply made up of nutrient arteries within the medullary cavity and periosteal arteries. Bleeding at the time of injury results in the development of a fracture haematoma. At the fracture surfaces there is disruption of the Haversian systems together with osteocyte necrosis. This can be dependent on the degree of stripping of the periosteum and the degree of displacement and comminution.

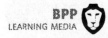

Inflammation

The haematoma at the fracture site stimulates the release of histamine from mast cells together with other various cytokines (see *Chapter 2: Acute Inflammation*). This results in chemotaxis and increased capillary permeability, leading to formation of a fibrin clot. The fibrin stimulates influx of neutrophils, lymphocytes and macrophages which release cytokines (interleukin-1, 6) including various growth factors (platelet derived, fibroblast) forming granulation tissue.

Repair

The granulation tissue develops reducing strain at the fracture ends. Initially cartilage forms until blood supply is improved when new bone is laid down. This initial cartilaginous phase is known as a *soft callus* which differentiates into woven bone (hard callus) with time. This process is referred to as *endochondral ossification*, whereby chondrocytes calcify and die leading to angiogenesis and woven bone deposition by osteoblasts. In cases where the periosteum is incompletely damaged, a bridging external callus develops, while in more substantial injuries fibrous tissue forms from the organised haematoma which stimulates deposition of new bone. An internal callus forms from the medullary canal restoring cortical continuity. Healing is slow therefore it is essential for internal fixation devices to be retained until this is complete.

Remodelling

Once the fracture is bridged, the new bone is remodelled. Any excess callus is removed and the osteoid (woven) bone is remodelled into lamellar bone. Angulation and shape are restored and bone is laid down in areas of greater stress. This process can continue long after the fracture heals clinically (up to seven years). Remodelling is greatest in children where alignment and angulation can be corrected to conceal the initial injury.

Factors affecting fracture healing

General factors

- **Age**: With increasing skeletal maturity the speed at which bones unite decreases. A similar principle exists for bone remodelling.
- **Nutrition and drug therapy**: Poor nutrition and general health slow the rate of heeling. Certain drugs such as steroids and NSAIDS can also delay healing together with smoking.
- **Bone pathology**: Pathological fractures, in pre-existing disease (malignancy, osteoporosis) heal more slowly. Similarly healing is quicker in cancellous in comparison with cortical bone due to a higher turnover of active cells. Upper limb fractures generally heal faster than lower limbs.

Local factors

- **Fracture site**: Excess separation of bone fragments after a fracture or interposition of soft tissue within the gap can cause delays in healing. Similarly, excess mobility at the fracture site leads to disruption of the bridging callus, also affecting the vascularisation of the haematoma.
- **Disturbance of blood supply**: Perhaps one of the most important factors is the blood supply. Any disruption can have significant effects on the healing of a fracture and can lead to avascular necrosis. Examples include intracapsular fractures of the neck of femur and fractures of the scaphoid bone.
- **Type of fractures**: Most displaced and comminuted fractures heal rather slowly. Avascular fragments of splintered bone require resorption and more time to remodel. Transverse fractures take more time to heel than spiral fractures due to more displacement of periosteum.

- **Infection**: Infections commonly delay healing preventing union. This is due to a prolonged inflammatory response together with strain on cellular activity. In the presence of prostheses bacteria generate biofilms limiting the effect of antimicrobials.
- **High dose irradiation**: Previous radiation exposure causes a reduction in the cellularity together with long-term changes within the Haversian system, increasing the risk of poor union.

Management of fractures

The primary aims of fracture management are to achieve sound bony union without any long-term deformity, and to restore function to normal, allowing the patient to resume previous activities as quickly as possible.

Primary survey and general assessment

- All patients should be assessed initially according to the Advanced Trauma Life Support (ATLS) protocol and any life-threatening conditions managed.
- An initial overall clinical examination should be performed to detect concerns and immediate management instituted.
- The priority should be to check for any airway or breathing issues. Anaesthetic support should be present early. Any suspicions of tension pneumothorax or haemothorax should be managed immediately.
- Severe external haemorrhage should be controlled with packing / bandaging and in some cases pneumatic tourniquet (limited time).
- The patient should be assessed for signs of internal haemorrhage with lower limb fractures causing loss of up to 1 litre of blood and pelvic fractures 2–3 litres. Immediate vascular access must be obtained and resuscitation commenced. Cross match blood should be ordered however O negative blood may be required sooner.
- Imaging will be required to investigate for any head injury (reduced consciousness, history) or visceral injury. This may result in the need for urgent surgery or transfer to a specialist centre.
- Immediate management of the fracture site include preventing movement by splinting, correcting deformity in case of neurovascular compromise or threatened skin, dressing of open fractures with administration of antibiotics.
- In cases of minimal displacement, reduction can be useful in preventing long-term complications.

Specific management of fractures

- Relative stability of the fracture can be achieved using:
  - Plaster fixation: This is the commonest form of support for a fracture, moulded to fit the contours of the affected region. Generally transverse fractures have axial stability in casts while oblique fractures may displace.
  - Continuous traction: This can be maintained for several weeks to maintain reduction in certain cases. This method is commonly used for femoral shaft fractures.
  - External fixation: This method allows the bone fragments to be held in place by percutaneous pins. This method is useful in cases of open fractures where the state of the skin limits the use of internal fixation.
  - Intramedullary nails: These prevent angulation and can provide rotational stability if used with locking screws.

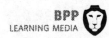

- Absolute stability with internal fixation prevents any motion between the fracture surfaces under load. The low strain allows primary bone healing to continue without formation of external callus. Dynamic compression plates and lag screws can be used to achieve compression across fragments.
- In cases of open fractures, a thorough debridement should be performed and skin cover issues considered. Associated surrounding soft tissue injury can often be severe leading to significant postoperative oedema requiring close observation. Close care to taking swabs and the early administration of antibiotics and tetanus prophylaxis must be undertaken. In cases of severe open injuries with gross comminution of bone, muscle and neurological damage a primary amputation is sometimes required.

Disorders of bone union

Some fractures are slow to unite in spite of optimal treatment.

Delayed union

Some of the fractures fail to unite in expected time due to intrinsic factors, local infection, a reduced blood supply or poor technique.

Non-union

The healing process ceases to be active if there is a wide separation of the bone ends, poor blood supply, or infection, or an adverse biomechanical environment. They are two types of non-union:

- **Hypertrophic**: Inadequate stability of the fracture leads to hypertrophic non-union, with normally viable bone ends that appear sclerotic and flared with excessive callus formation looking like an 'elephant's foot'. The fracture gap fills with cartilage and fibrous tissue with good blood supply and immobilisation usually results in union.
- **Atrophic**: There is a fault in bone biology leading to atrophic non-union. The fracture gap is filled with fibrous tissue. Rigid fixation with intra-fragmentary compression and elimination of the fracture gap is necessary possibly with the assistance of grafts. Recombinant human bone morphogenetic proteins are now commercially available and are licensed for use in such difficult cases.

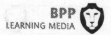

Further reading

- Anderson, I. (2003) *Care of the Critically Ill Surgical Patient*. 2nd edition. London: Hodder Arnold Publication.
- Ayub, K, Imada, R, Slavin, J. Endoscopic retrograde cholangiopancreatography in gallstone-associated acute pancreatitis. *Cochrane Database Syst Rev* 2004 18; (4): CD003630.
- CCM Tutorials.com (2011) *Critical Care Medicine Tutorials*. Available at: www.ccmtutorials.com.
- Dellinger, RP, Levy, MM, Carlet, JM, *et al*. Surviving Sepsis Campaign: International guidelines for management of severe sepsis and septic shock. *Crit Care Med*, 2008 36: 296–327.
- Dushianthan, A, Grocott, MPW, Postle, AD, Cusack, R. Acute respiratory distress syndrome and acute lung injury. *Postgrad Med J* 2011; 87: 612–622.
- Guyton, AC, Jones, CE, Coleman, TG (1973) *Physiology: Cardiac Output and its Regulation*. 2nd edition. Philadelphia: WB Saunders.
- Jackson, DM. The diagnosis of the depth of burning. *B, J Swg*. 1953; 40:588.
- Luks, A M. *A Primer on Arterial Blood Gas Analysis*. University of Washington, 2008 Available at: http://courses.washington.edu./med610/abg/abg_primer.html.
- Manrique, A, Jooste, EH, Kuch, BA, *et al*. The association of renal dysfunction and the use of aprotinin in patients undergoing congenital cardiac surgery requiring cardiopulmonary bypass. *Anesth Analg* 2009; 109(1): 45–52.
- NICE (2008) CG65 *Perioperative hypothemia (inadvertent): full guideline*. Available at: guidance.nice.org.uk/CG65/Guidance/pdf/English.
- Petrov, *et al*. Early endoscopic retrograde cholangiopancreatography versus conservative management in acute biliary pancreatitis without cholangitis: a meta-analysis of randomized trials. *Ann Surg* 2008; 247(2): 250–7.
- Sovensen, SPL. *Biochem Z*. 21:131 (1909); 22: 352 (1909).
- Starling, EH (1918) *The Linacre Lecture on the Law of the Heart*. London: Longmans, Green and Co.
- Stoutter, G, ed. (2007) *Cardiovascular Haemodynamics for the Clinician*. Chichester: Wiley-Blackwell.
- Strandness, DE, Sumner, DS (1975) *Haemodynamics for Surgeons*. New York: Grune and Stratton Inc.
- *Surviving Sepsis Campaign* Available at: www.survivingsepsis.org.
- UK Working Party on Acute Pancreatitis. UK guidelines for the management of acute pancreatitis. *Gut* 2005; 54: 1 – 9.
- Wallace, AB. The exposure treatment of burns. *The Lancet* 1951; 257: 501-504.
- Whitfield, AGW. The total lung volume and its subdivisions. A study in physiological norms. III. Correlation with other anthropometric data. *Brit. J. Soc. Med* 1950; 4(3): 113-136. Available at: www.ncbi.nlm.nih.gov/pmc/articles/PMC1037250/pdf/brjsocmed00015-0002.pdf.

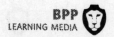

Chapter 5

Communication skills
(Giving and receiving information)

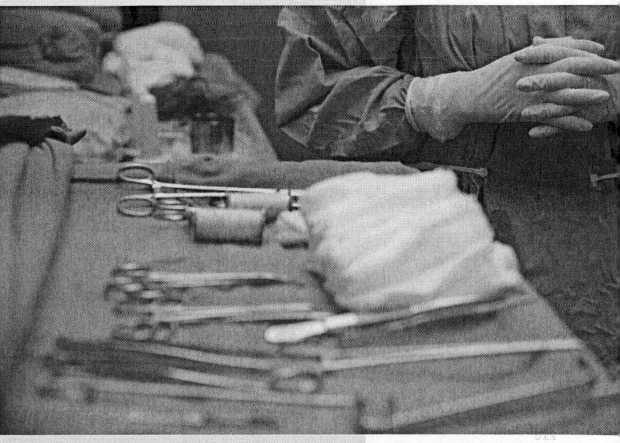

Overview

Successful clinical practice in surgery requires sound surgical knowledge, strong history taking and examination techniques, effective problem-solving abilities and good interpersonal communication skills. In this examination station of MRCS Part B, along with the candidates' surgical knowledge, their non-technical skills are also assessed: their professionalism and ability to demonstrate sensitivity to patients' and relatives' individual needs; their effectiveness in extracting the required information during consultation; and their efficiency in clearly transmitting this information to another colleague or healthcare professional.

This chapter introduces some concepts integral to developing good communication and provides frameworks to be used as skeletons for specific consultations, on various clinical or ethical topics related to surgical practice. These ideas can add to the basic communication skills already learnt to aid you to manage more complex communications with patients and relatives (see Chapter 6 – *History taking* for further information).

Introduction

Significant changes have been seen in the roles of health professionals over the last decade. With changes to the infrastructure of the working team within units, particularly the shift systems and the need for effective handover, and the formalisation of multidisciplinary teams for various specialties, the focus on improving communication skills continues to grow.

Despite the NHS Plan of 2000 reporting 90% of the public are satisfied with work performed by doctors, an increase has been seen over the last few years in the complaints made by patients regarding their doctors' communication. At present, communication issues constitute one of the main reasons for complaints to doctors: a report by the British Medical Association in 2004 declared that patients were less likely to complain about a doctor if the latter communicated well. With such outcomes, it is clear that improvements are needed in the communication methods adopted by health professionals and quality assurance systems need to be established.

Benefits of good communication	Barriers to good communication
Improves doctor-patient relationship Aids patient recall of information and compliance May improve patient health outcomes Patient centred approach promoting better quality of care Likely to reduce the incidence of clinical error May prevent emotional / psychological morbidity for health professionals	Lack of understanding of the structure of conversational interaction Lack of training in communicational skills Undervaluing the importance of communication Negative attitudes of doctors towards communication Lack of knowledge about the condition / illness Inconsistency in providing information Human factors; tiredness, stress Personality differences between doctor and patient

Table 5.1. Benefits / barriers to good communication.

Changes in the health system

The Darzi report highlighted changes within the NHS over the last decade. First, the exponential increase in information available to patients through various sources has certainly impacted on their expectations. Second, there have been significant changes in the demographics of the population and diseases themselves influencing the doctor-patient relationship. Third, the White Paper of 2000 highlighted the dissatisfaction felt by some of the population and thereby restructured the National Health Service to a patient-centred approach. Patients are now more involved in the decision-making process further altering the relationship. Finally, a change in the working patterns of junior doctors with the introduction of the European Working Time Directive has affected the continuity of care received by the patients together with the training received by the junior doctors. The above changes and move towards a patient-centred consultation has led to the development of various models to demonstrate the newer clinical interview.

McWhinney describes a more patient-centred clinical method allowing the physician to see the illness through the patient's eyes. This method encourages openness and understanding of the patient's specific unique expectations and fears. This information should be integrated with the clinical framework involving the signs, symptoms, investigations and differential diagnosis of the patient. With this integration a more specific explanation and plan can be offered to the patient in language they can understand and specific issues or concerns can be addressed.

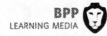

1. Explore disease and patient's illness experience (feelings, ideas, function and expectations).
2. Comprehend the whole person (individual and family).
3. Seek common ground regarding the goals of management.
4. Incorporate health prevention and promotion- suggestions for lifestyle modifications.
5. Enhance doctor-patient relationship.
6. Set realistic priorities, allocate resources appropriately.

Table 5.2. The six interactive components of the patient-centred clinical method.

Format of MRCS Part B communication skills section

Together with the broad content areas examined by the OSCEs, four domains have been identified which encompass the knowledge, skills and competencies of a surgeon. These domains are in keeping with the General Medical Council's Good Medical Practice framework and are assessed by the 18 OSCE stations. Two of these domains, communication and professionalism, are particularly relevant to the communication skills stations and are described below. (See also *Candidate Instructions and Guidance Notes: MRCS Part B Objective Structured Clinical Examination OSCE May 2010.*)

Communication

This refers to the ability of the clinician to assimilate information, identify what is important and convey it to others clearly, using a variety of methods; the capacity to adjust behaviour and language (written/spoken) as appropriate to the needs of differing situations; and the ability to actively and clearly engage patient / carer / colleague(s) in open dialogue.

Professionalism

This involves the demonstration of effective judgement and decision-making skills; the consideration of all appropriate facts before reaching a decision; the capacity to make the best use of information and think beyond the obvious; being alert to symptoms and signs suggesting conditions that might progress or destabilise; being aware of own strengths / limitations and knowing when to ask for help; the ability to accommodate new or changing information and use it to manage a clinical problem, to anticipate and plan in advance, to prioritise conflicting demands and build contingencies, to demonstrate effective time management; being aware of the need to put patient safety first.

The examination aims to assess the candidates on their communication skills in a clinical setting. Similar to the other OSCE stations, the scenarios will be those commonly encountered in busy surgical departments by the appropriate level trainee. There will be considerable variety between the scenarios trying to take the candidate out of their comfort zone and so it is essential to adhere to the basics of communication and remain professional at all times. Three parts are currently forming the communication skills section; information gathering, information giving and written communication.

Information gathering

The candidate will be provided with a short synopsis of the scenario in advance. The information will explain the basic details of who the candidate is, the patient's name and details and the expected task. The task may involve taking a history from a patient and relaying the information back to a Consultant, in this case, the examiner. The candidate will be allowed a few short minutes to prepare and then be escorted into the room; there the candidate is greeted by an examiner who may reiterate the format of the station and allow them to commence.

Tips for the candidate

- Make sure you have learnt the patient's name!
- You will not be introduced to the patient by the examiner so always start with this.
- Time will be short, so maintain a structured consultation allowing the patient or relative adequate time to talk.
- At the end of the consultation, close it as you would normally and then present your findings to the examiner in a concise fashion, answering any questions relating to diagnosis, investigations or management.
- While it is important to maintain a structure to the consultation, do concentrate on the patient's / relative's responses as often there is an underlying issue such as specific anxiety or a significant previous history. This often needs to be coaxed out gently using professionalism and empathy.
- Marking will include the communication skills used with the patient / relative in putting them at ease and gathering all the necessary information together with presenting the information in a logical and clinically orientated manner back to the Consultant / examiner.

Information giving

The candidate will be provided with a short synopsis of the scenario in advance containing the relevant information as mentioned above. The tasks in this station may include breaking bad news to a patient or relative or referring a patient to another hospital out of hours. The candidate will be allowed a few short minutes to prepare and then be escorted into the room, greeted by the examiner as above.

Tips for the candidate

- Introduce yourself to the patient or relative.
- Be accurate with the clinical information given to the patient / relative.
- Be prepared for an emotional or other unusual response from the patient / relative; there will be a specific issue within the consultation upon which you will be marked eg handling a distressed patient.
- Close the discussion as you would normally, summarising the discussion and plan and checking the patient / relative has no further questions.
- In all cases the idea is to push the candidate into a slightly uncomfortable environment either by the nature of the problem in front of them or the behaviours of the patient / relative. Make sure that, should the situation go beyond your competencies, you should recognise the need for further support by a senior and do not be afraid to mention this.

Written communication

This task involves the candidate being provided with information regarding a patient and they must construct an appropriate letter regarding the patient to another health professional. Examples include discharge summaries to General Practitioners or referrals to Consultants from another specialty. The task incorporates both of the above stations requiring a thorough analysis of the notes to incorporate the correct information in the discharge summary / referral letter together with a concise letter providing the other health professional with the necessary information including the diagnosis, treatment received, complications, medications and planned follow up.

Calgary-Cambridge framework

This is one of the most commonly utilised frameworks for communication by health professionals, including five distinct parts: initiating the session, gathering information, building the relationship, explanation and planning and closing the session. These are detailed below along with relevant tips for the candidate that aim to establish successful communication.

1. Initiating the session

This aims to establish initial rapport.

- Greeting: Welcome patient and obtain name.
- Introduction: Introduce oneself and clarify role.
- Demonstrate interest, respect and concern for patient's comfort.
- Identify the reason for the patient's attendance.
- Patient's agenda: Identify the problem the patient wishes to discuss. (How may I help you today?)
- Listen attentively to patient's opening sentence.
- Screening: Check and confirm list of problems.
- Agenda setting: Negotiate agenda taking both the patient's and doctor's needs into account.

2. Gathering information

This aims to explore the current problems.

- Narrative thread: Encourage patient to tell their story in own words, clarifying reason for presenting now.
- Questioning: Use both open and closed questioning moving appropriately from one to the other.
- Listen attentively to patient allowing them to finish sentences and natural pauses for thought.
- Facilitate patient's responses both verbally and non-verbally eg use of encouragement, silence and paraphrasing.
- Pick up on verbal and non-verbal cues.
- Use concise easily understood questions, avoiding medical jargon.
- Clarify patient's statements that are vague or unclear.
- Establish dates and sequence of events.

It is essential to focus on understanding the patient's perspective.

- Determine and acknowledge the patient's ideas and concerns.
- Expectations: Determine what goals the patient had expected.
- Feelings and thoughts: Encourage expression of patient's feelings and thoughts.
- Determine the effect of the problem on the patient's life.
- Pick up on verbal and non-verbal cues (body language, facial expressions).

In order to provide structure to the consultation:

- Summarise at the end of a specific line of inquiry to verify interpretation, ensure nothing important was omitted and demonstrate understanding.
- Signposting: Progress from one section to another by using transitional statements.
- Structure the consultation in a logical sequence.
- Attend to timing, keeping interview to task.

3. Building the relationship

In order to develop rapport:

- Demonstrate appropriate non-verbal behaviour: eye contact, posture and position, facial expressions.
- The use of notes or computer should not interfere with dialogue or rapport.
- Acceptance: Acknowledge patient's views and feelings.
- Empathy and support: Express concern, willingness to help.
- Sensitivity: Manage sensitive and disturbing topics sensitively including when associated with physical examination.

It is paramount to involve the patient in the decision-making process.

- Share thinking with patient to encourage patient's involvement.
- Explanation: Explain rationale for questions or parts of physical examination that could appear to be non-sequiturs.
- Examination: Explain process and ask permission. Ensure the presence of a chaperone if indicated.

4. Explanation and planning

Ensure that the correct amount and type of information is discussed.

- Chunks and checks: Provide information in assimilable chunks checking for understanding.
- Assess the patient's starting point: Ask for the patient's prior knowledge early on when giving information; discover the extent of patient's wish for knowledge.
- Ask the patient what other information would be useful ie aetiology, prognosis.
- Give explanation at appropriate times, avoiding giving information or advice prematurely.

In order to aid accurate recall and understanding:

- Organise the explanation into a logical sequence.
- Use explicit signposting: 'There are three important points to discuss'.
- Use repetition and summarising to reinforce information.
- Clarify language avoiding jargon.
- Use visual methods to convey information: diagrams.
- Check patient understanding: ask patient to restate in own words.

In order to achieve a shared understanding, incorporate the patient's perspective.

- Explanation should be related to patient's illness framework.
- Provide opportunities and encourage patient to contribute by asking questions, expressing doubts.
- Pick up verbal / non-verbal cues: be aware of when too much information is given, or distress is caused by the information.
- Elicit patient's beliefs, reactions and feelings towards the information given.

Planning – shared decision-making

- Share your own thoughts, ideas and dilemmas.
- Involve the patient by making suggestions rather than orders or directives.
- Encourage the patient to contribute their thoughts and preferences.

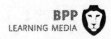

- Negotiate a mutually exclusive plan.
- Offer choices and encourage the patient to make decisions.
- Check with the patient that they accept the plan and all concerns have been addressed.

5. Closing the session

Finally

- Summarise the session briefly and clarify the plan.
- Contract with patient the next steps for patient and physician.
- Safety netting: Explain possible unexpected steps and what to do if the plan is not working.
- Final checking: Ensure the patient agrees and is comfortable with the plan and ask if any corrections are required.

Breaking bad news

Bad news is defined as any information that adversely and seriously affects an individual's view of their future. This task can be difficult for a clinician having to perform it numerous times throughout their career and even more stressful for inexperienced junior doctors. From the patient's perspective such discussions can impact on their comprehension of information, which in turn will help them make important decisions on their quality of life. For this reason a structured format can be useful to help reduce stress levels for doctors and ensure that patients receive the correct necessary information. This process aims to achieve four specific goals:

- Gather information from the patient.
- Provide information in accordance with the patient's requirements.
- Support the patient by reducing the emotional impact.
- Develop an agreed upon treatment plan.

A recommended structured format for a 'breaking bad news' interview (signposted as SPIKES – the acromym standing for Set up, Perception, Invitation, Knowledge, Emotions/Empathy, Strategy/Summary) involves the following principles.

1. Setting up the interview

Mental rehearsal can help reduce the stress associated with such tasks. Also, setting the appropriate environment (such as a private room with sufficient seating for family members and sufficient allocated time for the discussion) can aid achieving the planned goals.

2. Assessing the patient's perception

Prior to discussing the findings and diagnosis one should first assess the information and perception of the patient and close family members. This can be achieved by asking open ended questions to get a feel for the patient's insight and understanding and to look for any denial.

3. Obtaining the patient's invitation

Many patients express a definite desire to receive full information regarding their condition. Sometimes however, certain patients do not wish to have the full information regarding their diagnosis and prognosis; in such cases offer to answer any specific questions or talk to any family member the patient wishes you to.

4. Giving knowledge and information to the patient

Warning the patient that you have bad news can sometimes lessen the shock and can facilitate processing of the information. Avoid unnecessary jargon in the discussion and find a balance between being too blunt and too subtle. Provide the information in small chunks allowing processing and checking understanding intermittently.

5. Addressing the patient's emotions with empathetic responses

Responding to the patient's and relatives' emotions is an extremely difficult task. The emotional responses can vary from one extreme of silence to another of anger. Pay attention to identify the response and allow them sufficient time to express the emotion. Then let them know your connection to the response by showing empathy.

6. Strategy and summary

Patients with a clear plan for the future can feel less anxious. Check with the patient that they are ready to proceed with that part of the discussion. Present the treatment options to the patient allowing a shared decision-making process to take place. Clarify details to ensure no misunderstandings. Identify and agree upon specific goals the patient may have such as symptom control.

Examples of Scenarios

Information giving (Scenario 1)

An 81-year-old lady presents to the hospital with a one-day history of severe left iliac fossa abdominal pain associated with vomiting. She has a history of COPD managed at home with inhalers. On examination she is tachycardic and hypotensive. Abdominal examination reveals marked tenderness and peritonism in the left iliac fossa. An erect chest X-ray is performed confirming the presence of free air within the abdomen. On commencing your night shift you are asked to review the patient with a view to consenting her for an emergency laparotomy.

Preparation

Start by reviewing the patient together with all the documentation related to the patient's admission so as to clarify the potential diagnosis and therefore planned procedure. Next ensure the correct environment is available for the consultation. There may also be family members who wish to be involved in the communication.

Initiating the session

Introduce yourself to the patient clarifying your role. Check the patient's details and their preferred name. Outline the aim and format of the consultation.

Gathering information

Start by exploring what information the patient and family have received to date regarding the admission and investigations performed. Also explore their understanding of the significance of these results and their understanding of the plan.

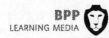

Building rapport

This is a difficult task. There will naturally be a lot of emotion and anxiety here. Pay attention to the patient's perspective as you progress noting any specific anxieties and expectations. There may be anxiety related to the patient's age and therefore fitness for surgery together with questions regarding her recovery not to mention the aetiology. Be sensitive and empathetic to the family allowing them time to digest the information you give and offer to answer any questions. With many family members present try to involve all in the discussion maintaining good eye contact with everyone.

Explanation and planning

Explain again the indication for surgery and the need for urgency. Describe the surgical procedure planned in detail starting from a short mention of the anaesthesia to the incision and procedure itself. It is useful to explain any drains, tubes etc the patient should expect to see on waking up and also a mention of where she may be transferred postoperatively – possibly critical care unit. Allow appropriate pauses for the information to be digested and answer questions as raised. Check frequently for understanding and use repetition and summarising regularly. Try to pre-empt specific anxieties so they can be discussed more in depth, eg the need for a stoma. Complications should be discussed including both general and specific to this procedure. In her case the history of COPD puts her at increased risk of respiratory complications which should be mentioned. Similarly all alternative management options with their risks / benefits should be mentioned so the patient can make an informed decision. Once satisfied check the details on the consent form with the patient and obtain the signature.

Closing

Summarise the discussion reiterating the diagnosis and urgency of the procedure. Clarify any points regarding the consent. Finish by giving an indication of timing of the surgery and take details of the next of kin to be informed.

Information giving (Scenario 2)

You are called to the general surgical ward in the middle of your night shift to review a 27-year-old lady. She underwent an elective laparoscopic cholecystectomy earlier that day. Over the course of the evening she has been complaining of increasing pain in the upper abdomen, requesting morphine every one hour. On examination she looks unwell. Her pulse rate is 115 beats/minute with a systolic blood pressure of 90 mmHg and she is pyrexical. Abdominal examination reveals an extremely tender right upper quadrant with localised peritonitis. Bloods are taken and fluids are commenced. Discuss the patient and plan with the Consultant on call.

Preparation

Before initiating such consultations it is often useful to take a couple of minutes to organise your thoughts. Once you have assessed the patient and ensured they are stable, spend a little time reviewing the case notes and recent investigations of the patient so as to ensure you are up to date. *In this particular case, look at the operation note to identify any difficulties and recent blood tests.* Making a call to the Consultant in the night to seek advice or assistance is often necessary. However the most important step to plan such a consultation is to know what you wish to achieve from the call in advance. In this particular case there is high risk of a post-cholecystectomy bile leak or haemorrhage. Your concern should be whether the patient needs to go back to theatre and therefore you need to present the relevant information so that the Consultant can make a decision.

Initiating the session

Make sure you contact the correct Consultant. Introduce yourself and explain your role. Outline the aim of the consultation.

Information giving

Provide the Consultant with a structured chronological history of the patient. Start with the initial presentation (elective / emergency). Describe any significant comorbidity and the operation details. Move to the postoperative course ending with the patient's current clinical state. Try to pre-empt the questions he/she will want to ask incorporating them into your synopsis.

Building rapport

Developing rapport is a difficult task when you have woken a Consultant up at three o'clock in the morning! The best you can do is to provide an accurate, concise clinical picture of the patient. The Consultant may ask you how unwell the patient is or your thoughts regarding the urgency of planning theatre / investigations so be confident in your opinion.

Planning

Once provided the full information a plan can be proposed. Clarify any points and summarise the plan at the end. If you disagree with an aspect of the plan be prepared to negotiate politely. Bear in mind the consultant on the other end of the phone cannot see the patient, you can.

Closing

Close by summarising any remaining points including clarifying any need for repeat communication before thanking them for their assistance.

Information gathering (Scenario 3)

A 39-year-old gentleman presents to your outpatient clinic with a few weeks' history of rectal bleeding. There has been no other associated symptom. He is otherwise fit and well working for an IT company. He is anxious about the aetiology of the bleeding. Please take a clinical history from the gentleman.

Preparation

This consultation involves taking a thorough history from the patient in a standard structured fashion. Focus should be directed towards aiming to identify the cause and severity of the bleeding together with the exclusion of any specific red flag symptoms. (See Chapter 6: *History taking – Lower gastrointestinal bleeding.*)

Initiating the session

Introduce yourself to the patient, clarifying your role. Check the patient's details and their preferred name. Outline the aim and format of the consultation. Ask the patient to outline their problem using an open ended question – What brings you to see us today? I understand from your GP you have suffered some bleeding? Often there may be more than one concern, so it is important to allow the patient to initially disclose their information uninterrupted. Once established this can be summarised back to the patient before moving on to gather further information.

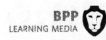

Gathering information

Spend time exploring the problem – in this case rectal bleeding. Identify the nature of the bleeding together with severity, frequency and other associated symptoms. Work slowly through the structured history using more closed questions as you progress.

Building rapport

Pay attention to the patient's perspective as you progress, noting any specific anxieties and expectations. There may be anxiety related to the possibility of malignancy or even the potentially required investigations. Summarise small subsections in the history along the way to confirm details and aid and improve rapport. Maintain good eye contact along with other verbal and non-verbal behaviour patterns. During the history taking share your thoughts with the patient to allow their involvement.

Explanation and planning

Once the history is complete, it is useful to relay a short summary back to the patient to check specific details and further confirm your attention. Following this further information should be offered to the patient regarding the possible diagnoses highlighting the important ones. A brief mention of the treatment options can also be useful while introducing the plan to the patient, although it would be unwise to start discussing surgery without confirmed diagnosis; always wait for histologic confirmation of lesions where malignancy is suspected. Second, a brief description should be offered of the investigations available and the reason for considering them to aid confirmation of the diagnosis. Naturally there can be some concern regarding the more invasive investigations (colonoscopy / sigmoidoscopy) so look out for this and try to alleviate this by expanding with a description and mention of risks. Once you have suggested your management plan try to involve the patient to contribute their thoughts. They may wish to negotiate specific aspects of the plan so be prepared to discuss alternatives.

Closing

At the end, give a brief summary of the plan checking that the patient agrees. Offer some assistance and clarify recommended actions regarding any interval changes in the patient's condition while awaiting the investigations (eg call GP, attend A&E, liaise with specialist nurse or Consultant's secretary). Finally, answer any remaining questions.

Further reading

- Baile WF *et. al.* SPIKES – A six-step protocol for delivering bad news: application to the patient with cancer. *Oncologist* 2000; 5(4): 302–11.

- British Medical Association, Board of Medical Education (2004). *Communication Skills Education for Doctors: An Update, November 2004.* London: British Medical Association.

- Stewart, M, 2001. 'Towards a global definition of patient centred care', *BMJ*, vol. 322, no. 7284, pp. 444–445.

Chapter 6
History taking

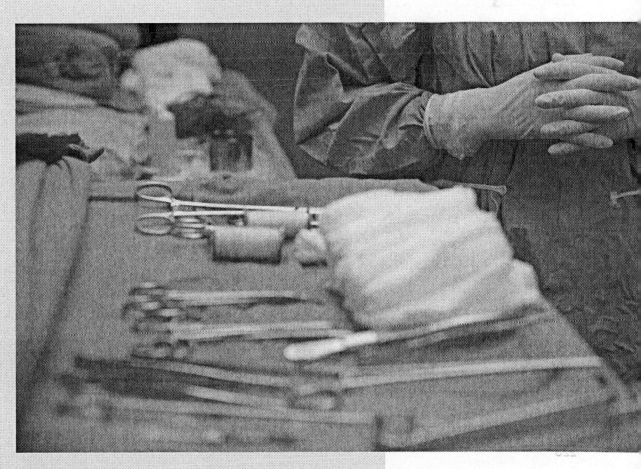

Overview

There has been an increased focus on communication skills in both undergraduate and postgraduate education over the last few years. Communication and professionalism make up two of the four domains examined in the MRCS Part B OSCEs in accordance with the General Medical Council's Good Medical Practice guidelines. A thorough and accurate medical history is often critical in identifying the aetiology of the patient's presenting complaint. Certain studies suggest that in up to 82% of cases the diagnosis can be made before proceeding to clinical examination. Naturally this is dependent on the ability of the clinician to elicit the necessary information. The history should follow a structured format commencing with questions surrounding the patient's presentation, previous medical history including significant investigations, drug and allergy history, social and family history and a full review of systems. The candidates need to introduce themselves at the start and ensure the environment is correct for the consultation planned. They should aim to develop initial rapport and commence the consultation with more open questions following up later with closed questions. Clear non-technical language must be employed avoiding medical jargon. As emphasised by recent national initiatives, the patient should also be involved in all discussions as steps in their care pathway. (See Chapter 5 *Communication Skills* for further tips.)

Haematuria

This refers to the presence of red blood cells in the urine.

It can sometimes be confused with other causes of red discolouration of the urine (food, myoglobinuria). Haematuria can be broadly classified as nephrological or urological in origin. Gross haematuria is often considered a sign of malignancy until proven otherwise. In certain circumstances the nature of the haematuria can give an idea to the site of origin.

- Total haematuria: Blood throughout the stream implies a cause either in the bladder or upper urinary tract.
- Initial haematuria: Blood at the beginning of the stream only implies an anterior source (penile, urethral).
- Terminal haematuria: Blood at the end of the stream implies a cause in the bladder neck or prostatic urethra.

Screening studies have suggested that the prevalence of asymptomatic microscopic haematuria in the UK adult male population is around 2.5%. Risk factors for significant disease include smoking history, occupational exposure to chemicals (benzenes or aromatic amines), previous history of gross haematuria, age > 40 years, history of urological disease, previous frequent urinary tract infections, analgesic abuse and history of pelvic irradiation (Table 6.1). A large UK series reported that important disease (cancer, nephrological disease or stone disease) was diagnosed in 26.4% of patients evaluated for haematuria, with an incidence of cancer of 9.4% in patients with microscopic haematuria and 24.2% in patients with macroscopic haematuria.

History

The following features have to be evaluated while obtaining history of haematuria.

- Is haematuria microscopic, macroscopic, are there any clots?
- Are there any other changes in urine (smoky, brown discolouration, crystals / stones)?
- Is it painful? Associated pain usually suggests inflammation, infection or obstruction, whereas painless haematuria is associated with malignancy or tuberculosis. Loin pain suggests renal disease, abdominal pain can be found with acute intermittent porphyria and suprapubic pain is commonly found in bladder disease.
- Determine the onset, course (intermittent or progressive) and duration of symptoms.
- Are there associated *urinary* symptoms (dysuria, hesitancy, poor stream, terminal dribbling, frequency, incontinence, nocturia, stangury)?
- Are there any associated *general* symptoms, such as vomiting, itching, lethargy (uraemia), weight loss, fever, arthralgia, rashes, other bleeding, respiratory symptoms (Goodpasture syndrome, Wegener's granulomatosis).
- Determine the effect of exercise on haematuria and inquire into recent trauma (abdominal, flank trauma, pelvic fractures) or recent biopsies.
- Past medical history: Is there a previous history of urinary disorders, urolithiasis, urinary tract infections, bleeding disorders or renal failure?
- Drug history: Anticoagulants, chronic analgesics, antihypertensives, oral contraceptive pill, or recent contrast medium.
- Social history: Smoking, alcohol, recreational drugs, recent contact with tuberculosis (TB), recent travel abroad (TB, schistosomiasis), occupation (exposure to alanine dyes).
- Family history: Polycystic disease, benign familial haematuria, haemolytic anaemia.

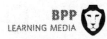

Haematuria	

General
     Anticoagulant therapy
     Sickle cell disease
     Haemophilia
     Thrombocytopenia
     Strenuous exercise
 Kidney
     Carcinoma
     Stones
     Trauma
     Glomerular disease
     Tuberculosis
     Embolism
     Polycystic kidneys
     Renal vein thrombosis
	Ureter
	     Stones
	     Tumour
	 Bladder
	     Inflammatory
	     Tuberculosis, schistosomiasis
	     Stones
	     Trauma
	     Carcinoma
	 Prostate
	     Benign prostatic hypertrophy/carcinoma
	 Urethra
	     Stones, Trauma, Tumour

Non-haematuria	
Haemoglobinuria, myoglobinuria, porphyria, beetroot	

Table 6.1. Causes of red urine

Diagnostic work up

- Haematology: Full blood count (anaemia, polycythaemia, infection, thrombocytopaenia), erythrocyte sedimentation rate, haematinics, clotting screen, group and save.
- Biochemistry: U&Es (renal failure), LFTs (malignancy), C-Reactive Protein , Ca $^{2+}$ (calculi, malignancy), Creatine PhosphoKinase (rhabdomyolysis), Prostatic Specific Antigen (prostatic carcinoma), autoimmune screen (glomerular disease).
- Urinalysis: Microscopy (proteinuria and casts indicate a renal cause, white cells and organisms indicate infection), 24-hour urinary creatinine and protein, early morning sample urine microscopy, exfoliative cytology (three voided samples to maximise diagnosis, useful for diagnosing bladder tumours).
- Microbiology: Urethral swabs.
- Radiology:
  - Kidneys, ureters and bladder (KUB) X-ray for renal calculi: struvite, cystine and calcium stones are radio-opaque (90%) while uric acid stones are radiolucent.
  - CXR, if suspected malignancy or infection (metastases, tuberculosis).
  - Renal ultrasonography: It can differentiate cystic versus solid lesions, and can diagnose kidney trauma, urinary tract obstruction, calculi.
  - CT scan KUB: Diagnostic of trauma, obstructive uropathy and staging of tumour.
  - Intravenous urogram (IVU): For obstructive uropathy, calculi, tumour, tuberculosis.
- Cystoscopy: It is the gold standard for clinically detectable lesions of the lower urinary tract. It can be used to distinguish between infection, tumour, and stone (diagnostic, therapeutic, surveillance). The procedure carries a risk of urinary tract infection of approximately 5%.
- Ureteroscopy: Can assess for causes of obstruction, tumour (offer biopsy option).
- Selective renal angiography: Can reveal vascular malformations, tumour.
- Renal biopsy: For diagnosis of tumour, glomerular disease.
- Prostatic biopsy: For the diagnosis of prostatic carcinoma / infections.
- DMSA scan (technetium dimercaptosuccinic acid): It is used for the preoperative assessment of distribution of renal function; it can diagnose renal scars, congenital anomalies of the kidneys and ureters, and renal masses.

Urolithiasis

Epidemiology and risk factors

Renal tract stones are a common disorder with an approximately 10% risk of Caucasian men developing a stone by the age of 70. In the absence of treatment, the risk of recurrence for calcium oxalate stones is 10% at one year. There is higher prevalence in males (3:1) with peak incidence between 20–40 years. A positive family history is identified in 25% of patients. Increased incidence is reported in hot climates due to the more concentrated urine. A diet high in animal protein is also believed to be associated with calculi formation. Precipitating factors for stone formation include dehydration, cystinuria, diet, hyperparathyroidism, urine stasis, chemotherapy (excess uric acid), infection and gout.

Classification of stones

Calcium stones (oxalate / phosphate)

This is the commonest form of stones making up approximately 70% of calculi. A predisposing factor in formation is supersaturation of the urine with calcium. Causes described are idiopathic hypercalcuria, primary hyperparathyroidism (commonest cause – solitary adenoma), hyperoxaluria, and renal tubular acidosis. Management of calcium stones is based on prevention of further formation. Methods include increasing oral fluid intake, limiting dietary protein and thiazide diuretics to promote renal calcium resorption.

Uric acid stones

These stones account for approximately 5–8% of all stones. Dietary purines are metabolised to uric acid. Patients are found to have increased production of uric acid although the cause is not known. The urine is acidic and often of low volumes. Investigations include urinary pH testing and monitoring of uric acid levels. Such stones are radiolucent and can form large staghorn calculi. Treatment includes increasing oral fluid intake, alkalisation of the urine to dissolve the stones and allopurinol to reduce the production of uric acid.

Struvite stones

These stones are related to infection and are composed of magnesium ammonium phosphate making up between 15–20% of stones. Certain urease secreting bacteria such as Proteus mirabilis and Ureaplasma urealyticum are common causes. The majority of staghorn calculi are such infection stones. Presenting symptoms usually include loin pain, dysuria and fever with other systemic symptoms. Management options include percutaneous nephrolithotomy and extracorporeal shock wave lithotripsy for stone removal and antibiotics to prevent further formation.

Cystine stones

These represent approximately 1–2% of all stones, occurring in patients with cystinuria (autosomal recessive). The stones are often large and multiple and are radio-opaque. Investigations include urine analysis for cystine crystals and amino acid chromatography. Treatment includes oral fluids, reducing dietary methionine (fish, meat) and alkalisation of the urine.

Treatment of calculi

- Conservative: Stones smaller than 4mm in size often pass spontaneously.
- Extracorporeal shock wave lithotripsy: Effective for stones < 2cm.
- Flexible ureteroscopy + fragmentation: Indicated in cases of failed lithotripsy.
- Percutaneous nephrolithotomy: First line treatment for staghorn calculi and stones > 3cm.
- JJ stent insertion to decompress obstructed ureters from ureteric stones.
- Open extraction of stones.
- Percutaneous nephrostomy: For obstructed infected kidneys, impaired renal function.

Erectile dysfunction

This is the persistent inability to maintain an erection sufficient for sexual intercourse.

Epidemiology

It is associated with several conditions and can have a significant impact on the patient's quality of life. Studies within the UK focusing on men between the ages of 18 to 75 years have demonstrated a rate of 39% for lifetime erectile dysfunction and a current prevalence of 26%. A steep age related increase is shown.

Risk factors

Penile erection is a complex physiological process under hormonal and neurovascular control. Risk factors for erectile dysfunction are very similar to the recognised risk factors for cardiovascular disease – sedentary lifestyle, obesity, hypercholesterolaemia, smoking and metabolic syndrome. Erectile dysfunction itself is also a recognised cardiovascular risk factor conferring a risk equivalent to a moderate level of smoking. Based on this premise a thorough assessment of a patient with erectile dysfunction can uncover undiagnosed diabetes, dyslipidaemia or identify cardiac disease.

History

A thorough history for a patient presenting with erectile dysfunction includes four main categories.

Sexual history

It is important to clarify which of the five phases are affected – arousal, erection, orgasm, ejaculation and refractory period.

- Are you able to achieve an erection suitable for intercourse?
- How hard are the erections – scale?
- Is maintaining the erection an issue?
- Do you experience nocturnal or morning erections?
- Do you experience painful or premature ejaculation?
- Frequency of sexual intercourse?
- Partner issues?
- Affect on quality of life?
- Treatments attempted previously?

Medical history

- Previous medical history, pelvic surgery, trauma, pelvic radiotherapy.
- History and risk factors of cardiac disease.

Drug/social history

- All medications taken regularly, including non-prescription medication.
- Specific medications – antihypertensives, cholesterol lowering drugs, antidepressants, antipsychotics, 5 alpha-reductase inhibitors (finasteride).
- Previous steroid or testosterone therapy.
- Smoking history.
- Illicit drugs.
- Alcohol and caffeine intake.

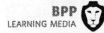

Psychological history

Purely psychogenic erectile dysfunction is rare however there is often a psychological component identified. Almost all men with severe depression suffer from erectile dysfunction.

- Predisposing factors – lack of sexual knowledge, previous abuse.
- Explore stresses either related to home or employment.
- Any symptoms or signs of depression – insomnia, lethargy, low mood.
- Difficulties within a relationship.
- Family or social pressures.
- Any trigger events.
- Any changes to sexual desire.
- Any anxiety related to performance.

Diagnostic work up

- Haematology: FBC, erythrocyte sedimentation rate, haematinics, clotting screen, group & save. Glycated haemoglobin (cardiovascular risk assessment).
- Biochemistry: U&Es, LFTs, CRP, lipid profile.
- Prostate specific antigen (if relevant history).
- Serum free testosterone.
- Serum prolactin.
- Serum FSH / LH.
- ACTH (synacthen) stimulation test.
- Urinalysis: Microscopy to exclude a genitourinary cause.
- Radiology:
    - Duplex ultrasonography to assess vascular function of the penis.
    - Ultrasonography of the testes to exclude any abnormality.
    - Transrectal ultrasonography to exclude any pelvic or prostatic abnormality.

Erectile dysfunction	
Neurological	**Drugs**
Spinal disease Neuropathies Pelvic surgery	Alcohol Antidepressants Antihypertensives Oestrogens Anticholinergics H_2 antagonists
Endocrine	**Other**
Diabetes mellitus Cushing's disease Addison's disease Hypothyroidism Hypogonadism	Phimosis Peyronie's disease Chronic renal failure Cirrhosis Malignancy Depression/ anxiety
Vascular Aortoiliac disease (Leriche's syndrome) Diabetic vascular disease	

Table 6.2. Causes of erectile dysfunction

- Injection of prostaglandin E1: This outpatient investigation includes the injection of prostaglandin E1 directly into the corpora cavernosa and to assess rigidity after ten minutes. While it can help to evaluate the vasculature, a positive result may still be found with mild vascular disease. It can also be utilised to assess penile deformities to aid planning of surgical correction.
- Angiography: It can be useful for planning vascular procedures / reconstruction, particularly following trauma.
- Nocturnal penile tumescence and rigidity: Nocturnal and early awakening erections are physiological and associated with REM sleep patterns. This test measures the natural event monitoring force and duration to exclude organic dysfunction.

Treatment of erectile dysfunction

Treatment options should take into consideration the possible associated cardiovascular disease.

- Risk factor modification by controlling lipidaemia and diabetes, weight loss, smoking cessation, increase exercise.
- Management of potential hormonal deficiencies: hypogonadism, hyperthyroidism, hyperprolactinaemia.
- Phosphodiesterase-5 inhibitor therapy (sildenafil): This is the commonest first line treatment commenced for patients, unless contraindicated. They function by increasing arterial flow to the penis causing smooth muscle relaxation, vasodilation and erection. Studies have reported 75% of sexual attempts resulted in sexual intercourse with treatment. Efficacy rates are reduced in diabetics and those following radical prostatectomy. Some people found to be refractory to treatment can be combined with prostaglandin E1 injection.
- Vacuum erection devices: This technique uses a cylinder over the penis pumping air out to create a vacuum. Once an erection is achieved a constricting ring is placed around the base. Vacuum devices are reported as effective regardless of the aetiology with satisfaction rates of 35%. Adverse effects include local pain and bruising. Contraindications include anticoagulant therapy or bleeding disorders.
- Intercavernous injection therapy (alprostadil): This is a highly effective therapy providing an excellent result in most men. It can also be used following nerve injury or radical prostatectomy. However its invasiveness render it unfavourable to some.
- Surgery: In some cases where patients have developed erectile dysfunction secondary to trauma to the pelvic arteries, revascularisation procedures can be planned using the epigastric vessels. This treatment however is only offered to healthy individuals with no evidence of generalised vascular disease.

The final potential procedure offered to patients refractory to other therapies involves the placement of a penile prosthesis which may take the form of either a semirigid or inflatable implant.

Back pain

Back pain is one of the most frequent presentations to general practitioners and orthopaedic clinics. A thorough clinical assessment is essential to exclude any red flag (malignancy) conditions. Similarly the identification of yellow flag (psychosocial stress factors) is also important in patients not showing improvement to minimise chronic pain and disability.

History

- Identify the primary site of pain and radiation (legs / abdomen).
- Character of pain: Aching, stabbing, burning, worse in the morning (ankylosing spondylitis)?
- Onset of symptoms: Circumstances, speed of onset (sudden trauma /disc lesion), progressive (degenerative).
- Intensity of pain, at rest, during movement /exercise.
- Duration of symptoms – is there night pain?
- Limitation of movements.
- Precipitating factors – is the pain related to movement / exercise, is it aggravated by coughing / straining (sciatica)?
- Associated symptoms:
  - Paraesthesiae, 'pins and needles' or numbness.
  - Symptoms of spinal cord compression, bladder / bowel disturbance, saddle anaesthesia, leg weakness, gait abnormality, erectile dysfunction.
  - Fever, weight loss, malaise, altered bowel habit, skin changes.
  - Abdominal pain, urinary symptoms (dysuria, haematuria – ureteric colic), menhorrhagia/ dysmenorrhoea.
- Past medical history: Previous back pain / surgery, abdominal aortic aneurysm, pancreatitis, malignancy, arthritis, osteoporosis, trauma, diabetes, immunosuppression.
- Drug history: Analgesia taken, hormone replacement therapy, steroids, immunosuppressive drugs, antiacid medication.

ACQUIRED	
Infective	**Degenerative**
Tuberculosis Discitis Osteomyelitis Spinal/epidural abscess	Osteoarthritis Intervertebral lesions
Neoplastic	**Metabolic**
Primary – multiple myeloma Secondary – Breast / thyroid / kidney / bronchus / prostate	Osteomalacia Osteoporosis
Inflammatory	**Referred pain**
Rheumatoid arthritis Seronegative spondyloarthritides – psoriatic, ankylosing spondylitis, Reiter's arthritis	Abdominal aortic aneurysm / dissection Pancreatitis / pancreatic lesion Renal calculus / pyelonephritis Penetrating peptic ulcer Rectal / uterine tumours
Traumatic	**Other**
Vertebral fractures Ligamentous injuries	
CONGENITAL	
Spina bifida / Kyphoscoliosis / Spondylolisthesis	

Table 6.3. Aetiology of back pain

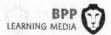

- Social history: Smoking, alcohol intake, recreational drugs, recent travel (tropical), occupational hazards, regular level of exercise, time off work, effect on sleep / mood.
- Family history: Malignancy, ankylosing spondylitis / colitis.

Diagnostic work up for back pain

- Haematology: FBC – assess for anaemia (malignancy), increased WCC (infection).
- ESR (malignancy, myeloma, tuberculosis).
- Biochemistry: U&Es (renal disease), LFTs (biliary tree obstruction, Paget's disease, malignancy), CRP (infection, inflammatory disease), Ca^{2+} (bone malignancy, primary or secondary), PSA.
- Immunology: Rheumatoid factor, HLA-B27 (ankylosing spondylitis).
- Plasma protein electrophoresis (myeloma).
- Microbiology: Blood cultures, tuberculosis screen.
- Urinalysis: Bence-Jones proteins (myeloma).
- CXR – Primary / secondary tumour
- Spine X-rays: Fractures, osteoporosis, osteoarthritis, Paget's disease (sclerotic lesions), myeloma (punched out lesions), secondary deposits, osteomyelitis.
- US abdomen: Abdominal aortic aneurysm, renal lesion.
- CT scan: Aortic aneurysm, abdominal malignancy.
- MRI: Disc lesions, degenerative changes, space occupying lesions.
- Technetium scan (bone scan): Secondary tumours, 'hot' spots.
- Bone marrow aspirate (haematologic malignancies).

Lower back pain – NICE guidelines (Adapted from NICE, 2009)

(Early management of persistent non-specific lower back pain)

Persistent or recurrent lower back pain is defined as non-specific low back pain that has lasted for more than six weeks but less than 12 months. Non-specific low back pain is tension, soreness and / or stiffness in the lower back region for which it isn't possible to identify a specific cause of the pain.

Principles of management

- Keep the diagnosis under review at all times.
- Promote self management – physical activity / exercise.
- Offer drug treatments as appropriate to manage the pain and help keep people active: Paracetamol, NSAIDs (consider side effects), weak opiates (consider dependence), tricyclic antidepressants, strong opiates (short term for people in severe pain).
- Offer one of the following treatments taking patient preference into account:
  - Structured exercise programme: eight sessions over up to 12 weeks, group supervision or one-to-one (aerobic activity, muscle strengthening, postural control).
  - Manual therapy including spinal manipulation, up to nine sessions over 12 weeks.
  - Acupuncture: Up to ten sessions over 12 weeks.
  - Consider offering another of these options if the chosen treatment does not result in satisfactory improvement.

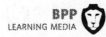

Constipation

Definition

Patients have varying perceptions of the definition of constipation. Many describe constipation as either straining, the passage of infrequent stool or hard pellet like stools.

The Rome III criteria (Longstreth *et al.*, 2006) describe functional constipation as two of the following in any 12-week period over the last 12 months:

- Fewer than three bowel movements (BMs) per week.
- Hard stool in more than 25% of BMs.
- A sense of incomplete evacuation or anorectal obstruction in more than 25% of BMs.
- Excessive straining in more than 25% of BMs.
- A need for digital manipulation to facilitate evacuation.

Epidemiology and risk factors

Colorectal functions are not significantly affected by the aging process. Constipation in older people is therefore not a result of aging, but is instead related to an increase in promoting factors such as chronic illnesses, immobility, neurological and psychiatric conditions, and certain drugs.

Risk factors for constipation include:

- Age: Infants and children and people over the age of 55.
- Recent abdominal or perianal / pelvic surgery.
- Late pregnancy.
- Limited mobility.
- Inadequate diet (low fibre).
- Medication (polypharmacy), especially in the elderly.
- Laxative abuse (normal long-term use is not a problem).
- Travel.

History

- Onset of symptoms: Speed, progression (sudden onset may indicate obstruction), duration.
- Is the change in bowel habit recent or long standing? Was there constipation at birth and during childhood?
- Is there a regular pattern in a week?
- Is patient passing any faeces or flatus?
- Is the urge to defecate present? (No urge could indicate colonic inertia disorder).
- Has there been any recent change in size or shape of stools? (Pellets, toothpaste, Bristol classification.) (See Further reading – *Bristol Classification of stool*).
- Are there any associated gastrointestinal symptoms? (Abdominal or anal pain, abdominal distension, rectal bleeding, mucus discharge, vomiting.)
- Are there any systemic symptoms? (Weight gain / loss, lethargy, intolerance to cold, hair changes.)
- Evaluate for any precipitating factors such as recent immobility, recent change in diet.
- Past medical history: Colonic carcinoma, diverticular disease, hypothyroidism, spinal cord disease, neurological disorders, psychiatric disorders, irritable bowel syndrome, recent surgery (anal surgery). Include all previous gastrointestinal investigations.

- Drug history (Table 6.6): Opiates, antidepressants, recent change to medication, previous laxative abuse, and current laxatives.
- Social history: Alcohol intake, smoking, recreational drugs, recent travel, occupation.
- Relevant family history (Hirschprung's disease, colonic carcinoma).

Congenital	
Hirschprung's disease	
Acquired	
Obstruction	**Painful anus**
Colonic carcinoma (strictures) Adhesions Hernias Diverticular disease (strictures) Pelvic masses – extrinsic compression	Strangulated haemorrhoids Fissure-in-ano Rectal prolapse
	Adynamic bowel
	Spinal cord injury Paralytic ileus
Drugs	**Other**
Opioids Anticholinergics Laxative abuse Iron salts Antidepressants / anticonvulsants	Myxoedema Hyperparathyroidism Dietary causes – low fibre Depression / anxiety Immobility Autonomic neuropathy Parkinson's disease / multiple sclerosis Slow transit constipation / pelvic floor dysfunction

Table 6.4. Aetiology of constipation

Diagnostic work up of constipation

- Haematology: FBC (anaemia, diverticulitis), ESR (raised in malignancy, inflammation).
- Biochemistry: U&Es (dehydration in obstruction), LFTs (metastatic spread, decreased albumin – starvation), CRP, Ca^{2+} (malignancy, hypercalcaemia), thyroid function tests, Glucose (diabetic autonomic neuropathy).
- Radiology:
  - AXR – obstruction (erect CXR if indicated – stercoral perforation)
  - Barium enema – diverticular disease, malignancy, redundant sigmoid colon
  - US abdomen and pelvis – ovarian pathology, pregnancy, fibroids
  - CT scan – staging of malignancy, pelvic masses
  - MRI – spinal trauma, disease, complex pelvic disease
- Sigmoidoscopy / colonoscopy to exclude malignancy, inflammatory bowel disease, diverticular disease, Hirschprung's disease (rectal biopsy – absence of ganglion cells).
- Colonic transit studies (radiopaque markers).
- Anorectal physiology (manometry and electromyography).

Management of constipation

Classify the patient's type of constipation according to following classification system:

Constipation type	Clinical findings
Normal-transit constipation, constipation predominant IBS	Pain and bloating Feeling of incomplete evacuation No pathology at clinical examination
Slow-transit constipation	Slow colonic transit with normal pelvic floor function
Evacuation disorder	Prolonged/excessive straining Difficult defecation even with soft stools Patient applies perineal/vaginal pressure to defecate Manual manoeuvres to aid defecation High basal sphincter pressure (anorectal manometry
Idiopathic/organic/secondary constipation	Known drug side effects, contributing medication Proven mechanical obstruction Metabolic disorders—abnormal blood tests

Table 6.5. Classification of constipation

- For uncomplicated normal-transit constipation without alarm symptoms:
  - Commence treatment by increasing fibre, use milk of magnesia
  - Add lactulose or polyethylene glycol
  - Add bisacodyl or sodium picosulfate
  - Adjust medication as needed (Table 6.6)
- In treatment-resistant constipation, specialised investigations can identify a cause and guide treatment. Perform routine blood tests (including thyroid function tests), and colonic anatomic studies to rule out organic causes.
  - The majority of patients will have a normal/negative clinical evaluation and may meet the criteria for constipation-predominant IBS. These patients will probably benefit from treatment with fibre and/or osmotic laxatives.
- If treatment fails, continue with specialised testing: Radiopaque marker study for slow transit colon, anorectal manometry and balloon expulsion test for evacuation disorders and defecography for anatomic defects.
- Treatment of slow transit colon requires aggressive laxative programs with fibre, milk of magnesia, bisacodyl/sodium picosulfate, adding prucalopride or lubiprostone if necessary and finally lactulose polyethylene glycol if no improvement.
- In refractory constipation, a few highly selected patients may benefit from surgery.

– Aluminium antacids
– Antimuscarinics (e.g. procyclidine, oxybutynin)
– Antidepressants (most commonly tricyclic antidepressants)
– Antiepileptics: carbamazepine, gabapentin, oxcarbazepine, pregabalin, phenytoin
– Sedating antihistamines
– Antipsychotics
– Antispasmodics: dicycloverine, hyoscine
– Calcium supplements
– Diuretics
– Iron supplements
– Opioids
– Verapamil

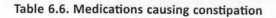

Table 6.6. Medications causing constipation

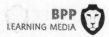

Diarrhoea

Definition

Diarrhoea may be defined in terms of stool frequency, consistency, volume, or weight. Patients' conceptions of diarrhoea often focus around stool consistency. An agreed upon definition is: diarrhoea is the abnormal passage of loose or liquid stools more than three times daily and / or a volume of stool greater than 200g/day. Note faecal incontinence is often misinterpreted as diarrhoea.

History

- Define diarrhoea from patient perspective – watery, loose or frequent.
- Onset of symptoms (speed of onset, progressive), duration, previous episodes.
- Associated urgency, tenesmus or faecal incontinence.
- Colour and consistency of stools (pale coloured, difficult to flush, offensive suggest steatorrhoea and malabsorption).
- Any blood or mucus (mixed in with stool or coating).
- Associated symptoms: Vomiting, abdominal pain, lethargy, weight loss, fever, arthralgia, rashes, jaundice or mouth ulcers.
- Precipitating factors: Recent foreign travel, unusual meals (others affected), contact with individuals with similar symptoms, recent hospital admissions (Clostridium difficile).
- Past medical history: Any previous diarrhoea or inflammatory bowel disease, previous abdominal surgery (bowel resection) or radiotherapy, thyroid disease.
- Drug history: Laxatives, recent antibiotics, change in regular medications, treatment already received for diarrhoea.
- Social history: Foreign travel, alcohol intake, sexual history (HIV related diarrhoea).
- Family history: Inflammatory bowel disease, gastrointestinal malignancy, coeliac disease.

Infective		
Bacterial	**Viral**	**Parasitic**
Campylobacter	Rotavirus	Giardiasis
Shigella	HIV-related	Entamoeba histolytica
Salmonella		
Vibrio cholera		
Yersinia		
Staphylococcus aureus		
Clostridium difficile		
Inflammatory		
Crohn's disease		
Ulcerative colitis		
Diverticular disease		
Neoplastic	**Malabsorption**	**Drugs**
Adenoma	Short bowel syndrome	Alcohol
Carcinoma	Coeliac disease	Laxatives
	Blind loop syndrome	Magnesium-based antacids
	Radiation enterocolitis	Antibiotics
Endocrine	**Other**	
Diabetes mellitus	Cystic fibrosis	
Thyrotoxicosis	Pancreatic dysfunction	
Carcinoid syndrome	Anxiety	
Addison's disease	Post gastric surgery	
VIPoma		
Zollinger-Ellison syndrome		

Table 6.7. Causes of diarrhoea

BPP
LEARNING MEDIA

Diagnostic work up for diarrhoea

- Haematology: FBC (anaemia, increased WCC), ESR.
- Biochemistry: U&Es (dehydration), LFTs (malignancy), CRP, Ca^{2+} (malabsorption), albumin (malabsorption), amylase (pancreatic insufficiency), TFTs (thyrotoxicosis).
- Immunology: Coeliac screen (anti transglutaminase antibodies have superseded the previously used antigliadin, antiendomysial and antireticulin antibodies).
- Microbiology: Blood cultures, stool culture and microscopy, HIV serology.
- Faecal fats (malabsorption), faecal elastase, pancreolauryl test (pancreatic function).
- Radiology:
  - AXR – inflammatory bowel disease (toxic megacolon), chronic pancreatitis (calcification).
  - US abdomen (liver malignancies, carcinoid).
  - Small bowel follow-through with fluoroscopy, CT enteroclysis or MRI enteroclysis (Crohn's disease).
  - CT abdomen: pancreatic dysfunction.
  - Barium enema (less commonly for evaluation of carcinoma, diverticular disease, inflammatory bowel disease).
- Endoscopy:
  - Rigid sigmoidoscopy, flexible sigmoidoscopy, colonoscopy (inflammatory bowel disease, diverticular disease, carcinoma, pseudomembranous colitis) with biopsies.
  - Small bowel enteroscopy – capsule endoscopy or double balloon enteroscopy (Crohn's).
  - OGD and duodenal biopsy (Coeliac disease).
  - ERCP, if pancreatic abnormality identified by above imaging, as appropriate.
- Selectively, within the appropriate clinical context: Serum calcitonin (medullary carcinoma of the thyroid), fasting serum gastrin (Zollinger-Ellison), Short SynACTHen test (Addison's disease) and 24-hour urine collection.

Chronic diarrhoea

It is one of the most common reasons for referral to an outpatient gastroenterology or surgical clinic. There is no agreed upon definition for the duration of symptoms that define chronic in comparison to acute. Many groups accept symptoms persisting for longer than four weeks to merit further investigations. Studies in Western populations have estimated a prevalence of 4–5%. A focused history must be taken to distinguish between organic and functional causes and distinguish inflammatory bowel disease from malabsorptive causes.

British Society of Gastroenterology 2003 for investigation of chronic diarrhoea

- All patients should undergo routine investigations including; liver and thyroid function test, vitamin B12 levels and a coeliac screen.
- In patients below the age of 45 years with symptoms suggestive of functional bowel disease and a normal examination and blood tests, a diagnosis of irritable bowel syndrome is appropriate.
- In patients below the age of 45 years with atypical symptoms and/or chronic diarrhoea, a flexible sigmoidoscopy should be performed as a first line.
- In patients above the age of 45 years with chronic diarrhoea a colonoscopy should be performed with biopsies.
- Antiendomysium antibody testing should be performed in cases of suspected coeliac disease. If negative an OGD can be performed with distal duodenal biopsies to investigate small bowel malabsorption.
- In cases of small bowel malabsorption with normal distal duodenal biopsies, small bowel imaging in the form of barium follow through or enteroclysis should be considered.

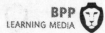

- Pancreatic causes of malabsorption should be investigated with CT imaging and faecal elastase or chymotrypsin.
- 99mTechnetium hexa-methyl-propyleneamine oxime (Tc- HMPAO) labelled white cell scanning can be used to investigate intestinal inflammation particularly for terminal ileal Crohn's disease.
- In more difficult cases of diarrhoea with normal investigations, inpatient assessment should be sought to include stool weight and osmolality, together with a screen for laxatives. Further hormone assays may be required eg VIP, 5-HIAA.

(Adapted from Thomas PD *et al* (2003))

Faecal incontinence

Definitions

- Faecal incontinence refers to the unintentional loss of solid or liquid stool, although some definitions include flatus.
- True anal incontinence is the loss of anal sphincter control leading to the unwanted or untimely release of faeces or gas.
- Faecal urgency also must be differentiated from faecal incontinence because urgency may be related to medical problems other than anal sphincter disruption.

Epidemiology

The reported prevalence of faecal incontinence in the general population is approximately 2–3%, although it can be underestimated due to reluctance of patients to report it. Amongst women three to six months post vaginal or caesarean delivery the prevalence may be as high as 25% and can be up to 50% in the nursing home population.

Aetiology

- Vaginal delivery (risk increases with number) with / without pudendal nerve injury.
- Congenital abnormalities such as spina bifida and myelomeningocele.
- Inflammatory bowel disease.
- Anal surgery: haemorrhoidectomy and sphincterotomy (internal sphincter injury).
- Diabetes mellitus.
- CVA.
- Spinal cord trauma.
- Degenerative disorders of the nervous system.
- Advanced age.

History taking

- Type and duration of faecal incontinence, frequency of incontinent episodes.
- Type of stool lost.
- Protective undergarment use.
- Impact of the disorder on the patient's life.
- History of associated trauma or surgery.
- Medications and dietary habits.
- Obstetric history (number of vaginal deliveries, prolonged second stage of labour, forceps delivery, significant tears, and episiotomy).

Clinical examination

- As per examination of the abdominal system in general (See Chapter 7).
- Also focused examination of the perineum, including vaginal examination and digital rectal examination (DRE) is necessary.
- During the DRE the sphincter tone is examined.
- Perineal sensation is also assessed with light touch.

Diagnostic work up

- Transanal or endoanal ultrasonography.
- Anal manometry, to evaluate the resting and squeeze pressures of the rectum and evaluate the rectoanal inhibitory reflex, rectal capacity, and rectal compliance.
- Electromyelogram: Helps evaluate the electrical activity generated by muscle fibres during voluntary muscle contraction, rest, and Valsalva-type activities.
- Evacuation proctogram involves imaging the rectum with contrast material and observation of the process, rate, and completeness of rectal evacuation under fluoroscopy.

Management

- Exclusion and treatment of systemic disease, if present.
- Medical therapy: Bulking agents and biofeedback (a behavioural technique that uses auditory or visual feedback to re-educate the pelvic floor musculature).
- Surgical treatment:
  - Injection of various materials (such as silicone) to augment the function of the internal anal sphincter.
  - Anterior overlapping sphincteroplasty.
  - Postanal repair to restore the anorectal angle and lengthen the anal canal.
  - Sacral spinal nerve stimulation is currently being the subject of increasing research with promising results.

Dysphagia

Definitions

Dysphagia refers to the difficulty in initiating a swallow (usually referred to as oropharyngeal dysphagia) or the sensation that foods and / or liquids are hindered in their passage from the mouth to the stomach (oesophageal dysphagia). Its incidence in acute care is considered as high as 33%; studies in nursing homes identify that between 30–40% of patients suffer from swallowing disorders.

Pain on swallowing is referred to as odynophagia, which does not interfere with the act of swallowing. It usually reflects a severe corrosive disease which may be caused by infectious agents such as Candida or CMV in immunocompromised patients, or caustic agents.

Oral phase	Oropharyngeal phase	Oesophageal phase
1. Food enters oral cavity 2. Mastication and formation of food bolus	3. Tongue elevated and bolus propelled to pharynx 4. Nasopharynx closed by soft palate 5. Larynx and hyoid bone move upwards 6. Epiglottis moves downwards 7. Respiration pauses	8. Relaxation of upper oesophageal sphincter 9. Food bolus passes to upper oesophagus 10. Contraction of oesophagus 11. Relaxation of lower oesophageal sphincter 12. Food bolus enters stomach

Table 6.8. Phases of swallowing

Oropharyngeal dysphagia

This high dysphagia is associated with difficulty in initiating swallowing. Oral dysphagia is often coupled with spillage or drooling of food from the mouth. Pharyngeal dysphagia is commonly linked with the sense of a food bolus within the neck and repeated swallowing or coughing. Associated symptoms include coughing, nasal regurgitation, choking, dysarthria (neurological causes), and halitosis (pharyngeal pouch).

Oesophageal dysphagia

This low dysphagia is caused by either mechanical causes or motility disorders. Patients with mechanical causes commonly suffer dysphagia for solids, which is progressive. Patients with motility causes suffer dysphagia for both solids and liquids which is not progressive.

History

* Assess the level of obstruction: Throat, suprasternal notch, sternum or chest.
* Onset of symptoms: Inflammatory causes such as GORD are often associated with retrosternal pain and develop gradually. Dysphagia associated with oesophageal carcinoma is usually of rapid onset. Achalasia causes intermittent dysphagia which worsens progressively.
* Duration of symptoms and course: Intermittent or progressive?
* Types of foods/liquids: As malignancy develops symptoms are initially for solids then liquids, whereas with motility disorders (achalasia) both liquids and solids.
* Precipitating and relieving factors: Patients with GORD-related symptoms often describe worsening of symptoms on bending or lying down.
* Associated symptoms: Odynophagia, swelling in neck, halitosis, nocturnal asthma, coughing or choking, heartburn, vomiting, haematemesis, weight loss, anorexia, voice changes, change in bowel habit, weakness.

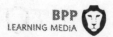

Congenital	
Oesophageal atresia	
Acquired	
Intraluminal	**Intramural**
Foreign body	Inflammatory stricture – GORD, caustic, candidiasis
Food bolus	Carcinoma – oesophageal, gastric cardia
Polypoid lesion	Infective – CMV, HSV, HIV, Candida
	Plummer – Vinson syndrome
	Achalasia
	Scleroderma
	Irradiation
Extramural	**Neuromuscular disorders**
Goitre (retrosternal extension)	CVA
Paraoesophageal hiatus hernia	Bulbar palsy
Mediastinal tumours – bronchial, lymphadenopathy	Guillain-Barre syndrome
Thoracic aortic aneurysm	Myasthenia gravis
Dysphagia lusoria	Motor neurone disease
Left atrial enlargement	
Pharyngeal pouch	

Table 6.9. Aetiology of dysphagia

- Past medical history: Peptic ulcer disease, proton pump inhibitor (PPI) treatment, previous endoscopy, systemic disorders, radiation therapy, neurological history (CVAs).
- Drug history: NSAIDs, proton pump inhibitors, Helicobacter Pylori eradication therapy.
- Social history: Smoking, alcohol intake.
- Family history: Oesophageal carcinoma.

Diagnostic work up for dysphagia

- Haematology: FBC, ESR, haematinics. Anaemia may be noted with malignancy or Plummer-Vinson syndrome. A raised ESR is found in scleroderma.
- Biochemistry: U&Es (dehydration), LFT (liver metastases/nutrition), TFT (goitre), CRP.
- Immunology: Autoantibody screen for scleroderma.
- ECG: Left atrial enlargement.
- Microbiology: Throat swabs.
- Radiology:
  - CXR – foreign bodies, tumours, left atrial enlargement, goitre extension, thoracic aortic aneurysm.
  - Barium swallow – this is often used to distinguish between a mechanical cause or motility disorder – pharyngeal pouch, achalasia, stricture, external compression.
  - CT chest – diagnosis of goitre, staging of tumour, thoracic aortic aneurysm, dysphagia lusoria.
  - US Liver/CT abdomen for staging if carcinoma is confirmed.
  - Oesophageal endoluminal US, also for staging of carcinoma.
- OGD: Investigation of choice for diagnosing dysphagia, for removing foreign bodies or food boluses, distinguishing between benign and malignant strictures, Plummer-Vinson syndrome. Biopsies can be taken and strictures can be dilated.
- 24-hour oesophageal pH monitoring: A small probe is passed transnasally to 5cm above the lower oesophageal sphincter and attached to a portable device that records the amount of oesophageal reflux and a temporal correlation between symptoms and reflux is made.

Indications for ambulatory oesophageal pH moitoring (Adapted from BSG 2006)

1. Patients with symptoms clinically suggestive of acid gastro-oesophageal reflux, who fail to respond during a high dose therapeutic trial of a proton pump inhibitor.
2. Patients with symptoms clinically suggestive of acid gastro-oesophageal reflux without oesophagitis or with an unsatisfactory response to a high dose proton pump inhibitor in whom anti-reflux surgery is contemplated.
3. Patients with persistent acid gastro-oesophageal reflux symptoms despite anti-reflux surgery.

Oesophageal manometry: Used for assessing oesophageal motility. Can identify the location of the lower oesophageal sphincter for pH probe placement, assess peristaltic function for patients being considered for antireflux surgery and diagnose achalasia or diffuse oesophageal spasm.

Indications for oesophageal manometry (Adapted from BSG 2006)

1. To diagnose suspected primary oesophageal motility disorders (eg achalasia and diffuse oesophageal spasm).
2. To diagnose suspected secondary oesophageal motility disorders occurring in association with systemic diseases (e.g. systemic sclerosis).
3. To guide accurate placement of pH electrodes for ambulatory pH monitoring studies.
4. As part of the pre-operative assessment of some patients undergoing anti-reflux procedures.
5. To reassess oesophageal function in patients who have been treated for a primary oesophageal disorder (e.g. sub-optimal clinical response to pneumatic balloon dilatation) or undergone anti-reflux surgery (e.g. dysphagia following fundoplication)

*   Mediastinoscopy / bronchoscopy: In suspected invasive carcinoma.
*   Echocardiography: Atrial enlargement.
*   CT brain: CVA
*   Tensilon test / electromyography: Myasthenia gravis.

Achalasia

*   This is an idiopathic condition characterised by loss of peristalsis in the lower two-thirds of the oesophagus and dysfunctional relaxation of the lower oesophageal sphincter.
*   Prevalence: 1 per 100,000, usually between the ages of 30–60 years.
*   Aetiology: Neuromuscular abnormality consisting of elective loss of inhibitory nerve endings at the myenteric plexus level.
*   Symptoms: Gradual onset of dysphagia for solids and often liquids, substernal discomfort and regurgitation (nocturnal leading to coughing or aspiration).
*   Carcinoma develops in 3% of cases, usually a squamous cell carcinoma.
*   Investigations:
    *   Plain chest X-ray: Air-fluid level may be seen in a large oesophagus.
    *   Barium swallow: Oesophageal dilation and poor emptying with a 'bird's beak' tapering of the distal oesophagus (Figure 6.1).
    *   OGD: To assess the distal oesophagus and exclude a distal stricture or small infiltrating carcinoma.
    *   Oesophageal manometry: Absence of peristalsis, incomplete lower oesophageal sphincter relaxation, greater intraoesophageal pressures than gastric pressures.

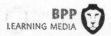

- Treatment:
  - Endoscopic injection of botulinum toxin into the lower oesophageal sphincter reduces the pressure and improves symptoms in 85% of patients. However, there is a high rate of relapse of symptoms (50% in six to nine months).
  - Pneumatic dilation of the lower oesophageal sphincter can provide long-term relief in 50–70% of patients. The main risk is perforation of the oesophagus (< 3%).

Endoscopic pneumatic dilation (PD) versus botulinum toxin injection (BTX)

Meta-analysis of six studies involving 178 participants: There was no difference in mean oesophageal pressures and remission rates between PD or BTX treatment at one month, but PD was more effective at six months. BTX was safer with no serious complications, while PD was complicated by perforation rate of 1.6%.

(Leyden JE, Moss AC, MacMathuna P. Endoscopic pneumatic dilation versus botulinum toxic injection in the management of primary achalasia. *Cochrane Database Syst Rev.* 2006: 18; 4.

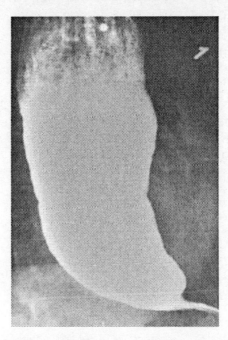

Figure 6.1. Barium swallow: 'Bird's beak' tapering of oesophagus in achalasia
Reproduced with permission from Maidstone Hospital

- Surgery: The Heller cardiomyotomy of the lower oesophageal sphincter and cardia of the stomach provides symptomatic relief in over 85% of cases. This procedure can often lead to significant gastro-oesophageal reflux so many surgeons opt to perform a fundoplication at the same time.

Barrett's oesophagus

An acquired condition characterised by columnar lined distal oesophagus due to intestinal metaplasia. This can progress to dysplasia and adenocarcinoma indicating the need for surveillance. Patients with Barrett's have a 30-fold increased risk of developing adenocarcinoma, approximately 1% per year. Gastro-oesophageal reflux is seen in approximately 10% of cases. Bile reflux seems to be an important aetiological factor. Usually patients are asymptomatic and the diagnosis is made at OGD: pink, velvety epithelium extending > 3cm above gastro-oesophageal junction.

Management includes lifelong acid suppression (PPI). Anti-reflux surgery may reduce progression to dysplasia and cancer. The aim of surveillance is to detect dysplasia before progression to carcinoma. 40% of patients with dysplasia have a focus of adenocarcinoma. Oesophagectomy for dysplasia has an 80% five-year survival.

Guidelines for the management of Barrett's columnar lined oesophagus (CLO) (Adapted from British Society of Gastroenterology, 2005)

- Patients should be explained the potential benefits and efficiency of surveillance also highlighting the risks associated with endoscopic surveillance including not all tumours are detected by endoscopic surveillance.
- The most effective time interval oncologically and financially is 2 years, with a risk of developing an adenocarcinoma at 1% per year.
- All surveillance endoscopies should include quadrantic biopsies every 2cm in the columnar region together with any suspicious lesions.

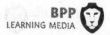

Upper gastrointestinal bleeding

Definitions

- Haematemesis: Vomiting of blood from the upper gastrointestinal tract, or occasionally after swallowing blood from a source in the nasopharynx; this may be frank blood or altered blood by gastric fluids that has 'coffee-ground' appearance.
- Melaena: Passage of black tarry stools due to acute upper gastrointestinal haemorrhage and occasionally from the small bowel or right colon.
- Haematochezia: Passage of frank blood per rectum.
  - Differential: True haematemesis has to be differentiated from blood arising from the respiratory tract; 'coffee-ground' vomiting is commonly confused with faeculent vomiting of intestinal obstruction.

Swallowed blood		Oesophagus	
Haemoptysis		Oesophageal carcinoma	
Epistaxis		Oesophageal varices	
		Reflux oesophagitis	
Stomach		**Drugs**	
Mallory-Weiss syndrome		NSAIDS	
Gastric carcinoma		Aspirin / Clopidogrel	
Peptic ulcer disease		Anticoagulants	
GIST (leiomyoma)		Steroids	
Vascular malformations (Dieulafoy's lesion)		Alcohol	
Hereditary haemorrhagic telangiectasia (Osler-Weber-Rendu disease)			
Acute gastric erosions			
Duodenum		**Others**	
Haemobilia		Thrombocytopaenia	
Duodenal diverticulae		Haemophilia	
Aorto-duodenal fistulae		Uraemia	
		Connective tissue disorders	

Table 6.10. Differential diagnosis of upper GI haemorrhage symptoms

Risk factors associated with poor outcome

- Age: Mortality increases with age.
- Comorbidity: Even one comorbidity doubles mortality, worse for cardiac failure and malignancy.
- Liver disease: Cirrhosis is associated with a higher mortality and need for intervention. Mortality for patients presenting with haematemesis due to oesophageal varices is 14%.
- Initial shock: Hypotension and tachycardia.
- Inpatients have a threefold increased risk of death.
- Haematochezia doubles the re-bleeding, mortality and surgery rates.
- Elevated blood urea is associated with a need for intervention.

History taking

- Onset of symptoms (speed, progression), and duration (number of episodes).
- Nature of blood (fresh / coffee ground), quantity.
- Is the bleeding effortless (varices)?
- Blood present in first vomit only (Mallory-Weiss tear)?

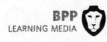

- Associated symptoms: Indigestion / heartburn, abdominal pain, dysphagia /odynophagia, rectal bleeding (fresh / melaena), altered bowel habit, lethargy, breathlessness, weight loss, anorexia.
- Past medical history: Previous gastrointestinal bleeding, peptic ulcer disease, bleeding disorder, liver disease, abdominal aortic aneurysm repair, malignancy, recent surgery / illness (Curling's ulcer), recent head injury (Cushing's ulcer).
- Drug history: Anticoagulant, NSAIDS, aspirin / clopidogrel, steroids, iron therapy, proton pump inhibitors / Histamine-2 receptor antagonists.
- Social history: Smoking, alcohol, recreational drugs, recent travel abroad, occupation (stress).
- Family history: Hereditary bleeding disorders, malignancy.

	Variable	0	1	2	3
Initial score criteria	Age	< 60 years	60–79 years	≥ 80 years	
	Shock	No shock SBP ≥ 100 mmHg, Pulse < 100	Tachycardia SBP ≥ 100 mmHg, Pulse ≥ 100	Hypotension SBP < 100 mmHg	
	Comorbidity	No major comorbidity		Ischaemic heart disease, cardiac failure, any major comorbidity	Renal failure, liver failure, disseminated malignancy
Additional criteria for full score (after endoscopy)	Diagnosis	Mallory-Weiss tear, no lesion identified and no stigmata	All other diagnoses	Malignancy of upper GI tract	
	Stigmata of recent haemorrhage	None or dark spot only		Blood in upper GI tract, adherent clot, visible or spurting vessel	

Maximum additive score prior to diagnosis = 7
Maximum additive score after diagnosis = 11

Table 6.11. Rockall score. This scoring system was designed to predict mortality based on clinical and endoscopic findings.

Diagnostic work up

- Haematology: FBC (anaemia), MCV (alcohol), ESR, haematinics, clotting screen (liver disease, anticoagulants, bleeding disorder), group and save / cross match.
- Biochemistry: Urea & electrolytes (urea to creatinine ratio rise), liver function tests (liver disease, haemobilia), amylase, glucose.
- ECG: Cardiac disease (Rockall scoring), cardiac ischaemia.
- Radiology:
  - Erect chest X-ray – perforation, chest lesion, aspiration.
  - US scan – aortic aneurysm, liver disease, portal hypertension.
  - CT thorax, abdomen pelvis – aortic graft infection, staging of carcinoma.
  - Barium swallow – malignancy, if OGD (below) not feasible.
  - Angiography – vascular malformations.

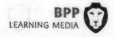

- OGD, with Helicobacter Pylori test and biopsies, for diagnosis (varices, oesophagitis, erosions, peptic ulcer disease, carcinoma), therapy (injection / clipping in active bleeding) and surveillance of lesions.

Management

The management of upper gastrointestinal bleeding will be summarised with that of lower gastrointestinal bleeding along with the pertinent guidelines.

Lower gastrointestinal bleeding

Lower gastrointestinal haemorrhage originates distal to the ligament of Treitz; however approximately 15% of patients with rectal bleeding will have an upper gastrointestinal source. Rectal bleeding remains a common presentation to hospital, with approximately 80% of cases resolving spontaneously. Despite haemorrhoids being a common cause, a thorough history and examination is necessary to identify the severity of bleed and any red flag symptoms.

Risk factors for increased mortality

- Increasing age.
- Inpatients (23% mortality in patients already hospitalised for another condition compared to 3.6% in patients admitted with rectal bleeding of new onset).
- Drugs (NSAIDs or aspirin).
- Comorbidities.
- Haemodynamic disturbance on initial presentation.

History

- Onset of symptoms, duration, frequency of episodes during the day.
- Composition of bleed: Fresh blood, dark (altered), melaena (tarry black), clots.
- Quantity of blood per episode.
- Is blood separate or mixed with stools?
- Where was blood noted – on the toilet paper, in the pan?
- Is it associated with defaecation (painful)?
- Precipitating factors: Passing a stool, trauma.
- Associated symptoms: Nausea /vomiting, mucus discharge per rectum, altered bowel habit (constipation – fissure, diarrhoea – inflammatory bowel disease, malignancy), pruritus ani, pain (abdominal, anal), urgency / tenesmus, sensation of lump around anus (haemorrhoids, rectal ulcer, prolapse), weight loss, fever, anorexia, dizziness, skin changes, urinary changes.
- Past medical history: Colorectal cancer, diverticular disease, inflammatory bowel disease, previous colonoscopy / sigmoidoscopy (polyps), peptic ulcer disease, alcohol abuse, haemorrhoids, coagulation disorder, ischaemic heart disease, recent surgery.
- Drug history: Anticoagulants, NSAIDs, recent antibiotics.

Small bowel	Colon and rectum
Aorto-enteric fistula Meckel's diverticulum Mesenteric infarction Intussusception	Polyps Carcinoma Diverticular disease Ischaemic colitis Inflammatory bowel disease Angiodysplasia Solitary rectal ulcer Rectal prolapse Irradiation proctitis
Anus	**Others**
Haemorrhoids Anal fissure Trauma Carcinoma	Significant haemorrhage from upper GI tract (ulcer disease) Bleeding disorder Anticoagulants Uraemia

Table 6.12. Aetiology of lower gastrointestinal bleeding

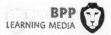

- Social history: Smoking, alcohol intake, recent travel (tropical).
- Family history: Colorectal malignancy, diverticular disease, inflammatory bowel disease, polyps.

Diagnostic work up

- Haematology: FBC (anaemia, leucocytosis of infective colitis, inflammatory bowel disease, ischaemic colitis), low platelets (bleeding disorder), clotting screen, group and save / cross match for transfusion.
- Biochemistry: U&Es, LFTs (hepatic failure with variceal bleed, malignancy), cardiac enzymes if appropriate (myocardial infarction).
- Arterial blood gases: Raised lactate (ischaemia), metabolic acidosis.
- ECG: Mesenteric ischaemia, atrial fibrillation (emboli).
- Endoscopy: OGD (to exclude upper gastrointestinal cause), sigmoidoscopy / proctoscopy (haemorrhoids, anorectal lesion, distal colitis, rectal ulcer) and colonoscopy (malignancy, diverticular disease, colitis, angiodysplasia).
- Mesenteric angiography (CT or invasive) / Technetium scan / Labelled red cell scan, if source not identified by endoscopy (looking for angiodysplasia / Meckel's diverticulum).
- Radiology: AXR (obstruction, toxic megacolon of inflammatory bowel disease) and US scan / CT (if suspected malignancy, for liver metastases and staging).
- Microbiology: Stool cultures (infective colitis).

Management of (non-variceal) gastrointestinal bleeding according to the Scottish Intercollegiate Guidelines Network (2008), adopted by BSG

- All patients presenting with **upper** GI bleeding should have an initial (pre-endoscopic) Rockall Score (RS) calculated.
  - If RS = 0, patient not for admission or for early discharge with outpatient follow up.
  - If RS > 0, endoscopy is recommended to assess bleeding risk.
  - Patients with a full (post-endoscopic) score of <3 have a low risk of re-bleeding/ mortality and can be considered for outpatient follow up.

  Decisions should not be based solely on the Rockall score but to include other clinical factors.
- Patients with acute **lower** GI bleeding

  Admission should be considered in patients with age 60 years, haemodynamic instability, evidence of gross rectal haemorrhage, a significant history of either NSAID or aspirin use or other significant comorbidity.
- For patients with acute **both upper and lower** GI bleeding:
  - Vigorous fluid resuscitation (crystalloid or colloid) is necessary for shocked patients and red cell transfusion administered after loss of 30% of the circulating volume.
  - Proton pump inhibitors (PPI) should not be used in patients with acute upper GI bleed prior to diagnosis by endoscopy.
  - Early endoscopy is necessary within 24 hrs of presentation.
- Pharmacological therapy for **upper** GI bleeding:
  - *Helicobacter pylori* examination is necessary and for those positive, eradication therapy for one week is necessary with PPI cover for a total of 4 weeks.
  - Patients with diagnosed ulcer who do not used NSAIDs should not be on long term PPI treatment.
  - For patients with major peptic ulcer bleeding, high dose PPI is necessary: 80 mg omeprazole/pantoprazole IV, followed by PPI infusion of 8 mg/hr for 72 hrs after haemostatic therapy at endoscopy.

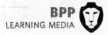

Jaundice

Jaundice is the yellow discolouration of the skin, sclera and other tissues due to accumulation of bilirubin. For jaundice to be clinically apparent, the bilirubin levels should be above 35 μmol/L.

History

- Onset of symptoms (speed), continuous or intermittent (Gilbert's syndrome)?
- Is it progressive, where was it noticed first?
- Precipitating factors: Recent travel, contacts, recent infections, unusual food.
- Associated symptoms: Abdominal pain, anorexia, weight loss, fever / rigors, vomiting / haematemesis, altered bowel habit, dark urine / pale stools, pruritus, rectal bleeding.
- Past medical history: Previous jaundice, blood transfusions, known gallstones, chronic liver disease, malignancy.
- Drug history: Any recent change in regular medications, oral contraceptive pill, recent antibiotics, paracetamol (overdoses), illicit drugs, vaccinations.
- Social history: Alcohol intake (CAGE questionnaire – see below), travel history, sexual history (HIV, hepatitis), occupational history.

> The CAGE questionnaire (Ewing 1984)
>
> 1. Have you ever felt you should **C**ut down on your drinking?
> 2. Have people **A**nnoyed you by criticising your drinking?
> 3. Have you ever felt bad or **G**uilty about your drinking?
> 4. Have you ever had a drink first thing in the morning to steady your nerves or to get rid of a hangover (**E**ye opener)?
>
> A total score of 2 'yes' or greater is considered clinically significant (sensitivity of 93% and specificity of 76%) for the identification of problem drinking.

- Family history of jaundice (haemochromatosis, Wilson's disease, haemolytic anaemia, Gilbert's disease), inflammatory bowel disease (primary sclerosing cholangitis), or respiratory disease (α1-antitrysin deficiency).

Diagnostic work up

- Haematology: FBC, ESR, haematinics, blood film, clotting screen.
- Biochemistry: U&Es, LFTs, albumin, CRP, amylase, glucose, fractioned bilirubin, serum copper and ceruloplasmin (Wilson's disease), paracetamol levels (in suspected intoxication), serum α1-antitrypsin (autoimmune hepatitis, cirrhosis).
- Serum alanine and aspartate aminotransferase levels correlate with the patients' body mass index. Elevated levels result from hepatic inflammation or necrosis. Alanine aninotransferase is more liver-specific. Elevated alkaline phosphatase levels are seen in cholestasis or infiltrative liver disease; if it results from hepatic dysfunction (in contrast to bone) the gamma glutamyl-transpeptidase (GGT) will also be found elevated.
- Urinalysis: See Table 6.14.
- Immunology: Autoantibody screen, antimitochondrial antibodies, tumour markers (CEA, α-fetoprotein, CA 19-9).

Pre-hepatic	
Congenital Gilbert's disease Crigler-Najjar syndrome Hereditary spherocytosis Sickle cell disease Thalassaemia	**Acquired** Autoimmune Malaria Haemolytic disease of the newborn
Hepatic	**Post-hepatic**
Viral hepatitis Autoimmune Drugs – paracetamol Alcohol, toxins Carcinoma – primary / metastatic End stage liver disease – cirrhosis, haemochromatosis, Wilson's disease	Gallstones Carcinoma of head of pancreas, ampulla of Vater Sclerosing cholangitis Cholangiocarcinoma Stricture (inflammatory, post procedure) Chronic pancreatitis Malignant lymphadenopathy at porta hepatis Mirizzi syndrome Congenital biliary atresia Guillain-Barre syndrome Myasthenia gravis Motor neurone disease

Table 6.13. Aetiology of jaundice

Biochemical parameter	Pre-hepatic	Hepatic	Post-hepatic
Blood			
• Unconjugated bilirubin	↑	N/↑	N
• Conjugated bilirubin	N	N/↑	↑
• Alkaline phosphatase	N	N/↑	↑↑
• Transaminases	N	↑	N/↑
Urine			
• Bilirubin	–	↑	↑
• Urobilinogen	N/↑	↑	↓↓

Table 6.14. Urinalysis and biochemistry in jaundice

- Microbiology: Hepatitis serology, CMV, EBV, blood cultures.
- Radiology:
  - CXR – enlarged heart (cardiac cirrhosis).
  - US scan – gallstones, dilated biliary tree, hepatic lesions, liver cirrhosis, pancreatic lesions. Biliary tree obstruction can be identified by ultrasound or CT scan with 90–95% sensitivity.
  - CT scan (± biopsy) – diagnosis and staging of pancreatic lesions (pancreatic protocol CT), cholangiocarcinoma, pancreatitis.
  - MRCP – non-invasive method for assessing the biliary tree and identifying stones, strictures or dilation (but less accurate at distinguishing benign from malignant strictures).
  - MRI liver – this is the most accurate method of diagnosing isolated liver lesions, fatty infiltration or iron overload.

- Invasive endoscopic / radiological procedures. (Reference is also made in Chapter 2: *Surgical pathology – Gallstone disease*.)
  - ERCP (Endoscopic retrograde cholangio pancreatography).
    Diagnostic value: stones in biliary tree, common bile duct stricture / tumour, peri-ampullary tumour, biopsy, brush cytology.
    Therapeutic value: stent insertion, sphincterotomy.
    Complications: pancreatitis (5%), perforation, bleeding and cholangitis.
  - PTC (Percutaneous transhepatic cholangiography) +/- biliary drain, if ERCP fails.
    Complications include biliary peritonitis and intraperitoneal haemorrhage.
  - Endoscopic US scan.
    Diagnosis of choledocholithiasis.
    Diagnosis and staging of small ampullary or head of pancreas lesions and assessment of resectability.
  - Liver biopsy – HCC.
    Percutaneous biopsy is the definitive test to diagnose and stage infiltrative liver disease or dysfunction. This can be performed under either ultrasound or CT scan guidance In cases of deranged clotting profiles or gross ascites, a transjugular approach can be adopted.
  - Lumbar puncture – leptospirosis.

Pancreatic cancer

Epidemiology

There has been a steady increase in the incidence of pancreatic cancer over the last few decades particularly in the Western world, and it is now the sixth most common cancer death in the UK. Approximately 80% of cases occur in the 60–80 year age group with presentation rare before the age of 45. The annual mortality rate from pancreatic cancer is almost identical to the incidence rate (11 per 100,000) as the prognosis is extremely poor. The one-year survival rate is generally low at around 12%, and less than 3% of patients survive to five years.

Risk factors

Proposed risk factors include cigarette smoking, high fat and protein diet, chronic alcoholic pancreatitis, obesity since early adulthood, diabetes mellitus, inherited pre-dispositions.

Histology

Ductal adenocarcinoma accounts for approximately 90% of tumours, with 80% occurring in the head of the pancreas gland. Lymph node metastases are present at the time of surgery in 40–75% of tumours < 2cm in size. The main presenting symptoms are pain, weight loss (90%) and jaundice, with nausea / vomiting and anorexia also common. Patients with carcinoma of the body or tail of the pancreas who present with jaundice will have developed hepatic or hilar metastases. Examination commonly reveals ascites, abdominal mass and supraclavicular lymphadenopathy.

Diagnostic work up

- US scan has 80–95% sensitivity for detecting cancer. It can also assess for gallstones, biliary tree dilation and hepatic metastases. Colour Doppler can be used to assess vascular invasion.
- Contrast enhanced CT scan: High sensitivity for detection of tumours (95%). In arterial and portal phases it can predict resectability in > 80% of cases by assessment of organ invasion, vascular involvement, lymph node metastases and hepatic metastases.
- MRCP can differentiate between chronic pancreatitis and cancer.
- ERCP: Useful for the diagnosis of ampullary tumours. Only lesions impinging on the pancreatic and common bile ducts can be histologically sampled. This technique also allows biliary stenting to relieve jaundice.
- Endoscopic ultrasound: High sensitivity in detecting small tumours, vascular invasion (resectability) and is used for biopsy.
- Laparoscopy: Useful for identifying liver and peritoneal deposits not picked up with other modalities.

Treatment

Resectional surgery

Approximately only 10–15 % of tumours are deemed suitable for resection at the time of diagnosis, based on tumour size, presence of metastases or ascites, invasion of superior mesenteric artery or portal vein. Four main types of operation are performed:

- Proximal pancreaticoduodenectomy with antrectomy (Whipple's procedure): Excision of head of pancreas and duodenum with end to side pancreaticojejunostomy, end to side

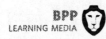

hepaticojejunostomy and gastrojejunostomy. Mortality in experienced centres is < 5%, with approximately 10% of patients developing diabetes and 30% requiring exocrine supplementation. Complications include haemorrhage, delayed gastric emptying, anastomotic and pancreatic leak, and pancreatic fistula.

- Pylorus-preserving pancreaticoduodenectomy: Less post-gastrectomy symptoms. Avoided in proximal duodenal involvement or when the pylorus is invaded.
- Total pancreaticoduodenectomy: For diffuse involvement of the gland without spread.
- Distal pancreatectomy: For lesions in the body and tail of the gland.

Adjuvant chemotherapy

Post-operative chemotherapy with gemcitabine has been shown to increase both overall and disease-free survival in patients who have undergone complete resection for pancreatic cancer.

Other treatment

Radiotherapy alone or combined with chemotherapy, biological therapy (vaccines, monoclonal antibodies, growth factor blockers) are currently subjects of ongoing research.

Palliative treatment

- In patients with biliary and / or gastric outlet obstruction the least invasive first-line option includes insertion of a biliary (metal) stent and a duodenal stent endoscopically. Complications of stent insertion include bleeding, perforation, pancreatitis, cholangitis and occlusion leading to recurrent jaundice.
- If stenting is not feasible, biliary drainage can be achieved via either a choledochojejunostomy or rarely cholecystojejunostomy. Prevention of duodenal obstruction can be succeeded by gastrojejunostomy or a duodenal bypass procedure (triple bypass: choledochojejunostomy, gastrojejunostomy and enteroenterostomy), open or laparoscopic.
- Pain control requires opiates. Neurolysis of the coeliac ganglia may provide significant, long-term pain relief in patients with refractory abdominal pain. A transthoracic / transabdominal approach is performed by invasive radiology or anaesthesiology, a transgastric approach using EUS-guided fine-needle injection, or intraoperatively.

Leg pain

Leg pain is a common complaint both in primary care and amongst referrals to outpatient clinics. The majority of cases are of orthopaedic or vascular origin.

History

- Primary site of pain: Unilateral / bilateral.
- Character of pain: Aching, stabbing, burning.
- Onset of symptoms: Circumstances, speed of onset (sudden – acute ischaemic / deep venous thrombosis / ruptured Baker's cyst), progressive, worse in morning / night, duration.
- Intensity of pain: At rest, during movement / exercise.
- Radiation to feet / buttocks / back.
- Limitation of movement: Distances, quality of life.
- Night pain- relieved by hanging leg off the side of the bed (ischaemic).
- Precipitating factors: Related to movement / exercise, any relation to walking uphill (spinal stenosis), coughing / straining (sciatica), recent trauma / puncture wound.
- Associated symptoms: Leg swelling, joint swelling, joint stiffness, back pain, abnormal gait, change in temperature (cold – ischaemia, hot – infection), redness, tenderness, puncture wound, numbness / pins and needles, muscle wasting, bladder / bowel disturbance, erectile dysfunction, palpitations, chest pain.
- Past medical history: Peripheral vascular disease, vascular surgery, ischaemic heart disease / cerebrovascular disease, DVTs / PEs, diabetes mellitus, hypertension, hypercholesterolaemia, recent immobility, ankylosing spondylitis.
- Drug history: Analgesics taken, beta blockers (can exacerbate claudication), oral contraceptive pill (DVT).
- Social history: Smoking, alcohol intake, recreational drugs, recent travel (flights), occupational hazards, regular level of exercise, time off work.
- Family history: Peripheral vascular disease, ischaemic heart disease, cerebrovascular disease, malignancy.

Infection	Trauma
Septic arthritis Osteomyelitis Cellulitis	Fractures Dislocations Haematoma Crush injuries
Inflammatory	Neoplastic
Rheumatoid arthritis Seronegative arthritides	Osteosarcoma Secondary deposits
Vascular	Degenerative
Intermittent claudication Acute – embolic / dissection Chronic – atherosclerotic / thrombotic Venous – deep vein thrombosis	Osteoarthritis Baker's cyst Meniscal lesions
Neurological	Others
Peripheral neuropathy Sciatica Spinal stenosis	Drugs (beta blockers exacerbate intermittent claudication) Gout / pseudogout Strenuous exercise

Table 6.15. Aetiology of leg pain

Diagnostic work up

- Haematology: FBC – anaemia (chronic disease, rheumatoid arthritis), increased WCC, ESR (inflammation, malignancy, infection), D-dimers (deep vein thrombosis).
- Biochemistry: U&Es (renal disorder), LFTs, Ca^{2+} (malignancy), CRP (infection or inflammatory disease), uric acid (gout), glucose (diabetes, peripheral vascular disease).
- Immunology: Rheumatoid factor, HLA-B27, autoimmune screen (vasculitis).
- Microbiology: Blood cultures (cellulitis, septic arthritis).
- Urinalysis: Glucose, protein (renal impairment).
- ECG: Atrial fibrillation (embolic episodes).
- Radiology:
  - Chest X-ray (lung metastases of malignancy), focused leg X-rays (fractures, osteoarthritis, rheumatoid arthritis, tumour, osteomyelitis, foreign bodies), spine X-rays (osteoarthritis, rheumatoid arthritis, tumours, osteomyelitis, osteoporotic fractures).
  - US joint (effusion).
  - CT scan / MRI spine (spinal lesions, disc prolapse, tumour).
  - Bone scan (malignancies, inflammation).
  - Duplex Doppler – peripheral vascular disease, DVT.
  - Arteriography (CT angiogram) – peripheral vascular disease.
- Nerve conduction studies (peripheral neuropathy).
- Joint aspiration if suspected septic arthritis.

Pyrexia of unknown origin

This is defined as:

- Temperature greater than 38.3°C (101°F) on several occasions, and
- More than three weeks' duration of illness, and
- Failure to reach a diagnosis despite one week of inpatient investigation.

History

- Onset of symptoms, duration, location.
- Course: Continuous or cyclical (patterns seen in malaria).
- Precipitating factors: Recent contact with people with illness / jaundice, recent contact with animals (Brucellosis), any recent injuries, symptoms of deep vein thrombosis.
- Relieving factors: Effect of paracetamol, any other medication taken.
- Associated symptoms: Dyspnoea, cough, jaundice, pain (chest, abdominal, joint, headache), altered bowel habit, night sweats, vomiting, weight loss, anorexia.
- Past medical history: Recent surgery (abdominal), prostheses (heart valves), immunosuppressive illness, transplant surgery, specific illnesses (inflammatory bowel disease, rheumatic fever).
- Drug history: Any regular medication, immunosuppressive medication, contraceptive pill (hepatoma), known allergies, recent vaccinations, over the counter medication.
- Social history: Recreational drugs, recent piercings / tattoos, recent contact with animals, occupation, sexual history.
- Travel history: Where and when did you travel, bites (mosquitoes, ticks, animals), visit to malarial zones, malarial prophylaxis taken, vaccinations before travel, food eaten abroad (seafood, raw meat), swimming in fresh water.
- Family history: Malignancies, immune disorders, inflammatory bowel disease, familial Mediterranean fever, family members with recent infections (tuberculosis).

Diagnostic work up

- Haematology: FBC for anaemia (chronic disease, malignancy), leucocytosis (infection, leukaemia), thrombocytopaenia; ESR (malignancy, tuberculosis, connective tissue disorders); D-dimers (deep vein thrombosis / pulmonary embolism), blood film (malaria, blood disorders).
- Biochemistry: U&Es (renal impairment), LFTs (biliary / liver disease), CRP, Ca $^{2+}$, tumour markers (CEA, CA 19-9, CA 125, PSA).
- Immunology: Rheumatoid factor, autoimmune profile, serum immune-electrophoresis (myeloma).
- Microbiology: Blood cultures (three sets), sputum culture (including acid-fast stain for tuberculosis), viral antibodies, stool culture and microscopy, Mantoux test (tuberculosis), serology for brucellosis, leptospirosis, Q fever.
- Urinanalysis: Microscopy and culture, urine glucose levels, microscopic haematuria (endocarditis, renal cell carcinoma), early morning mid stream urine tests (tuberculosis).
- Radiology: CXR – atypical pneumonia, malignancy, hilar changes (sarcoidosis, tuberculosis, lymphoma), tuberculosis.
- US abdomen: Intra-abdominal collections, malignancy.
- CT scan chest / abdomen: Malignancy, occult infection.
- MRI brain: Hypothalamic / pituitary lesions.
- Transthoracic or transoesophageal echocardiography (endocarditis).
- Lumbar puncture (meningitis).
- Antistreptolysin O titre (rheumatic fever).

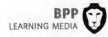

- Bone marrow aspirate (leukaemia, myeloma).
- Liver biopsy (hepatitis), renal biopsy (malignancy, glomerular disease), temporal artery biopsy (giant cell arteritis).

Infective			
Bacterial	**Viral**	**Parasitic**	**Fungal**
Abscesses Tuberculosis Subacute bacterial endocarditis Typhoid Rheumatic fever Brucellosis	HIV EBV Hepatitis	Malaria Toxoplasmosis	Histoplasmosis Candidiasis Aspergillosis
Inflammatory			
Crohn's disease Ulcerative colitis Ischaemic colitis Diverticular disease			
Neoplastic			
Lymphoma Acute leukaemia Renal carcinoma Hepatoma Pancreatic carcinoma			
Other			
Myocardial infarction Drug induced / allergy Transfusion reaction Alcohol withdrawal Deep vein thrombosis / pulmonary embolism Sarcoidosis Familial Mediterranean fever Postoperative complication (anastomotic leak)			

Table 6.16. Aetiology of pyrexia of unknown origin

Postoperative pyrexia

Pyrexia is a common symptom after surgery. Its significance depends on a number of factors including the time since surgery, the type or procedure performed and the clinical assessment of the patient.

Assessment of the patient should involve thorough history and examination looking for:

- Respiratory symptoms: Dyspnoea, cough, haemoptysis, purulent expectoration.
- Cardiac symptoms: Chest pain, dyspnoea, palpitations.
- Wound infection: Erythema, tenderness, temperature, discharge, dehiscence.
- Leg pain or swelling.
- Urinary symptoms: Dysuria, retention, frequency.
- Neurological: New onset confusion, neurological deficits.
- Abdominal examination: Distension, tenderness, vomiting, ileus.
- Surgical site infections, including infected cannulae, central lines, urinary catheters, epidural site, thrombophlebitis.

Diagnostic work up

Investigations should include: blood tests (FBC, U&E, LFTs, CRP, cardiac enzymes); urine dipstick followed by microscopy culture and sensitivity; sputum and blood cultures; chest and abdominal X-ray as appropriate (if abdominal distension is present and ileus is suspected); wound swab; arterial blood gas and ECG. Other problem-specific investigations that can be used are ultrasound / CT scans (abdominal collections), contrast enema (anastomotic leak), duplex scan of leg (DVT) and CT PA or Ventilation / Perfusion scan (suspected pulmonary embolism).

First 24 hours	Day 3–7
Systemic response to trauma / surgery Pre existing infection	Chest / urinary infection Wound infection Anastomotic leak Intra-abdominal sepsis
24–72 hours	**Day 7–10**
Pulmonary atelectasis Chest infection Urinary infection	DVT / PE Intra-abdominal sepsis

Table 6.17. Common causes of post-operative pyrexia

Further reading

- Bodger, K, Trudgill, N. (2006) *Guidelines for oesophageal manometry and pH monitoring* (British Society of Gastroenterology). Available at: www.gastroscan.ru/literature/pdf/bodger01.pdf.
- Bristol Classification of Stool: Lewis SJ, Heaton KW (1997). "Stool form scale as a useful guide to intestinal transit time." Scand J. *Gastroenterol* 32(9): 920–4.
- Ewing, JA. Detecting alcoholism. The Cage questionnaire. *JAMA*/1984 12; 252 (14) 1905–7.
- Leyden, JE, Moss, AC, MacMathuna, P. Endoscopic pneumatic dilation versus botulinum toxin injections in the management of primary achalasia. *Cochrane Database Syst Rev* 2006: 18; 4.
- Longstreth, GF, Thompson, WG, Chey, WD, Houghton, LA, Mearin, F, Spiller, RC. Functional bowel disorders. *Gastroenterology* 2006; 130(5): 1480–9.
- NICE (2009) *CG88 Low back pain*. Available at. www.nice.org.uk/cg88fullguidelines.
- Reigler, G, Esposito I, Bristol Scale Stool Form. A still valid help in Medical Practice and Clinical Research. Tech Coloproctol. 2001 Dec; 5(3): 163–4.
- Rockall TA, Logan RF, Devlin HB, Northfield TC. Selection of patients for early discharge or outpatient care after acute upper gastrointestinal haemorrhage. National Audit of Acute Upper Gastrointestinal Haemorrhage. *Lancet* 1996 Apr. 27; 347 (9009): 1138–40.
- Scottish Intercollegiate Guidelines Network (2008) *Management of Acute Upper and Lower Gastrointestinal Bleeding. A National Clinical Guideline.* [Online] Available at: www.sign.ac.uk/pdf/sign105.pdf.
- Thomas, PD, Forbes, A, Green, J, Howdle, P, Long, R, Playford, R, Sheridan, M, Stevens, R, Valori, R, Walters, J. Addison, G.M., Hill, P,. Brydon, G. *Guidelines for the investigation of chronic diarrhoea*, 2nd edition. *Gut* 2003; 52 (Suppl V): V1–V15. Available at www.ncbi.nlm.nih.gov/pmc/articles/PMC1867765/pdf/v052p000v1.pdf.
- Watson A *et al* (2005) *Guidelines for the Diagnosis and Management of Barrett's Columnar-lined oesophagus.* [Online] British Society of Gastroenterology. Available at: www.bsg.org.uk/images/stories/docs/clinical/guidelines/oesophageal/Barretts_Oes.pdf.
- World Gastroenterology Organisation (2011) World Gastroenterology Organisation Practice Guidelines: Constipation Available at: www.worldgastroenterology.org/assets/downloads/en/pdf/guidelines/05_constipation.pdf.

Chapter 7
Clinical examinations

Overview

In the clinical examination station the candidate's clinical acumen is evaluated under the stressful exam conditions and within very limited available time. Real patients or actors simulating surgical diseases are presented and the examiners are assessing the trainees with reference to a number of criteria: professionalism; rapport; polite and sympathetic manners; organised approach to a diagnostic problem; methodical and reproducible examination skills; and sound medical knowledge, relevant to common surgical pathology. A correct diagnosis is not the ultimate objective *per se*, but if it results from an organised and methodical clinical examination, it certainly leads to top marks!

In this chapter we list a thorough step-by-step guide to facilitate examination of the main organ systems, providing key information that supports the methodology of examination. Also provided are common topics of anatomy, surgical pathology, history taking and applied surgical science, relevant to the systems examined, with the underpinning evidence. These have been included for purposes of relevance and continuity of information but also because there may be similar opportunities for questions at the end of a clinical session on the exam day!

During the preparation period, as a candidate, you need to master a routine sequence of clinical tests for each system and follow it unfailingly. The importance of exercising this routine in everyday practice at work, in the emergency department or outpatient clinics, cannot be overemphasised. Practising in small groups of trainees on real patients who are willing to offer you some of their time, can be useful, as it can reproduce some of the stressful circumstances of the exam day, and can prove enjoyable for the patients as well!

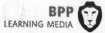

Arterial system

'Examine this patient's peripheral arterial system.'

History taking

- Assess for risk factors: Age, smoking, hypertension, diabetes, hyperlipidaemia, obesity.
- Identify comorbidities: Ischaemic heart disease, cerebrovascular ischaemia, abdominal aortic aneurysm, impotence, previous thromboembolic episodes, trauma, and Buerger's disease. Include previous cardiovascular surgery.
- Determine chronic symptoms: Pain (intermittent claudication, rest or nocturnal pain), skin ulceration, gangrene.
- Determine the localisation of pain (buttock, thigh, or calf muscles in claudication, forefoot in rest pain) and the severity of claudication by assessing the limitation of walking (march distance).
- Enquire about other neurological symptoms, such as paraesthesiae or numbness.
- Evaluate how symptoms affect the patient's quality of life.

Clinical examination

- Inspect and comment on any obvious general clinical signs (dyspnoea, cyanosis), operations (amputations) and bed-side indicators of risk factors (oxygen masks, drips, inhalers etc). If not instructed to focus on a particular area (i.e. lower extremities), start with the hands and work your way to the head, torso and then lower limbs.
- Hands: Inspect and palpate the patient's hands looking for nicotine staining, clubbing or digital ischaemia, estimating the temperature and capillary refill time (normal ≤ 2 seconds). Feel the radial pulse (lateral to the flexor carpi radialis tendon), describe its features (rate, rhythm, volume) and assess for radio-radial delay (coarctation or dissection of the aorta).
- Upper limb: Palpate the brachial pulse; for the right arm, support the patient's forearm in your left hand, with the patient's upper arm abducted, the elbow slightly flexed, and the forearm externally rotated; curl your right hand over the anterior aspect of the elbow to palpate along the course of the artery *just medial to the biceps tendon and lateral to the medial epicondyle of the humerus*. State you would check the arterial blood pressure.
- Face: Inspect for xanthelasmata on the eyelids and corneal arcus in the eyes (hyperlipidaemia).
- Neck
  - Inspect for scars of carotid surgery (along the anterior border of the sternocleidomastoid muscle) and assess the jugular vein pressure.
  - Auscultate both common carotids for bruits (behind and medial to the sternocleidomastoid muscle) and if present, auscultate the precordium to exclude transmission of an aortic stenosis murmur.
  - Gently palpate alternate carotid pulses (between sternocleidomastoid muscle and thyroid cartilage of the larynx by pressing against the prevertebral muscles posteriorly).
- Precordium: Inspect the chest looking for sternotomy or other scars, pacemaker boxes, obvious deformities or visible pulsation and offer to examine the cardiorespiratory system.
- Abdomen
  - Expose the patient as per any abdominal examination (see relevant section later).
  - Inspect for scars: a midline or transverse abdominal incision could indicate open abdominal aortic aneurysm (AAA) repair; a transverse iliac fossa incision combined with a groin incision is used for ilio-femoral bypass; bilateral groin incisions for endovascular repair of AAA or femoral-femoral crossover.

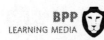

- Ask the patient to keep a deep breath and inspect for any visible abdominal pulsation.
- Palpate the abdomen as for any abdominal examination, focusing on deep palpation of the epigastrium for AAA, having warned the patient of the potential discomfort; if there is a pulsatile mass, then assess its expansibility, by placing your hands laterally on either side of the abdomen and move them progressively more medially, until the expansile pulsation is felt in the radial aspect of your index fingers. If an abdominal aortic aneurysm is palpated, above umbilicus as the aortic bifurcation occurs at L2 level, then determine its extension cephalad by assessing its superior border or to the iliac arteries by palpating the iliac fossae bilaterally for pulsatile masses.
- Auscultate the abdomen for bruits of the aorta (in the midline above the umbilicus), bilateral renal arteries (5cm away from the umbilicus at 10 and 2 o'clock positions), iliac arteries (in both lower quadrants) and femoral arteries (see below).
- Palpate for the femoral pulse bilaterally, assess for femoro-femoral and radio-femoral delay.

- Lower limbs: If instructed to examine the arterial system of the lower limbs, start from the abdomen as described above, and then proceed to the legs.
  - Inspect for lower limb scars: groin and medial thigh or knee longitudinal incisions are used for femoro-popliteal bypass, possibly with a saphenous vein harvest scar; these will invariably be present on legs of amputees as well, indicating previous attempts for revascularisation.
  - Comment on the skin colour (pallor or cyanosis with severe chronic ischemia). Gangrenous tissue appears permanently blue or black.
  - Look for ulceration or gangrene (dry/wet), inspecting the pressure points, heels, plantar surfaces and between ALL toes.
  - Determine the Buerger's angle (Buerger's test). With the patient supine, gradually raise and support both straight legs assessing the angle at which the legs (soles) become pale. Hold the legs in the air for a few seconds and ask the patient to swing around and suspend the legs off the side of the bed. Determine the time taken to regain colour; erythematous legs suggest reactive hyperaemia (compare sides) and indicate significant ischaemia of the lower limb.
  - Palpate the limbs assessing the temperature and capillary refill of the toes comparing both sides (normal ≤ 2 seconds).
  - Palpate both femoral pulses (below the inguinal ligament at midinguinal point), assessing for femoro-femoral and radio-femoral delay.
  - Palpate each popliteal pulse, by either keeping the knees extended at resting position or by flexing the knee to 120°; place both hands around the top of the calf, thumbs on the tibial tuberosity, and pull the pulps of the fingers against the proximal posterior tibia.
  - Palpate both posterior tibial arteries simultaneously, just behind the medial malleolus.
  - Palpate both dorsalis pedis pulses, lateral to the extensor hallucis tendon.
  - Auscultate the femoral arteries (midinguinal point) and the superficial femoral arteries (at a point two thirds down a line extending between the anterior superior iliac spine and medial knee joint) for bruits indicating luminal stenosis.
  - Calculate the Ankle-Brachial Pressure Index (ABPI).
  Using a Doppler probe, identify the pedal (dorsalis pedis and posterior tibial) and brachial pulses and measure the systolic (closing) pressures.
  ABPI = Systolic pressure of pedal artery / systolic pressure of brachial artery
  If different values obtained for each pedal artery, accept the highest value of two. Normal ranges between 0.9 and 1.1 (beware of diabetic patients who can have false high ABPI because of non compressible arteries). Intermittent claudication is likely with ABPI < 0.9 and with values < 0.5 significant ischaemia and rest pain is possible.
- Offer to perform neurological examination.

Surgical pathology

Abdominal aortic aneurysm

Aortic aneurysm is a permanent abnormal dilatation of the aorta by more than 50% of its normal diameter (> 3.0 cm). They can be classified as true or false (pseudoaneurysms). True aneurysms involve all three layers of the artery (intima, media and adventitia), while false aneurysms are collections of blood connecting with the lumen of the vessel.

Epidemiology

The most common abdominal aortic aneurysms are true aneurysms (90%). Their incidence increases with age and AAA rupture accounts for 10,000 deaths per year in the UK.

Aetiology

It is multi-factorial; genetic (familial clustering in 15–25% of cases), degenerative, inflammatory, mechanical, congenital and rarely as sequelae of Marfan syndrome, Ehlers-Danlos syndrome, Behçet disease, syphilis or long-term aortic dissection.

Clinical manifestations

The majority (75%) are asymptomatic.

The manifestations vary and may be secondary to:

- Compression on adjacent organs: Dysphagia, ureteric obstruction.
- Inflammation: Back pain and increased inflammatory markers.
- Rupture: Abdominal, back, flank or groin pain, syncope, unexplained hypotension, hypovolaemic shock.
- Fistulation into intestinal lumen: Massive gastrointestinal bleeding.
- Fistulation into inferior vena cava (shunting): Tachycardia, lower limb ischaemia and venous congestion, heart failure.
- Embolism from a mural thrombus: Acute lower limb ischaemia.

Diagnostic work up

- B-mode ultrasound scan (to detect and measure size),
- CT aorta (to detail the morphology).

Management

It depends on the size and symptoms of the aneurysm.

- Ruptured aneurysms: Immediate repair if comorbidities and physiological state of patient at presentation allow (mortality > 40%).
- Asymptomatic aneurysms: The risk of rupture is weighed against the perioperative risk of repair. Rupture risk appears to be directly related to aneurysm size as predicted by Laplace's law (Table 7.1).

The UK Small Aneurysm trial was a randomised multicentre controlled trial across 93 UK hospitals investigating the optimum management of small aortic aneurysms – early elective open surgery versus regular ultrasound surveillance. It demonstrated that small aneurysms (< 5.5cm) can be monitored safely under surveillance until they become 5.5cm, tender or grow by > 1cm/year.

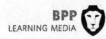

Diameter of aorta (cm)	Estimated annual risk of rupture (%)	Estimated five-year risk of rupture (%)
2–3	0	0 (unless AAA develops)
4–5	1	5–10
5–6	2–5	30–40
6–7	3–10	> 50
>7	>10	Approaching 100

Table 7.1. Annual risk of rupture of AAA based on maximum transverse diameter

Surgical options

Open repair

Procedure: Midline or transverse abdominal incision is employed. Small intestine and transverse colon are retracted to expose the retroperitoneum which is accessed, followed by isolation of both proximal and distal segments of the AAA. IV heparin is given, followed by clamping of the proximal and distal segments of the aneurysm. The aneurysm sac is opened and a prosthetic graft (tube or bifurcated) is used to reconstruct the aorta. The overlying aneurysm sac and the retroperitoneum are closed to cover the prosthetic graft and minimise potential exposure to bowel (fistula formation). The intestines are returned to the abdominal cavity followed by the closure of the abdominal fascia and skin.

Advantages	Risks
• No risk of recurrence or delayed rupture • No long-term imaging surveillance • Direct assessment of the circulatory integrity of the colon is possible • Explore for other abdominal pathologies	• Cardiac complications, myocardial infarction or arrhythmias (2–6%) • Renal failure or transient renal insufficiency (< 2%) • Ischemic colitis (5%, but higher in patients with a prior colon resection) • Graft infection (1–4%) • Intestinal adhesions, bowel erosion and aorto-enteric fistula

Table 7.2. Advantages and risks of open repair of AAA

Endovascular stenting

Procedure: An aortic stent graft is fixed proximally and distally to the non-aneurysmal aortoiliac segment, excluding the aneurysm from the circulation. Both common femoral arteries are accessed surgically or percutaneously. The renal arteries are located by angiography and the main body of the stent is inserted and deployed just below their level; the position of the internal iliac arteries is defined and the iliac limbs inserted just above the internal iliac ostia. Angiography is performed to confirm flow through the graft and exclusion of the aneurysm sac.

A percentage 30–40% of patients are not good candidates for endovascular repair, because of young age (<60 years – there is data on long-term durability); short (< 1.0 cm), conical or severely angulated proximal neck (the segment between the lowest renal artery and the sac); significant thrombus within the proximal neck; severe iliac disease with extensive strictures or severe tortuosity.

Advantages	Risks
• Minimally invasive • Short hospital stay • No need for ITU • Better for patients with COPD, less GI complications or herniae • Regional or epidural anaesthesia can be used, avoiding the risks associated with general anaesthesia in patients with severe cardiopulmonary dysfunction.	• Endoleak: Blood flow persists outside the lumen of the endoluminal graft but within an aneurysm sac due to incomplete stent graft exclusion of the aneurysm (up to 24%) • Rupture rate following an endovascular AAA repair < 0.8% • Stent graft thrombosis • Renal artery occlusion, due to improper stent graft positioning or migration • Graft limb separation or dislocation • Pelvic ischemia (buttock claudication, impotence, gluteal skin sloughing, and colonic ischemia) in patients who undergo preoperative coil embolisation of the internal iliac artery (prevalence 20 to 45%) • Groin haematoma and wound infection • Conversion to open

Table 7.3. Advantages and risks of endovascular repair of AAA

Types of endoleaks

- Type I: Attachment site leak
- Type II: Side branch leak caused by lumbar or inferior mesenteric artery
- Type III: Junctional leak (of overlapping endograft components)
- Type IV: Endograft fabric or porosity leak
- Type V: 'Endotension' or increasing aneurysm size without a visible leak

Evidence supporting endovascular repair

- The EVAR-1 study was a multicentre randomised trial comparing open to endoluminal repair on 1,082 patients at 34 centres in the United Kingdom using all available devices. Short-term mortality at 30 days was 4.7% in the open and 1.7% in the endoluminal group. The in-hospital mortality rate was also increased in the open when compared to the endoluminal group (6.2 to 2.1%).
- The EVAR-2 study was a multicentre randomised trial investigating whether EVAR improves survival compared to no intervention in patients unfit for open repair on 338 patients of 60 years or over with aneurysms of 5.5cm and above. EVAR had a considerable 30-day operative mortality (9%) with significant difference from the no intervention group. EVAR did not improve survival and was associated with a need for continued surveillance and re-intervention and increased costs.
- IMPROVE Trial – Immediate Management of the Patient with Rupture: Open Versus Endovascular repair: this is a multicentre randomised controlled trial comparing mortality from ruptured aneurysm in patients treated by endovascular or conventional open technique (in progress).

NHS Abdominal Aortic Aneurysm Screening programme

This commenced rolling out across the UK in 2009, with full implementation planned for 2013. The programme plans to invite men for ultrasound screening the year they turn 65. Men over the age of 65 can self refer to the programme providing they have not previously been diagnosed with an AAA.

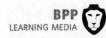

Acute limb ischaemia

Acute limb ischaemia refers to the sudden loss of limb perfusion commonly within two weeks of an initiating event.

Aetiology

Common causes include embolism, native vessel thrombosis, reconstruction thrombosis, trauma, and complications of proximal aneurysm.

The origin of emboli can be:

- Heart: in > 90% of embolic events, in atrial fibrillation, after cardioversion, from a mural thrombus overlying a myocardial infarction, within a dilated left ventricular aneurysm or cardiomyopathy, from diseased valves of rheumatic aetiology or bacterial endocarditis.
- Proximal aortic aneurysm.
- Deep venous thrombosis via a right-to-left communication (paradoxical embolus).

Arterial thrombosis is associated with hypercoagulable states (malignancy, polycythaemia, thrombocythaemia, factor V Leiden deficiency / deficiency of protein C or protein S / lupus anticoagulant).

Clinical manifestation

Classically, the '6 Ps': Pain, Pallor, Paraesthesiae, Paralysis, Pulselessness, Perishing cold limb.

Classification of severity

The management of ischaemic limb depends on the classification of severity and evaluation of limb viability according to the parameters shown in Table 7.4.

Classification	Viable	Threatened	Irreversible ischemia
	Not immediately threatened	Salvageable if promptly treated	Major tissue loss, amputation unavoidable
Capillary return	Intact	Intact, slow	Absent (marbling)
Muscle weakness	None	Mild, partial	Profound, paralysis (rigor)
Sensory loss	None	Mild, incomplete	Profound anaesthetic
Arteriovenous Doppler	Audible	Inaudible or audible	Inaudible

Table 7.4. Severity of limb ischaemia and viability

Management

- Investigations should be guided by the patient's clinical condition and access to resources, avoiding unnecessary delays.
- Expedient anticoagulation is necessary using intravenous heparin to prevent propagation of the clot into unaffected vascular beds.
- IV fluids, urinary catheter to monitor urine output, baseline blood tests including creatinine levels and hypercoagulable state work-up (before initiation of heparin, if there is sufficient suspicion of thrombosis).
- Arteriography, if feasible in a timely fashion, localises obstructions and helps determine the indicated type of intervention.

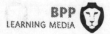

Intervention options

- Surgical embolectomy (can be performed under local or general anaesthesia): The groin is opened through a vertical or longitudinal incision, exposing the common femoral artery and its bifurcation. The artery is clamped and opened transversely over the bifurcation. Thrombus is extracted by passing a Fogarty balloon embolectomy catheter until satisfactory back-bleeding and antegrade bleeding is achieved. Embolic material often forms a cast of the vessel and is sent for culture and histologic examination. Completion angiography is advisable to ascertain the adequacy of clot removal. The arteriotomy is then closed and the patient fully anticoagulated.
- Bypass graft thrombectomy, revision or replacement for thrombosis of prosthetic bypass grafts with / without fasciotomy to circumvent reperfusion injury or compartment syndrome.
- Endovascular thrombolysis, especially for small vessel occlusion, unless contraindicated. (Contraindications: stroke, intracranial primary malignancy, brain metastases, intracranial surgical intervention, renal insufficiency, allergy to contrast material, cardiac thrombus, diabetic retinopathy, coagulopathy and recent arterial puncture or surgery.)

Complications of arterial revascularisation

These include compartment syndrome, ischaemic neuropathy, muscle necrosis, recurrent thrombosis, lower leg oedema and reperfusion syndrome (hypotension, hyperkalaemia, myoglobinuria and renal failure).

Acute compartment syndrome – lower limb

Definition

Acute increase of pressure within an unyielding osteofascial compartment, above the intravascular pressure resulting in capillary bed occlusion and tissue necrosis.

Aetiology

Common causes for compartment syndrome of the lower limb include trauma, revascularisation procedures, burns and exercise.

Clinical manifestations

Salient features include the presence of excessive limb pain, out of proportion to any injury and aggravated by passive muscle stretching, together with sensory loss due to nerve compression of the nerves coursing though the compartment (see Anatomy and contents of compartments of the leg in Table 7.5). The anterior compartment is most commonly affected, in which case numbness in the web space between the first and second toes is noted from compression of the deep peroneal nerve.

Investigations

Compartment pressure is measured by inserting an arterial line into the compartment and recording the pressure (> 20 mmHg is an indication for fasciotomy.)

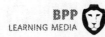

	Anterior	Lateral	Superficial posterior	Deep posterior
Muscles	Tibialis anterior Extensor digitorum longus Peroneus tertius Extensor hallucis longus Extensor digitorum brevis Extensor hallucis brevis	Peroneus longus Peroneus brevis	Gastrocnemius Plantaris Soleus	Tibialis posterior Flexor digitorum longus Flexor hallucis longus
Arteries	Anterior tibial artery	Anterior and posterior tibial branches of the popliteal artery		Posterior tibial artery Peroneal artery
Nerves	Deep peroneal nerve	Superficial peroneal nerve		Tibial nerve

Table 7.5. Anatomy and contents of the compartments of the leg

Management

It is a surgical emergency (CEPOD category 1) and requires

- Surgical release of compartment pressure by fasciotomies, debridement of necrotic muscle.
- Aggressive patient monitoring watching for rhabdomyolysis; it is necessary to monitor serum myoglobin, creatinine (risk of acute tubular necrosis and acute renal failure).
- Vigorous fluid resuscitation to maintain renal function, if required by forced saline diuresis, and alkalinisation of urine.

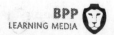

Chronic limb ischaemia

Definitions

- Chronic limb ischaemia is objectively proven lower extremity arterial occlusive disease and symptoms lasting for more than two weeks.
- Critical limb ischaemia is persistently recurring rest pain requiring analgesia for more than two weeks, or ulceration or gangrene of the foot in the presence of an ankle systolic pressure less than 50 mmHg or a toe pressure less than 30 mmHg in diabetic patients. (*The European Consensus Document*, 1989)

Clinical manifestations

The symptoms depend on the severity of ischaemia, as classified by Fontaine (Table 7.6).

Stage	Clinical
I	Asymptomatic
IIa	Mild claudication (at longer than 200 metres)
IIb	Moderate to severe claudication (at less than 200 metres)
III	Ischaemic rest pain
IV	Ulceration or gangrene

Table 7.6. Fontaine classification of chronic limb ischaemia

Aetiology

- Atherosclerosis (risk factors: smoking, diabetes mellitus, increasing age, family history, hyperlipidaemia, hypertension, raised level of homocysteine in serum, male sex).
- Thrombosis/emboli.
- Arteritis/vasculitis: Buerger's (thromboangitis obliterans), scleroderma, systemic lupus erythematosus, Takayasu's arteritis.
- Congenital anomalies: Persistence of the embryological sciatic artery, entrapment of popliteal artery (which lies medial to and not between the heads of the gastrocnemius, and is compressed by knee flexion); cystic adventitial disease (cysts develop in the adventitia of the artery causing intraluminal compression).
- Fibrosis: Fibromuscular dysplasia, retroperitoneal fibrosis or radiotherapy.
- Trauma, blunt and penetrating: Fractures and joint dislocations of the long bones are the most common causes.

Management

Conservative treatment

It involves risk factor modification, including smoking cessation, exercise, blood pressure control, good glycemic and lipid control, antiplatelet therapy with aspirin and selectively, oral prostanoids (misoprostol).

Operative intervention

Surgical interventions include revascularisation or amputation.

- Revascularisation
  For medically fit patients keen to undergo revascularisation, arteriography is performed for further evaluation and planning of revascularisation. At some centres, magnetic resonance angiography (MRA) is used as an alternative or supplement to arteriography to minimise the risk of dye exposure.

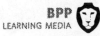

- *Angioplasty* or *stent placement* or *both*, is most successful with short, proximal lesions, such as those in patients with claudication.
- In critical limb ischemia with multilevel nature of the arterial occlusive disease *bypass surgery* is indicated, using either greater saphenous vein or prosthetic conduit.
- Primary amputation
  It may be indicated in certain patients, such as those with extensive tissue necrosis, life-threatening infection or lesions not amenable to revascularisation. The level of amputation should be one that has the greatest likelihood of healing while giving the patient the maximal chance for functional rehabilitation.

Decision-making

The choice of appropriate treatment depends on careful consideration of the relevant risks and benefits for patient health but also importantly on patient preference.

Carotid artery disease

Carotid artery disease refers to atherosclerotic stenosis of the carotid artery, which is a potentially treatable cause of:

- Ischaemic stroke: A focal or global loss of cerebral function of vascular aetiology lasting more than 24 hours.
- Transient ischaemic attack: A focal or global loss of cerebral function of vascular aetiology lasting less than 24 hours.
- Retinal infarction.

Epidemiology

About 150,000 new strokes occur in the UK each year. A patient with an asymptomatic 50% carotid stenosis has 1–2% per year risk of a stroke, which increases with the degree of stenosis and even further with the onset of symptoms. Once an ischaemic stroke has occurred the risk of further stroke is ~10% in the first year and ~5% in subsequent years.

Assessment of carotid artery stenosis

- Clinically: Carotid bruits are an unreliable guide to severity of stenosis.
- Imaging of the carotid arteries (see Table 7.7).

Diagnostic modality	Sensitivity*	Specificity*	
Duplex ultrasound	89%	84%	Allows assessment of flow at stenosis and imaging of arterial anatomy
CT angiography	77%	95%	
MR angiography	88%	84%	
Contrast-enhanced MR angiography	94%	93%	
Intra-arterial carotid angiography			1-2% risk of procedural stroke

* They refer to sensitivity and specificity of the method to diagnose stenosis 70–99%.

Table 7.7. Diagnostic methods assessing carotid artery stenosis

Management of carotid artery disease
- Medical management, including:
  - Stop smoking.
  - Pharmacological treatment of hypertension and diabetes.

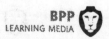

- Control of atrial fibrillation.
- Lipid-lowering agents.
- Antiplatelet therapy: Aspirin 75–150mg daily (dipyridamole, ticlopidine and clopidogrel are alternatives). It should be started once ischaemic stroke confirmed by CT and to patients with asymptomatic stenoses.
- Carotid endarterectomy: The common, internal and external carotid arteries are clamped and the plaque removed through a small arteriotomy. A shunt can be used to ensure cerebral blood supply during the procedure. Complications include bleeding / haematoma, stroke, hypoglossal nerve damage, hyperperfusion syndrome.

Evidence on management of carotid artery disease with carotid endarterectomy (CEA)

Symptomatic patients

The Carotid Endarterectomy Trialists' Collaboration (CETC) combined individual data from over 6,000 patients randomised in the ECST, NASCET and Veterans' Administration (VA) trials and concluded that for:

- Stenosis 70–99%: Maximum benefit is seen from surgery in significantly reducing the five-year risk of ipsilateral stroke (absolute risk reduction, ARR = 15.8%) and any stroke (ARR = 15.6%).
- Stenosis < 50%: Surgery conferred no significant benefit.
- Stenosis 50–69%: Small but significant benefit conferred by surgery in reducing the five-year risk of any stroke (ARR 7.8%) and ipsilateral stroke (ARR 4.6%).
- Near occlusion stenosis (string sign): No benefit from carotid endarterectomy (CEA).

Asymptomatic patients

- Asymptomatic Carotid Atherosclerosis Study (ACAS): 1,662 patients with more than 60% reduction in luminal diameter, randomised to either endarterectomy with medical treatment (aspirin 300 mg) or medical treatment alone. The study showed that the risk of ipsilateral stroke over a five-year period was reduced (5% v 11%) in the surgery group, but 2.3% had a stroke within 30 days of surgery (0.4% in the medical group).
- Asymptomatic Carotid Surgery Trial (ACST): 3,120 patients with more than 60% reduction in luminal diameter, randomised to either immediate or deferred carotid surgery. The results indicated that:
  - Risk of stroke within 30 days of surgery was 3.1%.
  - Risk of stroke over five-year period was reduced (6% v 11%) in surgery group.
  - Patients aged > 75 years do not gain significant benefit from CEA.

Evidence on percutaneous transluminal angioplasty and stenting (Carotid Artery Stenting, CAS)

- Cochrane review of 12 trials (2007): CAS is not superior to carotid endarterectomy, which remains the treatment of choice for suitable patients with carotid artery stenosis.
- International Carotid Stenting Study (ICSS) (2009): Multicentre trial, randomising 1,713 patients with symptomatic carotid stenosis > 50% to either carotid endarterectomy (CEA) or carotid artery stenting (CAS). The results showed that CEA is safer than CAS. (Prevalence of any stroke, death or peri-operative myocardial infarction, 8.5% for CAS v 5.1% for CEA.)

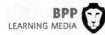

Venous system

'Examine this patient's lower limb venous system.'

History taking

Take a short history, focusing on:

- Presenting symptoms, effects on quality of life.
- Family history, obesity, pregnancy, use of oral contraceptive pill, occupation.
- Comorbidities, fitness for surgery.

Clinical examination

- Examine the patient in standing position and inspect for:
  - Obvious varicose veins, along the course of the long and short saphenous veins (see anatomy of superficial veins-to follow).
  - Inflammatory skin changes over the course of veins (superficial thrombophlebitis, i.e. sterile inflammation of the vein wall due to local thrombosis).
  - Skin changes indicating chronic venous disease, mainly over the 'gaiter area' (lower third of the leg circumference) and most commonly medially: Haemosiderin deposition (from degraded extravasated erythrocytes), eczema, oedema, lipodermatosclerosis (diffuse fibrosis of subcutaneous tissues, accentuated by chronic inflammatory changes), venous ulceration, 'atrophy blanche' (white scarring after healing ulcers).
- Palpate the varicose veins.
  - Determine whether they are firm, warm or tender (superficial thrombophlebitis).
  - Assess for presence of sapheno varix (varicosity at the saphenofemoral junction (SFJ), presenting as a compressible lump, reducible on supine position, with a cough 'thrill').
  - Perform the 'tapping test': If tapping the varicose veins proximally transmits a palpable thrill distally, this indicates valvular insufficiency along the course of the long saphenous vein.
  - Perform the Trendelenburg test, assessing for saphenofemoral incompetence. The patient lies down and the examined leg is raised to empty the veins. Exert pressure with fingers over the saphenofemoral junction and ask the patient to stand up while maintaining the pressure. If the veins do not fill immediately, but fill after release of finger pressure, this indicates incompetence of the SFJ only.
  - Tourniquet test: A variation of the Trendelenburg test that can assess different levels for saphenofemoral incompetence. Instead of controlling the SFJ by finger compression, a tourniquet is applied around the upper thigh to prevent saphenofemoral reflux. If the veins do not fill, this indicates that SFJ is the site of incompetence. If the veins do fill, we cannot comment on the SFJ, but there is definitely incompetence more distally. Thus the test is repeated at different levels below to identify more sites of valvular incompetence between the superficial and deep venous system.
  - Doppler examination: Identify the femoral artery and then move the probe inferomedially over the SFJ. Squeeze the calf which increases venous return with accompanying 'whooosh' sound on the Doppler. If this is followed by a sharp, short 'whosh' sound, this suggests a competent SFJ valve. If there is a prolonged second 'whooosh' this suggests regurgitation and therefore incompetence. This can be applied at the level of saphenopopliteal junction (SSPJ, lateral to the popliteal artery in the popliteal fossa) to assess for short saphenopopliteal valve incompetence. It is however more difficult to identify the SSPJ, as the short saphenous vein joins the popliteal at variable levels.
  - Evaluation of SFJ and SSPJ valvular incompetence and more accurate characterisation of varicose veins is achieved by duplex ultrasound scan.

- Complete the examination by offering examination of the arterial system and abdomen (to exclude intra-abdominal causes of peripheral venous hypertension).

Surgical pathology

Varicose veins

Varicose veins are abnormal tortuous dilated superficial veins.

Epidemiology

The incidence increases with age, equally common between the sexes, but female patients seek medical help more often.

Risk factors

Caucasian race, family history of varicose veins, obesity, pregnancy, oral contraceptive pill, occupations requiring long periods of standing.

Aetiology

Varicose veins are caused by superficial venous hypertension due to:

- Incompetence of venous valves between the deep and superficial venous systems, most commonly at the sites of saphenofemoral junction (SFJ), saphenopopliteal junction (SPJ) and the perforators (primary varicose veins).
- Disturbance in venous blood flow proximally (secondary varicose veins), as in pelvic vein thrombosis, external compression by pelvic masses, arteriovenous malformations.

Clinical manifestations

Dull ache relieved by elevation, unsightly appearance, itching, peripheral oedema, bleeding, superficial thrombophlebitis and skin changes of chronic venous insufficiency (described previously).

Investigations

Duplex ultrasound scan to determine the site of valvular incompetence, ensure patency of the deep venous system and exclude arteriovenous communication.

Management

Depends on symptoms and effect on quality of life.

- Conservative: Graduated compression stockings, leg elevation, exercise and avoidance of prolonged sitting or standing.
- Invasive, non-operative: Foam sclerotherapy, radiofrequency or photocoagulation (Laser) ablation (under local anaesthesia).
- Invasive, operative (under general anaesthesia): Varicose vein surgery is reserved for symptomatic patients with skin complications. It can involve ligation of the vein (long or short saphenous) near the site of incompetence and excision (for the long saphenous) by stripping through small skin incisions to reduce the risk of recurrence. Varicose veins can be avulsed through small stab incisions (phlebectomies), followed by compression bandaging.

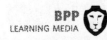

Complications of varicose vein surgery: Bleeding, femoral vein damage, bruising, healing fibrosis, wound infection (1%), temporary or permanent neuropraxia (causing skin numbness in 5–10% of patients), damage of the saphenous nerve (more common if LSV is stripped below the knee level) and of the sural nerve (during ligation of the short saphenous vein), recurrence (20% risk within five years).

Anatomy of the superficial veins of the lower limb

Long saphenous vein

It forms from the medial side of the dorsal venous arch of the foot, runs immediately in front of the medical malleolus at the ankle, closely to the saphenous nerve. At the knee, the vein passes a hand-breadth behind the patella, continues along the anteromedial aspect of the thigh and terminates at the groin, where it pierces the deep fascia of the thigh to enter the femoral vein. The surface marking of the saphenofemoral junction corresponds to a point a finger-breadth medial to the femoral pulse immediately distal to the skin crease of the groin.

Tributaries

* Just below the knee: Large anterior and posterior tributaries that receive perforators from the deep veins.
* In the thigh: Numerous tributaries, including a large perforator in the lower one-third of the thigh that communicates with the femoral vein in the subsartorial canal. Also the posteromedial and anterolateral veins of the thigh, 5–15cm below the groin.
* At the groin: Superficial external pudendal, superficial inferior epigastric, superficial circumflex iliac and thoracoepigastric veins (the latter connects the femoral vein with the lateral thoracic tributary of the axillary vein, a collateral pathway in IVC obstruction).

Short saphenous vein

From the lateral side of the foot it passes posterior to the lateral malleolus, continues lateral to the tendo calcaneus and then to the midline, ascending to the popliteal fossa, where it pierces the deep fascia to enter the popliteal vein, at a variable level.

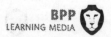

Breast examination

This is likely to be a patient with breast lump or post breast surgery.

History taking

Take a short history focusing on:

- Current presenting symptoms, local and general.
- Age.
- Family history of breast disease.
- Comorbidities, current medication, (assess fitness for surgery).
- Menstrual history (age of menarche, date of last menstrual period, hysterectomy and indications, menopause).
- Current or past use of oral contraception and hormonal replacement therapy.
- Parity, breast feeding, duration.
- Smoking.
- Past history of breast problems, previous surgery and investigations.

Clinical examination

- Establish rapport and take consent.
- Ensure patient comfort and privacy and secure the presence of a chaperone.
- Use antiseptic hand gel.
- Patient should lie on the examination couch, with the top half of the body exposed and raised at 45° to the legs.
- Inspect from the front for:
  - Symmetry of the breasts.
  - Signs of breast cancer-related treatment, such as
    - Surgical scars on the breasts, axillae, trunk and back (reconstruction surgery).
    - Signs of radiotherapy to the anterior chest wall, such as India ink marks, skin discolouration, telangiectasiae.
  - Skin abnormalities, such as puckering, peau d'orange (oedema because of invasion of cancer cells into breast lymphatics), nodules, ulceration.
  - Nipple abnormalities, such as retraction or inversion, discolouration, deviation, obvious discharge or duplication (accessory nipples). Also, look for erythema, encrusted and oozy non-itchy skin resembling eczema that indicates Paget's disease of the nipple.
  - Visible upper limb lymphoedema, enlarged lymph nodes, distended veins.
- Ask patient to raise both arms above her head to accentuate skin puckering and reveal scars in the infra-mammary fold or intertrigo.
- Ask patient to press both arms against her waist in order to tense the pectoralis muscles and make a swelling more prominent.
- Palpate the normal breast first. Use the flat of the fingers, rotate patient so that the breast sits flat on chest wall and examine the nipple, areola, the four quadrants of the breast and the axillary tail. If a lump is detected, determine its features.
- Examine the axillae and supraclavicular fossae for lymphadenopathy. Palpate the right axilla with your left hand, using your right hand to support the patient's right arm in 90° abduction. Systematically palpate the four walls of the axilla and its apex for lymph nodes, which, if detected, should be described.
- Examine the abdominal system, respiratory system and spine for signs of metastatic disease.

Differential diagnosis of a breast lump

- Benign: Normal glandular tissue, hamartoma, cyst, fibroadenoma, tubular adenoma, intraductal papilloma, fibroadenosis, periductal mastitis, abscess.
- Malignant: Carcinoma.

Anatomy
Anatomy of the axilla

It is a schematically pyramidal region lying between the medial aspect of the upper arm and the lateral thoracic wall. It has an apex, a floor and four walls:

- Apex: This has a triangular bony boundary, formed anteriorly by the posterior surface of the clavicle, medially by the external surface of the 1st rib and posteriorly by the superior scapular border.
- Base: Skin, superficial fascia and a thick layer of the axillary fascia.
- Anterior wall: Pectoralis major, pectoralis minor, the subclavius muscle and clavipectoral fascia. The pectoralis major forms the anterior axillary fold.
- Posterior wall: Above by the subscapularis muscle and below by the teres major and latissimus dorsi muscles, which form the posterior axillary fold.
- Medial wall: The upper 4 ribs and serratus anterior muscle.
- Lateral wall: Humerus (the intertubercular sulcus in particular) and the tendon of the long head of biceps.
- Contents:
  - Axillary vessels (artery and vein).
  - The infraclavicular part of the brachial plexus.
  - The axillary lymph nodes (apical, central, anterior, posterior, lateral groups), also classified with respect to the pectoralis minor as level I (below), level II (behind) and level III (above).
  - Intercostobrachial nerve and some lateral branches of some intercostal nerves.
  - The axillary adipose tissues and areolar tissue.
  - The axillary tail of the breast.

Blood supply of the breast

- Perforating branches of the internal thoracic artery.
- Pectoral branch of the thoracoacromial artery.
- Lateral branches of the posterior intercostal artery.
- Lateral thoracic artery.

Lymphatic drainage of the breast

(This is particularly relevant to the surgical staging and management of breast cancer.)

The lymphatic vessels of the breast form two plexuses.

- Subareolar plexus of Sappey: drains into the axillary group of lymph nodes.
- Submammary lymphatic plexus.

The lymphatic drainage of the breast follows the blood supply and runs in two sets:

- The superficial lymphatics drain the skin of the breast except the nipple and areola.
- Deep lymphatics drain the parenchyma, stroma, the nipple and areola of the breast.

About 75% of the lymph of the breast drains to the axillary group of lymph nodes, 20% drains into the parasternal group (internal mammary nodes) and 5% into the posterior intercostal nodes. Finally, the lymph of one breast can also drain to the opposite breast.

Examination of the groin and scrotum

This could be a patient with a lump in the groin or a swelling extending to the scrotum (male).

History taking

Take a short history focusing on:

- Age.
- Occupation (involving abdominal muscle straining or weight lifting).
- Comorbidities predisposing to hernia (persistent coughing, prostatism or constipation).
- Local symptoms (swelling, pain, tenderness, discharges and skin changes).
- General symptoms (change in bowel habit, intestinal obstruction symptoms).
- Fitness for surgery.

Clinical examination of the groin

- Establish rapport and obtain verbal consent.
  Ensure patient comfort and privacy and use antiseptic hand gel.
- Expose the abdomen, groin and genitalia. Examine patient erect first.
- Inspect from the front for:
  - Scars from previous surgery in recurrent herniae (transverse / oblique inguinal scars/ laparoscopic port scars).
  - Sinuses (stitch sinus or mesh infection).
- If lump not apparent, ask patient to cough or to point to the area of tenderness, if any.
- If lump present, describe as per any lump: 'a 3cm × 5cm (size) ovoid (shape) swelling at the right groin (site) with no skin changes, scars or sinuses...'
- Palpate the lump from the side with the ipsilateral examining hand and the other hand supporting patient's back, describing the palpable features of the swelling: '...it is soft in consistency, non tender, has normal temperature, smooth surface and well defined edges, and is compressible and non-pulsatile. It is originating from under the skin (layer of origin), and is not fixed or tethered to it (the skin moves easily above it and does not pucker)...'
- Demonstrate relation of the lump to important surface landmarks: anterior superior iliac spine (ASIS), pubic symphysis and inguinal ligament.
- Demonstrate expansile cough impulse (lump increases in size with cough and not just moves) which is the pathognomonic sign of a hernia.
- Palpate the scrotum (male) from the front to assess expansion to scrotum (inguinoscrotal hernia) or demonstrate dual pathology. A hernia should be separate from the testis, its superior border would not be felt ('not possible to get above it') and it would not normally transilluminate, unless it contained colon distended with air (see '*Examination of the scrotum*' below).
- Establish from history whether the lump is normally reducible and if so, position the patient supine and ask him to reduce it himself. Re-demonstrate the landmarks: ASIS, pubic tubercle (2–3cm lateral to the pubic symphysis or at the origin of the adductor longus tendon), inguinal ligament, the superficial and deep inguinal ring (above the midpoint of the inguinal ligament).
- The point through which the hernia reduces determines the type of hernia: an inguinal hernia reduces through a point above and medial to the pubic tubercle whereas a femoral hernia below and lateral to it.
- Once the hernia is reduced, attempt to control it by placing two fingers on the deep inguinal ring. If the hernia is held reduced while the patient coughs or stands up, it is probably an indirect inguinal hernia; if not, it is probably a direct hernia.

- Finally, watch the hernia reappear during patient coughing to reconfirm the findings.
- The hernia can then be auscultated, percussed or transilluminated to attempt determine its contents.
- Examine the contralateral side.
- Perform examination of the abdomen (assess intra-abdominal pathology that would predispose to hernia, ie masses, ascites), rectum (prostate) and cardiorespiratory systems (fitness for surgery).
- Summarise the findings and state the diagnosis.

Clinical examination of the scrotum

The examination of the scrotum can be part of the examination of the abdomen and groin and vice versa.

- Examine the patient supine or standing.
- Inspect groin and scrotum, looking for incision scars, sinuses, swellings.
- You should note that scrotal incisions may be difficult to see as they are made in the median raphe in between the two hemiscrotums.
- Palpate both testes, one at a time. Examine the normal contour; identify the epididymis and ductus deferens. The surface of testis is firm and regular and any lumps or irregularity are abnormal.
- If a scrotal swelling is present, you have to answer four questions in order to successfully characterise it:
  - Is it tender?
  - Is it separate from the testis?
  - Can you get above it (or otherwise, can you feel the superior border)?
  - Does it transilluminate?
- Finally, percuss (if lump does not look inflamed) and auscultate (listen for bowel sounds in suspected hernia containing bowel loops).
- Continue to examine the rest of the abdomen and groin, if not done already.

Examine the inguinal lymph nodes (this is relevant to problems of the scrotal skin and penis and not of the testes; the testicular lymph drainage occurs to the para-aortic lymph nodes).

Surgical pathology

Differential diagnosis of lump in the groin

(Think structures and layers of origin.) Lipoma, inguinal hernia, femoral hernia, vaginal hydrocele, hydrocele of the cord or the canal of Nuck, lipoma of the cord, undescended testis, lymphadenopathy, sapheno varix, femoral artery aneurysm, psoas abscess.

Abdominal wall hernia refers to the protrusion of an organ or contents of the abdominal cavity through its containing wall; it consists of the *sac* and its *content*s, protruding through the narrowest part of the sac, the *neck*.

Risk factors for abdominal wall hernia

- Congenital: Fetal hydrops, ambiguous genitalia, urethral abnormalities, extrophy of bladder, cryptorchidism.
- Birth-related: Prematurity, low birth weight.
- Hereditary: Muccopolysaccharidoses, cystic fibrosis, connective tissue disorders.
- Increased abdominal pressure: Liver disease with ascites, continuous ambulatory peritoneal dialysis, prostatism, constipation, strenuous exercise, abdominal aortic aneurysm.

Classification

- Types of abdominal wall hernia, classified according to anatomical position of the neck (in order of frequency in adults):
  - Common – inguinal, umbilical and paraumbilical, incisional, femoral, epigastric herniae.
  - Rare – spigelian, obturator, lumbar and gluteal herniae.
- Classification of abdominal wall herniae according to reducibility:
  - Reducible – hernia contents return to peritoneal cavity either spontaneously or by manipulation.
  - Irreducible – hernia contents cannot be reduced; these are further classified into:
    - Incarcerated – Irreducible hernia with no ischaemia of the contents.
    - Strangulated: Hernia contents are ischaemic with impending necrosis and inflammatory surrounding tissue changes; if the bowel is contained it is usually obstructed. Specific types of strangulated hernia include the Richter's hernia, where a knuckle of antimesenteric bowel wall is strangulated without causing luminal obstruction, and the Maydl's hernia (hernia en-W), where two adjacent loops of bowel are contained in the sac, with strangulation of the intra-abdominal intervening portion. Signs suggestive of strangulation include pyrexia / tachycardia, raised inflammatory markers, increasing tenderness, and increasing acidosis.

Inguinal hernia

Inguinal hernia occurs in 2% of full-term and in 10% of pre-term infants. In adults, it has peak incidence in the sixth decade and is ten times more common in men than women.

Classification

- Indirect: The contents and sac travel through the deep ring of inguinal canal, *laterally* to the inferior epigastric vessels, along the inguinal canal. Persistent patent processus vaginalis in adult life is a proposed contributing factor.
- Direct: The sac protrudes through the posterior wall of inguinal canal, *medially* to the inferior epigastric vessels, through the Hesselbach's triangle. (See also Chapter 1: *Anatomy – the inguinal canal*.)
- Pantaloon hernia: Simultaneous presence of both a direct and an indirect sac straddled by the inferior epigastric artery.
- Sliding hernia (Hernia en-glissade): Viscus protruding through the abdominal wall forms part of the sac (could be direct or indirect).

Complications of herniae

- Local discomfort from lump / swelling, pain, reduction en-masse (reduction of hernia but contents remain strangulated within the neck of the sac), irreducibility, incarceration, intestinal obstruction, perforation, strangulation with necrosis of hernia contents, peritonitis, sepsis, involvement in peritoneal disease process (mesothelioma, metastatic disease, endometriosis), mortality (in strangulation).
- The risk of strangulation varies between types of hernia, ranging from 3% for direct inguinal hernia to 40% for femoral hernia.

Management

Surgery is the definitive treatment, aiming to restore the functional integrity of the laminar musculoaponeurotic structure of the groin. The timing, hospital setting, surgical technique and materials vary depending on the type of hernia, symptoms at presentation and patient fitness.

- Painful irreducible (strangulated) groin hernia: Emergency operation. Consider non-mesh repair because of risk of infection.
- Femoral hernia: Urgent surgery (high risk of strangulation).
- Non strangulated, incarcerated groin hernia: Urgent operation.
- Symptomatic inguinal hernia: Elective surgery. If primary unilateral, the evidence supports that laparoscopic repair is associated with less post-operative pain and earlier return to work, but has no difference regarding recurrence rates compared to the open mesh repair (Table 7.8).
- Asymptomatic, small direct, easily reducible: Consider observation in unfit patients, but bear in mind that the risk of incarceration is estimated to be 0.3–3% per year and that operative mortality for strangulated hernia surgery is greater than 5%, higher than of elective hernia repair which is less than 1%. The evidence from two randomised controlled trials (RCTs) is not conclusive.

Surgical treatment options for inguinal hernia repair

The repair of an inguinal hernia can be performed via an open or a laparoscopic technique.

Open repair

Open repair can be performed under general or local anaesthetic. There have been several variations in the method employed to repair the musculoaponeurotic defect and the currently most popular are:

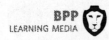

- **Tension-free (Lichtenstein) mesh repair:**
An oblique or transverse 6–8cm skin incision is deepened down to the external oblique aponeurosis; this is opened along the direction of its fibres from the pubic tubercle to the deep inguinal ring to form two leaves. The ilioinguinal nerve is exposed and protected and the spermatic cord is gently freed, avoiding damage to the external spermatic or cremasteric vessels. The upper leaf of the external oblique aponeurosis is cleared from the underlying internal oblique muscle to prepare the space for the prosthetic mesh. An indirect sac is searched for and if present, it is separated from the cord structures. The sac can then be reduced or opened; if opened, the contents are reduced and the sac is transfixed and amputated. With a direct hernia, the posterior wall should be plicated with an inverting suture. The mesh is prepared by trimming and creating lateral tails. The cord is retracted, allowing placement of the first non-absorbable suture above and medial to the pubic tubercle, ensuring adequate mesh coverage medial to the pubic tubercle. The stitch is continued laterally along the lower edge of the mesh and the inguinal ligament to just beyond the deep ring. The lateral end of the mesh is cut to create two tails and the larger upper one is pulled beneath the cord. The upper portion of the mesh is sutured to the internal oblique muscle. The upper tail is sutured to the lower tail and to the inguinal ligament creating a 'new' deep ring for the spermatic cord. Closure by layers follows of the external oblique aponeurosis and skin.

- **Shouldice repair**

- **Plug repair**

Laparoscopic technique

Laparoscopic technique is performed under general anaesthetic only. Smaller incisions are made and less postoperative pain is encountered. Recovery has been shown to be quicker with an earlier return to normal function. Two main methods of laparoscopic approach for inguinal hernia repair are recognised:

- **Transabdominal preperitoneal prosthetic repair (TAPP):**
Under general anaesthesia a pneumoperitoneum is safely created. The camera is placed through the umbilical port and the abdominal cavity visualised. Two further instrument ports (at midclavicular lines) are inserted under direct vision. The preperitoneal space is then entered by incising the peritoneum transversely anterior to the defect. Flaps are then developed and the hernia sac reduced. Once the anatomy is completely defined, the mesh (15 × 10cm) is fashioned and inserted adjacent to the pubic symphysis and behind the internal ring. The mesh is stapled in place and if necessary the process is repeated on the contralateral side. The peritoneum is then closed either by stapling or sutures.
(See also the video at WeBSurg www.websurg.com/ref/TAPP-vd01es1867.htm)

- **Totally extraperitoneal prosthetic repair (TEP):**
This technique involves the creation of an extraperitoneal space. Under general anaesthesia an infraumbilical incision is made and deepened to the anterior rectus sheath. A balloon dissector is inserted and the balloon is inflated carefully to create a pre-peritoneal space under the rectus muscle. A blunt port and a laparoscope are inserted and the space is extended using a sweeping action. Further ports are inserted under direct vision along the midline. Dissection is continued carefully identifying the spermatic cord and inferior epigastric vessels. Care should be taken to avoid making a hole in the peritoneum. A mesh is inserted and fixed as above. In some cases certain surgeons do not use staples as once the gas is removed the mesh remains in place.
(See also the video at WeBSurg www.websurg.com/ref/Laparoscopic_right_inguinal_hernia_TEP-vd01en1422e.htm)

NICE Guidelines overview – laparoscopic surgery for inguinal hernia repair (Adapted from NICE, 2004)

Summary of recommendations:

- Inform patients about the risks and benefits of each type of operation (open, TEP, TAPP) and consider the anaesthetic risks.
- Consider the optimum procedure for individual patient taking into account the surgeon's experience with each procedure.
- Laparoscopic surgery for inguinal hernia repair by TAPP / TEP should only be performed by specially trained surgeons regularly performing such procedures.

	Laparoscopic	Lichtenstein
Morbidity	28%	28%
Bowel injury	0.1%	0.06%
Bladder injury	0.1%	0%
Vascular injury	0.1%	0%
Wound infection	1 %	2.7%
Groin haematoma	13%	16%
Seroma	12%	9%
Urinary retention	3%	3%
Inguinal paraesthesia	4%	8%
Chronic pain	7%	13%
Testicular problems	0.6%	0.8%
Mean time to work	15 days	21 days
Recurrence	5%	2.7%

Table 7.8. Comparison of outcomes between laparoscopic and Lichtenstein repair methods

Femoral hernia

The incidence of femoral hernia is 2.5–4 times higher in females than males in the UK, although inguinal hernia is still the commonest hernia in females.

It is rarely large in size and can be difficult to detect, particularly in obese patients. It is usually not reducible, with no cough impulse, containing fat and, less frequently, bowel. Richter's type of hernia occurs more commonly in femoral herniae.

The proposed aetiology involves a defect in the transversalis fascia allowing insinuation of fat into the femoral canal and peritoneal protrusion. This is facilitated by increased abdominal pressure and atrophy of iliopsoas and pectineus muscle tissue with older age.

Surgical approaches to a femoral hernia

The aim is to remove the peritoneal sac, repair the fascia and reinforce the aponeurosis. The parietal repair is achieved by suturing the medial inguinal ligament to the pectineal ligament with a non-absorbable suture, taking care not to damage or compress the femoral vein, which lies immediately laterally.

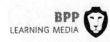

293

- **Crural or low approach (Lockwood):** Oblique incision in the groin about 1cm below and parallel to the medial two-thirds of the inguinal ligament. The sac is identified within the subcutaneous tissue, cleared, opened, then transfixed and excised. This approach is often reserved for elective cases.
- **Inguinal approach (Lotheissen):** The inguinal canal is opened as per inguinal hernia repair. The transversalis fascia forming the posterior wall is divided to gain access to the femoral canal from above. This approach enables an inguinal hernia, if present, and the femoral hernia to be repaired simultaneously, but predisposes to new inguinal hernia formation.
- **High extra-peritoneal approach (McEvedy):** This can utilise a midline vertical or transverse incision. The extraperitoneal space is opened by blunt dissection; the sac is found and evacuated. The peritoneum can be opened to inspect or resect contents. This approach is the most useful for strangulated herniae.
- **Laparoscopic (TAPP or TEP):** Allows good views of the femoral canal and provides the opportunity to repair a concurrent inguinal hernia; the experience is however still limited.

Complications of groin hernia repair

These are best discussed during the process of obtaining informed consent.

- General: Chest infection, thrombotic risk, visceral injury, cardiovascular complications.
- Specific: Wound haematoma, infection, damage to the cord, vas and testicular vessels, ischaemic orchitis with testicular atrophy, hydrocele (inguinal hernia), chronic pain, nerve injury, vascular injury, urinary retention, recurrence, mortality (higher in emergency repairs of strangulated hernias).

Examination of the abdominal system

The gastrointestinal and genitourinary systems are examined here, but any abnormalities of the cardio-respiratory systems should also be detected if present, as they can be important in patient management.

In the exam setting, it is particularly important that you pay attention to the exact wording of the examiner's instruction. If the instruction is 'examine this patient's abdominal system', start from the hands, upper extremity, then proceed to head, neck, and torso. If it is 'examine this patient's abdomen', just follow the instruction and focus on the abdomen.

Clinical examination

- Introduce yourself, establish patient comfort, obtain verbal consent to examine.
- Inspect from the end of the bed.
  - Assess patient's general condition and attitude.
  - Describe every relevant treatment sign around the bed (drips, catheters, drains, drugs, pumps etc; though it is less likely to have an acutely unwell patient in the new MRCS Part B exam)
- Examine both of the patient's hands, assess the capillary refill time (normal ≤ 2 sec) and look for signs of abdominal disease:
  - Digital clubbing: proliferation of soft tissue around the ends of fingers or toes, without osseous change) that can be associated with:
    1. Pulmonary aetiology: Lung cancer, cystic fibrosis, interstitial lung disease, idiopathic pulmonary fibrosis, sarcoidosis, pleural mesothelioma, pulmonary metastases.
    2. Cardiac aetiology: Cyanotic congenital heart disease, right-to-left shunting and bacterial endocarditis.
    3. Gastrointestinal diseases: Ulcerative colitis, Crohn's disease, liver cirrhosis.
    4. Malignancies: Thyroid cancer, lymphoma, leukaemia.
  - Peripheral cyanosis (a dusky or bluish tinge to the fingers and toes, indicating hypoxaemia or peripheral vasoconstriction).
  - Leuconychia (abnormal white discolouration of the nails). It can be congenital or acquired, secondary to hypoalbuminaemia of chronic liver disease, renal failure, fungal infection or lymphoma.
  - Koilonychia (fingernail dystrophy in which they are flattened and have concavities with raised edges, also called 'spoon nails'). It can be caused by anaemia, hyperthyroidism, cachexia, glossitis and chemotherapy.
  - Beau's lines (horizontal lines of darkened cells and linear depressions of fingernails resulting from interruption in the protein formation of the nail plate). They can be associated with trauma, malnutrition, major metabolic condition, chemotherapy.
  - Palmar erythema (reddening of the palms of the hands affecting the thenar and hypothenar eminences, attributed to high oestrogen levels). It can be a normal finding, but also sign of chronic liver disease, pregnancy, thyrotoxicosis, rheumatoid arthritis, polycythaemia and rarely chronic febrile diseases and chronic leukaemia.
  - Dupuytren's disease (presence of nodules and cords in the palm of the hand progressing to fixed contractures of the metacarpophalangeal and interphalangeal joints), associated with diabetes mellitus, alcoholism, HIV infection, epilepsy, trauma, manual labour and cigarette smoking.
  - Test for flapping tremor (asterixis): Ask the patient to hold out their outstretched arms and hands while cocking their wrists back; in the presence of asterixis, there is a non-synchronised, intermittent flapping motion at the wrists. It is present in hepatic, renal, respiratory failure and salicylate overdose.

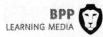

- Examine the upper extremities.
  - Assess the patient's radial pulse (see the section earlier on the examination of the arterial system) and state you would like to measure the blood pressure.
  - Look for scars of surgical arterio-venous fistula (forearm for radio-cephalic and arm for brachio-cephalic fistula) and palpate for the characteristic thrill. If present, end-stage renal failure is indicated and possibly renal transplantation (look for relevant scars).
  - Look for signs of liver disease:
    1. Muscle wasting (hypoalbuminaemia).
    2. Bruising (coagulopathy).
    3. Spider naevi: Cutaneous vascular anomalies occurring as a result of dilation of pre-existing vessels. They consist of a central arteriole with radiating thin-walled vessels. Compression of the central vessel produces blanching and temporarily obliterates the lesion. When released, the threadlike vessels quickly refill with blood from the central arteriole. The ascending central arteriole resembles a spider's body, and the radiating fine vessels resemble multiple spider legs). If more than five, they should trigger investigation of liver disease, but they are also common in children and in women using oral contraceptive pills.
    4. Scratch marks secondary to pruritus of jaundice.
- Examine the face and eyes.
  - Look for conjunctival pallor (anaemia), scleral jaundice, Kaiser-Fleischer rings (Wilson's disease), xanthelasmata of the eyelids (hyperlipidaemia, primary biliary cirrhosis, diabetes mellitus) and parotid enlargement (sarcoidosis, tuberculosis, alcoholism, myxoedema, Cushing's disease, diabetes / insulin resistance, liver cirrhosis, malnutrition).
- Examine the mouth and oral cavity.
  - Look for angular stomatitis (cheilosis, vitamin B deficiencies, iron deficiency), leucoplakia (adherent white plaques or patches on the mucous membranes of the oral cavity, including the tongue, associated with alcohol use), pigmentation of Peutz Jeghers syndrome, atrophic glossitis of the tongue (B12 or Fe deficiency), ulceration (Behçet's disease, Crohn's disease, coeliac disease).
- Examine the neck for cervical lymphadenopathy.
  - Look for abnormal lymph node at the left supraclavicular fossa (Virchow's node, Troisier's sign) indicating metastatic disease of gastrointestinal primary malignancy.
- Examine the chest.
  - Inspect the chest for spider naevi, gynaecomastia and loss of hair indicating high oestrogen levels of liver failure.
  - Look for thoracotomy scars (Ivor Lewis operation for oesophageal cancer) or even a sternotomy scar from heart surgery.
  - State you would examine the cardio-respiratory system to assess co-morbidities and fitness for surgery.
- Examination of the abdomen.
  - Inspect from the end of the bed and comment on the shape of the abdomen, the presence of distension (generalised symmetrical or localised asymmetrical) or visible peristalsis (bowel obstruction).
  - Ask patient to 'suck in and blow out tummy' to assess for peritonism and look for any prominent pulsation on deep inspiration (abdominal aortic aneurysm).
  - Comment on any scars or stomas; observe from closer distance, look for faint old appendicectomy scars, in the groins for hernia repair scars and small laparoscopic port scars. Turn patient on either side to look for nephrectomy scars extending to the loins (Figure 7.1).
  - Comment on skin striae (rapid weight gain, post partum, Cushing's or steroid use) or distended veins ('caput medusae' sign of portal hypertension or distended thoracoepigastric and lateral thoracic vein tributaries forming collateral circulation in inferior vena cava obstruction).

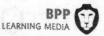

- Ask the patient to lift legs off bed or raise head to reveal divarication of the rectus muscle or other hernias (including incisional ones).
- Palpate the abdomen.
  - Kneel to the level of abdomen or elevate the bed (the examining hand and forearm should be aligned to maximise the sensitivity of the palpating hand). Focus on the patient's face when examining for signs of pain or discomfort.
  - Perform superficial palpation across all nine abdominal sections, starting away from you or away from the painful area, to assess tenderness and guarding.
  - Continue with deep palpation again following the same route, to detect abnormal masses. When in the epigastrium, palpate for abdominal aortic aneurysm. If an abnormal mass is palpated, determine its features as for any lump; these include general features such as its size, shape, surface, consistency, presence of any tenderness, its temperature, the layer of origin, any tethering to skin, any skin changes, and the direction of its movement in association to respiratory cycle; it also includes specific features such as pulsatility, transmitted or expansile (aneurysms), reducibility (herniae), transillumination (for thin-walled cysts) and auscultation (for contained bowel loops). In the case of identifying an abdominal aortic aneurysm, ascertain its size and position (in relation to renal arteries) if possible, check carefully for other aneurysms and assess the remaining peripheral vascular system.
  - Palpate for the liver: Start from the right iliac fossa and move your hand upwards while the patient takes deep breaths and determine the extent of the liver below the costal margin in the mid-clavicular line.
  - Percuss from the RIF upwards to determine the lower and upper borders of the liver.

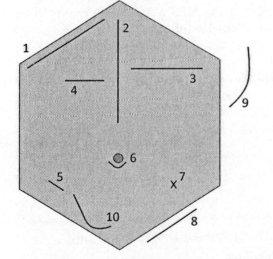

1. Kocher's incision – hepatobiliary surgery
2. Upper midline laparotomy – antireflux surgery
3. Transverse upper abdominal incision – splenic surgery
4. Ramstedt's pyloromyotomy incision – pyloric stenosis
5. Gridiron Incision – appendicectomy
6. Infraumbilical – umbilical hernia, laparoscopic surgery
7. Laparoscopic port site
8. Inguinal incision – hernia repair
9. Lateral thoracolumbar incision
10. Hockey stick incision – renal transplant

Figure 7.1 Common abdominal scars

Hepatomegaly is indicated by a mass descending below the right costal margin and costal angle that moves with respiration and it is not possible to get above it; also by dullness to percussion up to the level of the 8th rib in the mid-axillary line. Soft and tender hepatomegaly indicates hepatitis or heart failure; firm and irregular (nodular) liver is found in early cirrhosis, metastasis or hepatocellular carcinoma. (See Table 7.9 for causes of hepatomegaly.)

  - Palpate for the gall bladder below the liver edge; remember 'palpable gallbladder in the presence of jaundice is unlikely to be caused by gallstones' – Courvoisier's law. Tenderness with inspiratory catch at palpation of the right upper quadrant indicates cholecystitis (Murphy's sign). A similar manoeuvre in the left upper quadrant should not elicit the same response.

A distended gallbladder or gallbladder mass arises from below the tip of the right 9th rib, is smooth and hemi-ovoid in shape, moves with respiration, is dull to percussion and it is not possible to feel the space between mass and liver.

- Palpate for the spleen, starting from the right iliac fossa moving to the left upper quadrant and turning the patient slightly to the right.

Splenomegaly is indicated by a mass descending below the left 10th rib and enlarging in a line towards the umbilicus; it often has a palpable notch on the medial border, moves with respiration and is not possible to get above it; it is dull to percussion and can be brought forward by lifting the lower ribs but can not be felt bimanually or balloted. (See Table 7.10 for causes of splenomegaly.)

- Ballot for the kidneys: During deep patient inspiration, place one hand at the upper abdominal quadrant and one hand at the renal angle; the hand *below ballots* and the hand above palpates for abnormal enlargement of the kidney.

A renal mass lies in the paracolic gutter, moves with respiration cranio-caudally, can be felt bimanually, can be balloted and is not dull to percussion.

- Percuss all abdominal areas. In the presence of signs of liver disease look for ascites and demonstrate the horseshoe pattern of dullness, which shifts with the patient rolling to either side (shifting dullness), as well as the fluid thrill sign.
- Auscultate the abdomen for bowel sounds and aortic, renal and iliac bruits.
- Examine the groin, external genitalia and hernia orifices.
- State you would perform a digital rectal examination and examine the lower extremities for oedema (hypoalbulinaemia), toe clubbing and neurological deficits (peripheral neuropathy of alcoholism), perform a peripheral vascular examination and a urine dipstick test.

Surgical pathology

Organomegaly

The following tables (7.9, 7.10, and 7.11) present the common causes of organomegaly.

Smooth generalised enlargement	Localised swelling
Congestion due to cardiac failure Micronodular cirrhosis Reticuloses Hepatic vein obstruction (Budd-Chiari syndrome) Infective hepatitis Cholangitis Portal pyaemia Amyloidosis	Riedel's lobe Hydatid cyst Liver abscess Hepatocellular carcinoma
Nodular generalised enlargement	
Secondary carcinoma Macronodular cirrhosis Polycystic disease	

Table 7.9. Causes of hepatomegaly

Infection	Cellular proliferation
Bacterial – typhoid, typhus, TB Viral – glandular fever Protozoal – malaria, kala-azar	Myeloid and lymphatic leukaemia Myelofibrosis Pernicious anaemia Polycythaemia rubra vera Spherocytosis Thrombocytopenic purpura Myelosclerosis
Other causes	**Congestion**
Amyloidosis Gaucher's disease Felty's syndrome Angioma Lymphosarcoma	Portal hypertension Hepatic vein obstruction Congestive heart failure

Table 7.10. Causes of splenomegaly

Renal mass	Palpable gall bladder	Right iliac fossa mass
Hydronephrosis Pyonephrosis Perinephric abscess Hypernephroma Nephroblastoma Solitary cyst Polycystic disease	Obstruction of the cystic duct – Stone in Hartmann's pouch – Cholangiocarcinoma Obstruction of the common bile duct – Stone in common bile duct – Carcinoma of the head of the pancreas	Appendicitis Tuberculosis Carcinoma of the caecum Crohn's disease Iliac lymphadenopathy Psoas abscess

Table 7.11. More causes of organomegaly

Stomas

The term 'stoma' derives from the Greek word meaning mouth or opening.

Stomas can be formed electively or during an emergency procedure, according to the following indications (FLEDD):

- Feeding – gastrostomy (PEG) following neurological insult or upper GI/throat obstruction (tumours/trauma).
- Lavage – caecostomy, appendicostomy (for Antegrade Continence Enema - ACE procedure).
- Exteriorisation – when a permanent stoma is required (abdominoperoneal resection with end colostomy or panproctocolectomy with end ileostomy) or where anastomosis is not possible (contaminated abdomen – Hartmann's procedure).
- Diversion – to protect distal anastomosis (defunctioning loop ileostomy) or urinary diversion following cystectomy.
- Decompression – gastrostomy.

	Ileostomy	Colostomy
Site	Usually Right sided (RIF)	Usually Left sided (LIF)
Surface	Spout to protect skin	Flush with skin
Discharge	Watery small bowel contents	Solid faeces
Surrounding skin	Can be excoriated, inflamed	Usually normal
Example temporary	Loop ileostomy following anterior resection	Hartmann's procedure
Example permanent	Panproctocolectomy	Abdominoperineal resection (APR)

Table 7.12. Differences between ileostomy and colostomy

Examination of a stoma

Assessing and describing the following features of a stoma should help to identify its type:

- Site: Ileostomies are commonly in the right iliac fossa and colostomies commonly in the left iliac fossa. Loop colostomies can also been seen in the upper abdomen (transverse colon) or even in the midline in certain cases.
- Calibre: Generally colostomies have the widest lumen (the loop colostomies are wider than the end colostomies), followed by ileostomies and then urostomies.
- Number of lumens: This may not always be so easy to determine as in a loop stoma one lumen may be retracted. Examples of 2 lumens include a covering loop ileostomy following anterior resection or a double-barrelled colostomy and mucus fistula following modified Hartmann's procedure.
- Surface: Check for a spout or whether the stoma is flush with the skin. Always think of prolapse or retraction.
- Contents: Comment on whether the contents are liquid stool, formed stool or urine.
- Scars: Look for any abdominal scars to suggest the procedure undertaken. There may be evidence of a previous stoma scar or a midline scar. The absence of any scars would suggest either a trephine defunctioning colostomy or alternatively a laparoscopic procedure. Look at the perineum to confirm whether the stoma is temporary or permanent (APR).
- Complications of a stoma are described in Table 7.13.

General	Local
Stoma diarrhoea (ileostomy) – can lead to electrolyte disturbances	Ischaemia / gangrene – because of injury to vessel or tight fascial defect
Nutritional disturbance – vitamin B deficiency	Prolapse / Intussusception – poor siting; it can be often reduced, but re-siting sometimes is required
Stones – with ileostomy formation the risk of gallstones and renal calculi increases	Stenosis – either technical reason or due to underlying disease
Short gut syndrome – significant fluid / electrolyte imbalance and manutrition	Retraction – can sometimes be managed with appliance, or in certain cases needs re-siting
Residual disease – Crohn's disease	Skin excoriation – seen with ileostomies
Psychosexual	Parastoma hernia – bowel in hernia sac can obstruct / strangulate

Table 7.13. Complications of stomas

Examination of the respiratory system

- Position the patient at 45° head-up, with the upper body exposed, ensuring the patient's comfort and privacy.
- Inspect from the end of the bed.
  - Assess the patient's level of consciousness (lower in hypoxaemia, CO_2 retention).
  - Assess the patient's colour (look for cyanosis) and overall build (cachexia).
  - Is the patient dyspnoeic, gasping for breath or sitting forward to support respiration?
  - Is the patient able to speak and complete full sentences?
  - Are there any audible breath sounds (wheeze or stridor)?
  - Look for use of accessory muscles of respiration (neck muscles), for intercostal recession (in-drawing of intercostals) and for tracheal tug on inspiration (indicates airway obstruction and non-compliant lung).
  - Ask the patient to cough (productive v. non-productive).
  - Look around the bed for an oxygen mask, nebulisers or inhalers, oxymeter, sputum pot. Describe the features of sputum, if present: mucoid, purulent, pink / frothy, haemoptysis.
  - Look for surgical scars (thoracotomy, sternotomy or abdominal incisions, old TB surgery scars).
  - Assess the respiratory rate (normal 12–14/minute).
  - Increased: pneumonia, anxiety, metabolic acidosis, pleuritic pain.
  - Decreased: narcotic overdose, hypoventilation associated with cerebral or respiratory disease.
- Assess the shape of the chest.
  - Look from the side for kyphosis and from the back for scoliosis.
  - Pectus excavatum (funnel chest): the sternum is depressed.
  - Pectus carinatum (pigeon chest): the sternum and the costal cartilages project outwards, can occur secondary to childhood asthma.
  - Barrel shaped (COPD).
- Are the chest movements symmetrical? (Diminished movement on one side indicates disease on that side.)
- Examine the hands for:
  - Clubbing (see section on *Examination of the abdominal system*).
  - Peripheral cyanosis, tar staining (smoking).
  - Small muscles wasting (*Pancoast tumour* impinging on the brachial plexus).
  - Wrist tenderness (hypertrophic pulmonary osteoarthropathy).
  - Asterixis (respiratory / renal / hepatic failure).
- Assess the radial pulse (bounding pulse in hypercarbia) and blood pressure. Decrease in systolic arterial pressure of more than 15mmHg on inspiration is associated with severe airway obstruction such as acute asthma.
- Examine the head and neck.
  - Face and eyes: Look for polycythaemia facies, conjunctival anaemia or Horner's syndrome signs (ptosis, myosis, enophthalmos and anhydrosis) of Pancoast tumour.
  - Assess for hoarseness of voice.
  - Look in the mouth for central cyanosis.
  - Assess the JVP, which is raised in *cor pulmonale* (right heart failure secondary to chronic lung disease), in superior vena cava obstruction secondary to bronchial carcinoma, in pulmonary embolism and in tension pneumothorax.
  - Palpate the neck to determine the trachea is central (equal distance to each sternocleidomastoid muscle). Tracheal deviation can be caused by a collapsed lung, fibrosis, pleural effusion and pneumothorax.

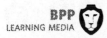

- – Look for tracheal tug and contraction of the sternocleidomastoids (accessory muscles).
  - – Examine the cervical lymph nodes.
- Palpate the apex beat (to assess for mediastinal shift).
- Palpate the chest assessing for expansion: Place your fingers around the chest on both sides, with the thumbs meeting in the midline and watch them moving apart with each inspiration (it should be > 5cm at the level of the nipples, symmetrical). Reduced expansion indicates consolidation, pleural effusion, pneumonectomy, lobe collapse or pneumothorax.
- Assess the tactile vocal fremitus at different levels, bilaterally (if increased it indicates consolidated lung; if it is diminished, it indicates that air, fluid or thickened pleura separates the lung from chest wall).
- Percuss at several levels including in the axilla and clavicles (comparing two sides). The percussion note can be:
  - – **Resonant**, for normal lungs.
  - – **Dull**, in solid lung (consolidation) or pleural thickening.
  - – **Stony dull**, in the presence of fluid (pleural effusion).
  - – **Hyper-resonant**, for hyperinflated lungs (emphysema or pneumothorax).
- Auscultate the chest (patient breathing with mouth open).
  - – Vesicular breathing: normal.
  - – Bronchial breathing: consolidation and upper level of pleural effusion.
  - – Diminished breath sounds: thickened pleura, air or fluid.
  - – Added sounds:
    - • **Crackles**: These refer to inspiratory sounds of airways opening. The coarser the crackle the larger the obstructed airway; the later in inspiration the more distal the obstruction.
    - • **Wheeze**: Vibration of airway wall as air passes an airway narrowed to the point of closure. The lower the pitch, the larger the airway. High pitched polyphonic wheezes indicate multiple distal 'airway narrowing' as in asthma. Low pitched monophonic wheeze suggest a single larger airway narrowing e.g. tumour, foreign body.
    - • **Stridor**: Monophonic inspiratory wheeze from a narrowed airway out of the thorax usually the trachea.
    - • **Pleural rub**: Inflamed pleural surfaces rubbing but can be heard with effusion.
- Offer to examine the abdomen, looking for hepatomegaly of right heart failure (*cor pulmonale*) or metastatic disease. Also the lower extremities, looking for ankle oedema, cyanosis or toe clubbing.
- Additional tests:
  - – Chest X-ray
  - – Oxygen saturation with an oxymeter.
  - – Peak expiratory flow rate.
  - – Arterial blood gas.
  - – Sputum pot examination, microscopy and culture.

Surgical pathology

Postoperative pulmonary complications

The following respiratory abnormalities can complicate surgical procedures and patients need to be warned of them during the consent process; additionally, preventive measures and active monitoring is required to minimise their effect on patient outcomes:

Postoperative hypoxia

Postoperative hypoxia results from impairment in either ventilation or perfusion to alveoli. Alveolar ventilation impairment is usually secondary to hypoventilation (airway obstruction, opiates), bronchospasm, pneumothorax or arteriovenous shunting (collapse, atelectasis). Alveolar perfusion impairment can be due to ventilation-perfusion mismatch (pulmonary embolism), impaired cardiac output, pneumonia or pulmonary oedema.

Atelectasis

This refers to the absence of air from part of the lung, mainly caused by bronchial obstruction by sputum or a foreign body or alveolar hypoventilation. Recognised risk factors include high BMI, COPD, age > 60 years and upper GI surgery. It manifests with postoperative pyrexia, usually presenting at about 48 hours with tachycardia and tachypnoea. Clinical signs include reduced air entry, dullness on percussion and reduced breath sounds. The diagnosis is confirmed by a chest X-ray (consolidation and collapse). Treatment includes intensive chest physiotherapy, nebulised bronchodilators, antibiotics for associated infection, adequate analgesia, early mobilisation and in certain cases continuous positive airway pressure (CPAP).

Pneumonia

This is acute infection of the lower respiratory tract characterised by pleuritic chest pain, cough with purulent expectoration, rigors and fever.

- Clinical criteria for pneumonia include a new or progressive lung infiltrate and at least two of the following: hyper– or hypothermia, elevated white blood cell count, purulent tracheal secretions or sputum, and worsening oxygenation.
- Classification (according to the origin of the insulting pathogen):
  - **Community-acquired pneumonia**: Patient with a first positive bacterial culture obtained ≤ 48 hours after hospital admission and lacking risk factors for healthcare-associated pneumonia.
  - **Health care-associated pneumonia**: Patient with a first positive bacterial culture obtained ≤ 48 hours after hospital admission and any of the following:
    a. Admission source indicates transfer from another healthcare facility.
    b. Receiving hemodialysis, wound, or infusion therapy as an outpatient.
    c. Prior hospitalisation for ≥ 3 days within the past 90 days.
    d. Immunocompromised state due to underlying disease or therapy.
  - **Hospital-acquired pneumonia (HAP)**: Patient with a first positive bacterial culture obtained > 48 hours after hospital admission.
  - **Ventilator-associated pneumonia (VAP)**: Mechanically ventilated patient with a first positive bacterial culture obtained > 48 hours after hospital admission or tracheal intubation, whichever occurred first.
  - **Postoperative pneumonia**: HAP or VAP occurring in a postoperative patient.

Aspiration pneumonitis

This results from aspiration of material into the lungs from regurgitation of gastric or oesophageal content or from material emanating from the oropharynx (rare).

- Risk factors: Large gastric or oesophageal residual volumes, poor function of the oesophagogastric sphincter and depressed or absent protective laryngeal reflexes.
- More common organisms: Staphylococcus aureus, Pseudomonas aeruginosa and other Gram-negative enteric organisms. These patients are more likely to develop aspiration. Pneumonitis, resulting in pulmonary oedema and severe hypoxaemia.

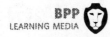

- Aspiration of gastric contents results in a chemical pneumonitis, resulting in pulmonary oedema and severe hypoxaemia.
- Treatment: The mainstay of treatment involves oxygen supplementation, monitoring and fluid resuscitation. Antibiotic therapy is not initially indicated in aspiration pneumonitis; it should be considered if the condition does not start to improve within 48 hours. Corticosteroids have been found to be of limited benefit in aspiration pneumonitis or aspiration pneumonia.

Pneumothorax

Pneumothorax is the presence of air within the pleural space. It results from disruption of the parietal, visceral or mediastinal pleura or spontaneous rupture of a sub pleural bleb. *Tension pneumothorax* occurs when pleura forms a one-way flap valve, drawing air into the pleural space during inspiration and preventing it from leaving during expiration. It can lead to significant deterioration in cardio-pulmonary status with patients showing signs of laboured respiration, cyanosis, hypotension and tachycardia. This is a medical emergency requiring urgent decompression.

Spontaneous pneumothorax	Traumatic pneumothorax
Primary No identifiable aetiology but risk factors are recognised: • Smoking • Tall, thin stature in a healthy person • Marfan syndrome • Pregnancy • Familial cases	**Aetiology – Thoracocentesis** • Trauma – penetrating and non-penetrating injuries • Rib fractures • Transthoracic or transbronchial needle aspiration biopsy • Thoracentesis • Central venous catheter insertion • Intercostal nerve block • Tracheostomy • Cardiopulmonary resuscitation • Positive pressure ventilation and ARDS in the ICU • High-risk occupation (eg, diving, flying)
Secondary	
Underlying pulmonary disorder: • Chronic obstructive lung disease • Asthma • Pneumonia (HIV/AIDS, Pneumocystis, Necrotising pneumonia) • Bronchogenic carcinoma • Metastatic malignancy • Chemotherapeutic agents • Tuberculosis • Cystic fibrosis (CF) • Inhalational and intravenous drug use • Interstitial lung diseases • Idiopathic pulmonary fibrosis • Sarcoidosis • Langerhans cell histiocytosis • Acute respiratory distress syndrome • Thoracic endometriosis (Catamenial pneumothorax)	

Table 7.14. Aetiology and classification of pneumothorax

Clinical manifestations

The following symptoms and signs are recognised:

- Acute onset of severe, stabbing chest pain, radiating to ipsilateral shoulder and increasing with inspiration (pleuritic) with associated sudden shortness of breath.
- Patient is diaphoretic, with shallow breathing to relieve pleuritic pain, cyanotic (especially with tension pneumothorax), tachypnoeic and tachycardic.
- There may be pulsus paradoxus, hypotension (often with tension pneumothorax).
- Asymmetric lung expansion is noted, along with mediastinal and tracheal shift to the contralateral side with a large tension pneumothorax.
- There are distant or absent breath sounds, hyperresonance on percussion, decreased tactile fremitus.
- Jugular venous distension is noted in tension pneumothorax.
- The mental status is altered because of hypoxia.

Diagnostic work up

- Chest radiograph: Linear shadow of visceral pleura with lack of lung markings peripheral to the shadow. Mediastinal shift toward the contralateral lung in larger pneumothoraces.
- Method to estimate the % of pneumothorax: Calculate the ratio of the transverse radius of the pneumothorax (cubed) to the transverse radius of the hemithorax (cubed) × 100.
- Cut-point between small and large pneumothoraces for the British Thoracic Society is 2cm.
- Lateral decubitus X-ray film, with the involved hemithorax positioned uppermost: for confirmation of a suspected pneumothorax that is not readily observed on standard supine anteroposterior radiograph.
- CT scan is used to: distinguish between a large bulla and pneumothorax; indicate underlying lung pathology; determine exact size of the pneumothorax, especially if it is small; and confirm diagnosis in patients with head trauma who are mechanically ventilated.
- Ultrasonography: It is increasingly used in the acute care setting as a readily available bedside tool, especially in ICU and emergency departments.

Management

- Spontaneous pneumothorax: The management depends on symptoms and the radiological size of the pneumothorax.
    - Small asymptomatic pneumothoraces (< 20%) may be followed with serial CXR.
    - Symptomatic but clinically stable: the British Thoracic Society (BTS) advocates for simple aspiration.
    - Haemodynamic instability is life-threatening and must be treated immediately with tube thoracostomy.
- Tension pneumothorax: Requires immediate needle aspiration by placing an adequate length cannula anteriorly through the second intercostal space in the mid clavicular line. This should be left in place until a fully functioning chest drain has been inserted.

Indications for insertion of chest drain
- Pneumothorax in any ventilated patient.
- Tension pneumothorax after initial needle decompression.
- Persistent or recurrent pneumothorax after simple aspiration.
- Large secondary spontaneous pneumothorax in patients over 50 years.
- Malignant pleural effusion.
- Empyema and complicated parapneumonic pleural effusion.
- Traumatic haemopneumothorax.
- Postoperative – for example, thoracotomy, oesophagectomy, cardiac surgery.

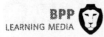

Surgery

Indications for surgery in pneumothorax include air leak persisting for more than 7–10 days, failure of lung re-expansion and recurrent spontaneous pneumothorax. The surgical options include partial pleurectomy; operative abrasion of pleural lining; resection of pulmonary bullae; and, for high risk patients, chemical pleurodesis with tetracycline.

Procedure: insertion of chest drain

Materials

- Chest drain, tubing, bottle with water, scalpel blade and handle, large clamps (Roberts).
- Packet of 0 or 1.0 silk suture on a curved needle, needle holder, scissors, tape, gauze.
- 1% or 2% lignocaine with or without adrenaline. (Dose: up to 3 mg/kg body weight for plain lignocaine, up to 7 mg/Kg body weight for lignocaine with adrenaline.) 20 ml syringe, 23-gauge needle for infiltration.
- Sterile prep solution: mask, gown and gloves.

Procedure

- Obtain informed consent where appropriate including the major steps of the procedure, major complications and their treatment and the necessity for repeated chest radiographs.
- Use mask, gown and gloves.
- Position patient with ipsilateral arm over head to 'open up' ribs.
- Prepare and drape the area of insertion.
- Widely anaesthetise the area of insertion with local anaesthetic, infiltrating the skin, muscle tissues, and right down to pleura.
- Insertion should be in the 'safe triangle' bordered by the anterior border of latissimus dorsi the lateral border of the pectoralis major, a line superior to the horizontal level of the nipple and the apex below the axilla.
- Make a 2cm incision through skin and subcutaneous tissues between the 4th and 5th ribs (to avoid injury of the liver or spleen), parallel to the rib margins, at the level of the anterior axillary line (to avoid injury of the long thoracic nerve). Continue the incision through the intercostal muscles, and right down to the pleura.
- Insert the clamp through the pleura and open the jaws, parallel to the direction of the ribs.
- Insert finger through your incision and into the thoracic cavity. Make sure you are feeling lung (or empty space) and not liver or spleen and that there are no previous adhesions.
- Grasp the end of chest drain with forceps (convex angle towards ribs), and insert it through the hole you have made in the pleura. **Do not use tubes with trocars.** After the tube has entered the thoracic cavity, remove the forceps and manually advance the tube in.
- Clamp the outer tube end with forceps and suture and tape the drain in place; attach tube to bottle with underwater seal. Watch the water column oscillating with respiration.
- Obtain post procedure chest X-ray to confirm position.
- Dress the wound and document procedure in patient's notes.

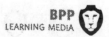

Examination of the neck and thyroid

Listen carefully to the examiner's instructions.

- 'Examine this patient's neck.' Focus on the neck.
- 'Examine this patient's thyroid' or 'thyroid status.' Start with examination of the thyroid gland, continue with rest of the neck, chest (for retrosternal goitre) and examine patient's eyes and extremities for peripheral signs of thyroid disease.

History taking

Enquire for:

- Features related to the neck lump (if one is visible) i.e. pain, discharge and rate of growth.
- Upper respiratory or gastrointestinal symptoms (sore throat, dysphagia, dysphonia, otalgia, nasal obstruction) and response to eating (increase in lump size indicates salivary gland lesion).
- General symptoms indicating systemic disease.
- Social history (smoking, alcohol use, occupation), family history, comorbidities.

Clinical examination

- Begin with the usual introductions, comfort assessment, consent to examine, hand hygiene.
- Position yourself opposite and at the same level with the patient who is sitting in a chair; this needs to be placed in such way in the room that you can easily move behind the patient during examination.
- Have a cup of water available.
- Expose the patient's head, neck and upper chest (do not hesitate to look under a long beard!)
- Inspect from the front:
    - Look for goitre, any asymmetrical swellings, skin changes, scars or sinuses.
    - Ask patient to open their mouth and stick their tongue out as far as possible. If a lump is present and moves on protrusion of the tongue, it is attached to the hyoid bone and therefore likely to be a thyroglossal cyst.
    - Ask patient to sip some water and then swallow: a lump attached to the larynx (thyroid tissue and thyroglossal cyst) will rise during swallowing.
- Palpate the neck from behind.
    - Ask patient to take a sip of water, hold it in their mouth and swallow when asked.
    - Feel the thyroid gland rise with swallowing.
    - Palpate each lobe of the thyroid. For the right lobe, ask patient to rotate their head mildly to the right side (relaxing the ipsilateral sternocleidomastoid muscle), press gently the left side to make the right lobe more prominent and palpate the right lobe evaluating all features of a lump. Repeat for the opposite side.
    - Determine whether the thyroid is diffusely enlarged or nodular.
    - Palpate for the trachea and establish its midline position.
    - Palpate the cervical lymph nodes.
    - Percuss over the sternum, from the notch downwards: dull percussion note indicates possible retrosternal goitre.
- Auscultate: listen for bruits over each lobe.
- Examine patient for systemic signs of thyroid disease.
    - **General appearance and composure:** Assess patient's clothing with respect to room temperature. Is patient hyperactive, restless and fidgety (hyperthyroid) or immobile and uninterested (hypothyroid)?

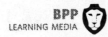

- **Examine the extremities.**
  1. Take the patient's hands and look for:
     a. Fine tremor (made more obvious by placing a sheet of paper on outstretched hands), increased sweating, palmar erythema, onycholysis (Plummer's nails) are associated with hyperthyroidism.
     b. Thyroid acropachy (soft tissue swelling and periosteal bone changes, usually occurring in the fingers, toes and lower extremities) and vitiligo are seen in association with autoimmune disorders such as Grave's disease.
     c. Coarse, dry skin, anaemia are seen in hypothyroidism.
  2. Examine the pulse rate and rhythm, blood pressure.
     a. Tachycardia or atrial fibrillation is found in hyperthyroidism.
     b. Bradycardia is noted in hypothyroidism.
  3. Assess for proximal myopathy, which can be present in either hyperthyroidism or hypothyroidism (more commonly adult myxoedema).
  4. Examine reflexes (decreased in hypothyroidism).
  5. Look for pretibial myxoedema (also known as thyroid dermopathy) of Grave's disease: localised lesions of the skin resulting from the deposition of hyaluronic acid, most often confined to the pretibial area, although it may occur anywhere on the skin.
- **Examine the patient's eyes.**
  1. Look for loss or thinning of hair on outer one-third of eyebrows and for periorbital oedema of hypothyroidism.
  2. Look for eye signs of Grave's disease (infiltrative ophthalmopathy):
     Strabismus, diplopia, exophthalmos (whiteness of sclera visible below the iris), proptosis (eye protrusion beyond level of supraorbtial ridge, best appreciated looking from the side), chemosis (conjunctival oedema).
  3. Lid retraction and lid lag (caused by sympathomimetic response of the eyelid muscles or proptosis or fibrosis in the superior rectus levator palpebrae superioris muscle complex). Ask patient to fix on your finger, held at least a metre away, and not move their head; move the finger slowly upwards and downwards, observing the movement of the patient's eyes and eyelids. Normally they should move simultaneously; in lid lag the lids move more slowly than the eye.
  4. Offer to test visual acuity and visual fields.

Skin and subcutaneous tissues	Embryonic remnants
– Epidermal (sebaceous) cyst – Lipoma	– Branchial cyst – Cystic hygroma – Dermoid cyst – Thyroglossal cyst
Lymph nodes	**Salivary glands**
– Acute infection – Chronic infection (tuberculosis, actinomycosis, syphilis and HIV) – Malignant (carcinoma, sarcoma, lymphoma or leukaemia), primary or secondary (Virchow's node in abdominal malignancy) – Sarcoidosis and autoimmune disorders	– Submandibular – Tail of parotid gland – Sublingual
Vascular	**Thyroid swelling**
– Carotid artery aneurysm – Carotid body tumour – Subclavian artery aneurysm	– Thyroid cyst – Neoplasia: benign adenoma, carcinoma – Goitre

Table 7.15. Differential diagnosis of neck lump (layers of origin and structures)

Orthopaedic examinations

In orthopaedic examinations, where joints are mainly assessed, the following sequence of actions is recommended:

- **Look** at the patient, the problem and any relevant indicators (aids, testing devices etc.)
- **Feel**, after asking about tender areas.
- **Move**, assessing active and passive movements of the joint.
- **Perform** special tests.

This sequence of actions is demonstrated for each examination below.

Examination of the hip joint

The patient must be adequately exposed (down to underwear) and is best examined standing first and then lying down. The following steps are recommended:

- Introduction, assessment of comfort, verbal consent, hand hygiene, as standard.
- With patient in standing position, comment on the presence of any walking aids.

Look

- From the front, for any obvious swelling, deformity, skin changes, scars, sinuses, pelvic tilt or antalgic position.
- From the side, for changes in the spine curvatures (kyphosis or lordosis) or scars.
- From behind, assessing any asymmetry of the shoulders, the alignment of the spine (scoliosis), the position of the pelvis (pelvic tilt) and any lower extremity malalignment (valgus / varus deformity of the knee).
- Assess the muscle bulk – particularly gluteal, hamstrings and quadriceps and comment on possible muscle wasting (old poliomyelitis, Charcot-Marie-Tooth) or hypertrophy (calf pseudo-hypertrophy in muscular dystrophy).
- Ask the patient to walk and assess the progression of phases of the gait cycle (stance, toe-off, swing and heel-strike) and the flexion / extension at all lower limb joints.

Abnormal gait patterns

- Trendelenburg gait: pelvic sway / tilt (waddling gait if bilateral)
- Broad-based (ataxia)
- High-stepping (loss of proprioception / drop foot)
- Antalgic (reduced stance phase on the affected side)
- In-toeing (persistent femoral anteversion)

Perform the Trendelenburg test

- Ask the patient if they are able to stand on one leg.
- Position yourself opposite to the patient; ask them to rest their forearms on your forearms and at the same time place your index fingers on patient's anterior superior iliac spines (ASIS) bilaterally. (In this way you ensure patient safety and protect them from falling).
- Ask the patient to raise the foot of the non-examined side from the ground, holding the hip joint at between neutral and 30° of flexion. The knee should be flexed sufficiently to allow the foot to be clear of the ground and therefore nullify the effects of the rectus femoris muscle. Watch the movement of the pelvis and position of ASIS of the opposite unsupported side.

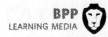

- Normal (Trendelenburg negative): The unsupported side of the pelvis remains at the same level as the side the patient is standing on, or it may even rise a little, because of powerful contraction of hip abductors on the stance leg.
- Abnormal (Trendelenburg positive): In the one-legged stance, the unsupported side of the pelvis tilts downwards, because of weakness of hip abductors on the stance leg. Also the patient may try to compensate by swinging his / her torso away from the unsupported side, ie towards the examined abnormal hip. The abnormal tilt can be noted immediately or after 30 seconds of one-leg standing (delayed positive test), which indicates abnormal fatiguability of the hip abductors.

Causes of positive Trendelenburg test

- Neurological disorders.
- Mechanical disorders.
  - Congenital dislocation of the hip.
  - Subluxating hips.
  - Coxa vara.
  - Slipped femoral capital epiphysis.
  - Perthes disease.
  - Arthritis of the hip.
  - Leg length inequality after hip arthroplasty.
  - Avulsion of the greater trochanter after hip arthroplasty.
  - Fractured neck of femur.
  - Avascular necrosis of the femoral head.
- Spinal disorders.
  - Ankylosing spondylitis.
  - Severe scoliosis.
  - Pain from nerve root irritation.

- With patient supine complete the inspection:
  - Comment on the quadriceps muscle bulk.
  - Measure the true and apparent lengths for each leg, using a tape measure, and compare the two sides.

The apparent leg length is measured from a fixed midline point (ie the umbilicus or xiphisternum) to the medial malleolus of each leg.
True leg length: from the anterior superior iliac spine to the medial malleolus.

  - If there are different apparent leg lengths and equal true lengths, the discrepancy is positional, usually because of tilted pelvis.
  - If there is true leg length discrepancy, it is secondary to bone shortening and you need to determine which segment is the cause:
    a. Below or above the knee?
       Perform the Galeazzi test: Ask the patient to flex hips to about 45° and knees to about 90°. Ensure that the heels are together on the couch, with medial malleoli touching. Look from the side to determine if the knees are at the same level. If one is proximal to the other, there is femoral shortening; if it is lower to the other there is tibial shortening.

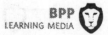

b. If it is above the knee, is it above or below the greater trochanter?
Draw a perpendicular from the side of the ASIS, measure the distance from greater trochanter to this line and compare the two sides.

Causes of limb length discrepancy:

- Fractures / dislocation of the neck of femur / femoral shaft / tibia.
- Avascular necrosis of the femoral head.
- Perthes disease, Developmental Dysplasia of the Hip (DDH), Slipped Upper Femoral Epiphysis (SUFE).
- Neuromuscular disorders (Poliomyelitis infection).
- In children – hemimelia, hemihypertrophy, vascular malformation, haemangioma, epiphyseal plate injury, Wilms' tumour.

Feel

Feel for any soft tissue swelling or tenderness along the iliac bone and greater trochanter.

Move

Assess active movements of the hip joint and determine if limited movement is caused by pain and, if not, assess range of passive movements. (See also Chapter 1: *Anatomy – The hip joint*.)

- Flexion.
- Extension (patient must be prone for this movement).
- Abduction and adduction: Place a finger on the ASIS contralateral to the hip being examined to identify the true movement at the hip joint (there can be significant compensatory movement of the pelvis).
- Internal and external rotation – perform both with the leg extended and flexed.
- (Rotation is often the first movement to be limited by pain in degenerative and inflammatory conditions.)
- Assess the power of the hip flexors and extensors.
- **Perform the Thomas test** to identify fixed flexion deformity:
Ask the patient to fully flex both hips and knees, bringing them up to their chest. Place your hand under the patient's lumbar spine, ensuring that the lumbar lordosis has been obliterated. Holding one leg flexed, ask the patient to extend the other fully; if there is fixed flexion deformity the femur will not fully extend and the angle between the bed and the femur is the degree of fixed flexion deformity. This is then repeated for the other leg.

Finally

Finally, offer to examine the joints above and below (spine and knee) and to perform a full neurovascular examination of the lower limb.

Surgical pathology

Fractures of the proximal femur

Epidemiology

The incidence is approximately 10 per 1,000 population in the UK; an increasing trend is noted due to increasing elderly population. They are more common in women.

Risk factors

- Increased risk of falls (concurrent medical illness, cognitive impairment, medications, alcohol).
- Decline of protective responses (confusion, dementia, neuromuscular disorders).
- Loss of local shock absorbers (muscle atrophy and loss of fat from hip region).
- Decreased bone strength (osteoporosis and relevant risk factors, primary or secondary malignant disease).

Clinical manifestations

- Inability to weight bear after a fall.
- Shortened and externally rotated leg, the greater trochanter is elevated on the injured side.
- Tenderness over the anterior and lateral aspects of the hip joint.
- Extremely painful movements (except in the case of an impacted type of fracture).
- If the fracture is spontaneous or with minimal energy trauma, it is likely to be pathological; in these cases patients may experience pre-fracture pain.

Diagnosis

- X-ray: Anteroposterior and lateral view of hip.
- If doubt about diagnosis, MRI scan is most accurate (shows bone marrow oedema).
- In cases of pathological fractures, further staging imaging may be required.
- Isotope bone scan is not specific.
- In doubtful cases waiting, mobilising and then repeating X-rays is not recommended as it runs the risk of displacement of an undisplaced fracture.

Classification

Fractures of the proximal femur are classified according to their anatomical position into *intracapsular*, *subcapital*, *transcervical* and *basal* (or basicervical). Differences between intracapsular and extracapsular fractures are presented in Table 7.16.

Classification of intracapsular fractures according to degree of displacement (Adapted from Garden 1961)

- Grade I: Incomplete fracture of the neck (impacted or abducted).
- Grade II: Complete fracture without displacement.
- Grade III: Complete with partial displacement (there is malalignment of the femoral trabeculae).
- Grade IV: Complete femoral neck fracture with full displacement. The proximal fragment is free and lies correctly in the acetabulum so that the trabeculae appear normally aligned.

Management

	Intracapsular	Extracapsular
Incidence	Less common	More common
Causative violence	Minimal rotation violence	Lateral violence
Clinical features		
• External rotation	Minimal	Fully externally rotated
• Local swelling	Nil	Marked local swelling
Complications		
• Non union	Common	Does not occur
• Malunion	Rare	Common

Table 7.16. Differences between intracapsular and extracapsular hip fractures

- History: Determine comorbidities, drugs, pre-fracture mobility, and social circumstances.
- Examination: Look for dehydration, cardiorespiratory disease, CNS impairment, perform mini mental test.
- Provide adequate pain relief.
- Blood tests to prepare for surgery: Full Blood Count, renal function tests, electrolytes, clotting screen, group and save, chest X-ray, ECG.
- Ensure hydration while patient is starved.
- Thromboprophylaxis: Mechanical / chemical.
- Definitive treatment: The mode of treatment depends on the anatomical classification of fracture and patient's fitness for surgery.
  1. Intracapsular fractures
     a. Conservative treatment: Rarely used, reserved only for impacted fractures. Consists of bed rest followed by partial weight bearing or unrestricted weight bearing. It is associated with high risk of displacement requiring arthroplasty (15%).
     b. Internal fixation: The fracture is reduced on table using traction, internal rotation and abduction or adduction guided by image intensifier. (The displacement risk is 5% for undisplaced fractures.) The fixation is performed with three cannulated partially threaded screws or a sliding hip screw with use of a derotation pin / screw.
     c. Arthroplasty: Options include either a hemiarthroplasty (cemented Thompson, cemented bipolar hemiarthroplasty or uncemented Austin Moore) or total hip replacement (this is considered in coexistent osteoarthritis, rheumatoid arthritis, Paget's disease, metabolic bone disease or damage to the acetabulum, but with inferior results compared to arthroplasty performed for osteoarthritis).

  Post-operative care: For elderly patients, no restriction on weight bearing. Follow up is usually required with X-ray to look for malunion, avascular necrosis or non-union. Complications of internal fixation of intracapsular fractures include early redisplacement, non-union, avascular necrosis, backing out of screws, and fracture around screw entry point.

  2. Extracapsular fractures
     The treatment options include:
     a. Extramedullary fixation: For trochanteric and high subtrochanteric fractures.
     b. Sliding (dynamic) hip screw method of choice (DHS): To allow compression of the fracture while maintaining the neck shaft angle of the femur.
        Complications of DHS fixation include:
        – Cut out of lag screw through the femoral head (2–10%).
        – Detachment of plate from femur (1–3%).
        – Non-union.
        – Avascular necrosis of femoral head (very rare).

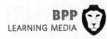

   c. Intramedullary fixation of extracapsular fractures with a *cephalomedullary nail*, for:
- Low subtrochantric fractures as biomechanically more stable than plates.
- Hip fracture with ipsilateral femoral shaft fracture.
- Pathological extracapsular fractures.

Complications

- Non-union: Failure of union of this fracture, due to improper reduction of imperfect internal fixation. The patient complains of pain and develops instability on walking.
- Avascular necrosis of the femoral head: A complication after any type of internal fixation. The patient presents with pain in the hip and limping. There is limitation of all movements of the hip with muscle spasm. Radiography shows patchy areas of increased density in the head of the femur.

General	Local	Social
Respiratory Cardiac DVT/PE TIA/CVA Pressure sores Urinary tract infection Gastrointestinal haemorrhage Mortality	Wound infection Wound haematoma Failure of fixation Loosening of prosthesis Dislocation of hemiarthroplasty Re-operation	Reduction in ADLs Reduction in mobility Reduction in residential status

Table 7.17. Complications of treatment of hip fractures

Examination of the knee joint

Look

Look from front, side, back, mention any noted walking aids / splints.

- Inspect patient while standing and walking.
- Look for asymmetry between two sides, sinuses, scars (ie vertical midline incision of knee arthroplasty, transverse scars on either side of patella for arthroscopy), skin erythema or any obvious swelling.

> **Differential diagnosis of knee swelling**
> a. Swelling confined to the limits of synovial cavity and suprapatellar pouch: Joint effusion, haemarthrosis, pyarthrosis, space-occupying lesion.
> b. Swelling extending beyond limits of knee joint: Infection, tumour, major injury.
> c. Local swelling: Prepatellar bursitis (housemaid's knee), infrapatellar bursitis (clergyman's knee), meniscus cyst, exostosis.

- Assess the position of the patella and the quadriceps muscle for wasting.
- Look from the front for varus or valgus deformity (measure the intermalleolar distance between two ankles if valgus) and from the side for fixed flexion deformity.
- Inspect the popliteal fossa for any swelling (Baker's cyst, semi-membranous cyst or popliteal aneurysm).
- Watch patient walking; look for antalgic gait and varus thrust (collapse into more varus in stance loading due to medial compartment osteoarthritis or lateral ligament laxity).

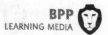

Feel

Feel, with patient lying supine:

- With the back of your hand, assess the temperature over the knee joint.
- Palpate for synovial thickening and any effusion in the knee:
  - **Perform the patellar tap test**: Squeeze any excess fluid from the suprapatellar pouch towards the knee by sliding your palm from the quadriceps to the patella. Jerk the patella quickly downwards; a 'click' indicates effusion, although small or very tense effusions can give negative test.

  - **Displacement test**: Evacuate the suprapatellar pouch as above. Stroke the medial side of the joint from the quadriceps to the tibia to displace any fluid laterally. Repeat on the lateral side and watch fluid filling the medial compartment.
- While watching patient's face, look for tenderness palpating:
  - The femoral condyles (knee bent).
  - The medial and lateral joint line (knee bent).
  - The medial and lateral collateral ligaments.
  - The patellar tendon and facets.
  - The tibial tuberosity (traction apophysitis in Osgood-Schlatters disease).
  - The popliteal fossa for any swelling.

Move

Assess the range of movements, active and passive (see Chapter 1: *Anatomy – The knee joint*).

- Extension (0°):
  - With patient sitting on the side of the examination bed, examine the extensor apparatus: Ask patient to extend knee while supporting the ankle and feeling the tone of quadriceps.
  - With patient supine, lift the leg supporting it at the heel to see if there is complete knee extension (to rule out fixed flexion deformity) or any degree of hyperextension.
- Flexion (> 135°): Ask patient to fully flex the knee, one side at a time; at the full active flexion ask the patient what is preventing further flexion (pain or stiffness). If there is no pain, assess if further passive flexion is possible.
- Repeat each movement for the opposite leg at the same time comparing symmetry.
- During passive flexion / extension of the knee place your palm on the patient's patella and feel for crepitus (osteoarthritis of the patello-femoral compartment).

Special tests

Position patient supine and ensure that there is no stiffness or pain at the hip joint.

- Assess the anterior knee stability (anterior cruciate ligament – ACL):
  Perform the anterior drawer test. Keep knee flexed to 90° and foot stable on the couch, then pull the proximal tibia forwards with both hands, assessing for abnormal anterior movement. Also, perform **the Lachman test**; hold the thigh firmly with your left hand from underneath, and the upper tibia with the right hand. Flex the knee slightly and assess for abnormal antero-posterior movement of the tibia on the femur.
- Assess the posterior knee stability (posterior cruciate ligament – PCL):
  Look for posterior sag; with both knees flexed, inspect from the side looking for posterior displacement of the tibia in relation to the femur. Also perform the **posterior drawer test**: push the proximal tibial backwards and assess for abnormal posterior movement.
- Assess for valgus and varus stress instability (for the medial and lateral collateral ligaments respectively):

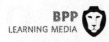

Hold patient's leg with both hands, placing your fingers bilaterally over each knee joint line, supporting the patient's foot under your axilla. Apply varus and valgus stress moving your body and using one hand as a fulcrum. Perform the test with the knee fully extended first and subsequently flexed at 30°. Watch and palpate for opening of the medial joint space during the valgus stress and laterally during the varus stress.

- Examine the menisci.

  Perform the McMurrays test: Flex the knee, take the foot with your right hand, internally rotate the leg and passively extend the knee, placing your left hand on the knee with fingers on both joint lines, while maintaining the internal rotation. If patient complains of lateral compartment pain or a 'click' is felt by your fingers, lateral meniscal injury is likely. The test is repeated with the leg externally rotated to assess the medial meniscus.

Examination of the shoulder

Look

- Inspect patient from the front, the side (patient standing) and above (patient sitting), looking for asymmetry, scars, sinuses, deltoid wasting, sternoclavicular (SCJ) or acromioclavicular (ACJ) joint deformity or swelling.
- From behind, look for rotator cuff wasting (supraspinatus and infraspinatus muscles), asymmetry in the shape and position of the scapulae (small and highly placed scapula in Sprengel's shoulder, skin webbing at the root of the neck in Klippel-Feil syndrome). Assess for winging of the scapula by asking patient to push their extended upper limbs against the wall (Table 7.18).

	Medial winging	Lateral winging	
Injured nerve	Long thoracic	Spinal accessory	Dorsal scapular
Muscle palsy	Serratus anterior	Trapezius	Rhomboids
Physical examination	Arm flexion; push-up motion against a wall	Arm abduction; external rotation against resistance	Arm extension from full flexion
Position of the scapula compared to normal	Entire scapula displaced more medial and superior	Superior angle more laterally displaced	Inferior angle more laterally displaced

Table 7.18. Neurogenic causes of scapular winging and physical examination
Martin *et al* 2007

Feel

- Palpate the SCJ, clavicle, ACJ, acromion, the glenohumeral joint, the spine of scapula and the biceps tendon in the bicipital groove of the humerus.
- Palpate the deltoid muscle and the rotator cuff muscles to assess for wasting.

Move

Assess the active (first) and passive (if active movements are restricted) range of movements, moving both arms at the same time:

- Forward flexion (0–165°), watching from the side, while patient swings arms forward and brings them above their head.
- Backwards extension (0–60°), watching from the side while patient swings arms backwards.

- Abduction (0–170°): watching from the back, to assess the *scapulothoracic rhythm*. Normally the glenohumeral (GH) to scapulothoracic (ST) motion ratio of total shoulder motion is 2:1, ie 180° of abduction consists of 120° of GH motion and 60° of ST motion.
    - If the range of movement is restricted, repeat passive abduction by holding the scapula fixed (placing your hand firmly on the shoulder) to evaluate the amount of glenohumeral movement: inability to abduct suggests that the previously noted movement was scapular rather glenohumeral).
    - Difficulty in initiating abduction indicates shoulder cuff tear.
    - Watch for painful arc: Pain that appears during abduction between 70–120° indicates shoulder cuff impingement at the acromion; if it appears after 120°, it indicates impingement and osteoarthritis at the acromioclavicular joint.
- Adduction (50°): Patient brings hand across chest to touch opposite shoulder with elbow flexed.
- Internal rotation (70°) and external rotation (100°) in abduction: watch from the side while patient abducts arms to 90°, elbows flexed to right angle and lowers the forearms from the horizontal plane (for internal rotation) and raises the forearms (for external rotation).
- Internal rotation in extension (70°): with patient elbows placed on the side of the body and flexed to right angle watch them move laterally.
- External rotation in abduction: patient palms are placed behind their head with the elbows pulled fully back.

Perform special tests

- To assess for impingement
    - **Neer's test**: Hold patient's scapula down, forearm pronated and forward flexion will cause pain indicating subacromial impingement.
    - **Hawkin's test**: With patient's arm in 90° forward flexion, internal rotation will cause pain, indicating impingement of the supraspinatus tendon against the coraco-acromial ligament. Crepitus can also often be detected at the subacromial bursa.
    - **Scarf test**: During forced cross body adduction in 90° flexion, pain at the extreme of motion is indicative of ACJ pathology.
- To assess for instability
    - **Sulcus sign**: Hold patient's arm at their side in a position of rest. Gently pull the arm downwards and look and palpate for a depression below the shoulder.
    - **Apprehension sign**: With the patient seated or supine, abduct arm to 90° and externally rotate the shoulder. The patient demonstrates apprehension that the shoulder will dislocate, and will often resist the activity.
- Examination of rotator cuff muscles
    - Supraspinatus strength **(Jobe's test)**: Patient arms abducted to 20°, elbows extended and thumbs pointing down; if there is pain in maintaining this position or weakness (patient cannot abduct further against your resistance) the test is positive indicating impingement.
    - Infraspinatus and teres minor: Resisted external rotation with the arms by side.
    - Subscapularis **(Gerber's lift off test)**: Ask patient to place their hand behind their back and push your hand away.
    - Biceps: Check for long head of biceps rupture. Also perform **Speed's test**; patient's supinated arm is flexed forwards against resistance; pain felt in the bicipital groove indicates biceps tendon pathology.
    - Deltoid: Test resisted abduction at 90°
    - Serratus anterior: 'Winging of scapula' test (described above).
- Finally examine the joints above and below (cervical spine and elbow) and assess the neurovascular status of the arm.

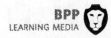

Surgical pathology

Rotator cuff disease – impingement syndrome

Impingement syndrome is caused by continuous abrasion of the rotator cuff muscles on the undersurface of the coracoacromial arch, with the anterolateral portion of supraspinatus being most vulnerable. It is usually reversible, but may lead to rotator cuff tear or even degenerative change in the glenohumeral joint ('rotator cuff arthropathy') if untreated.

Symptoms are more common in middle-aged and elderly patients often after a period of unaccustomed overhead overuse of the arm or injury. A painful arc of movement is noted between 60° to 120° of abduction, manifested by pain on overhead use of the arm. Passive movements are preserved, but the patient has positive tests for impingement (see above). Plain radiographs may be normal or may show sclerosis of subacromial bone.

Management

- Conservative: Relief of symptoms by subacromial injection of corticosteroid and local anaesthetic is diagnostic and therapeutic, although usually with only temporary relief (four to six weeks). Activity modification, non-steroid anti-inflammatory drugs and physiotherapy are useful adjuvant treatments.
- Surgical: Open or arthroscopic subacromial decompression, involving excision of the subacromial bursa (bursectomy) and removal of the anterior acromial spur (acromioplasty).

Rotator cuff tears

They are commonest in the middle-aged and elderly ('grey hair equals cuff tear'), resulting from chronic impingement or acutely after a shoulder injury. They manifest with pain and weakness when attempting to reach to the side or overhead. The supraspinatus and infraspinatus are usually involved, and inability to initiate abduction with selective weakness on resisted external rotation is usually pathognomonic.

Plain radiographs may show superior migration of the humeral head and degenerative joint disease of the shoulder or acromioclavicular joint. Ultrasound or MRI should be obtained to confirm the clinical diagnosis, assess the tear size and assess the extent of its retraction.

The management depends on the size and chronicity of the tear and patient's physiological status:

- Small or partial-thickness tears can often be treated conservatively or, if symptomatic, by open or arthroscopic repair of the cuff and subacromial decompression.
- Large symptomatic tears (> 2 cm) should also be treated surgically in those aged < 70 years with relatively acute tears.
- Massive tears (> 5 cm) are usually difficult to repair due to retraction of the muscle tendon. Pain may be relieved by decompression and partial repair of the cuff, or by transfer of the latissimus dorsi tendon (rare).

Adhesive capsulitis ('frozen shoulder')

This refers to chronic inflammation and fibrosis of the subsynovial layer of the shoulder capsule that reduces the range of active and passive movement of the shoulder. It is more common in the middle age.

Causes and risk factors

- Minor trauma
- Prolonged immobilisation of the shoulder
- More common in women and patients with heart disease or diabetes.
- Symptoms include severe debilitating pain that disrupts sleep. A marked limitation of shoulder movement is typical. The clinical course passes through an initial painful stage, followed by a stiff, and then a resolving 'thawing' phase. Selective loss of passive external rotation movement is diagnostic.

Management

The recovery of function can be long and the treatment options are:

- Conservative: Pain relief (NSAIDs), maintenance of range of movement by physiotherapy.
- Invasive, non-operative: Distension arthrography (injecting fluid to stretch the joint capsule).
- Operative: Manipulation under anaesthesia or, rarely, arthroscopic surgical release may be indicated in refractory cases, with physiotherapy starting immediately to retain the extra movement achieved.

Examination of the elbow

History taking

Enquire for:

- Patient age, duration of complaints, or time since onset of the elbow-related symptoms.
- Dominant side (as in every history-taking regarding upper extremity complaints); recent reversal of the natural dominance indicates severe impairment of function.
- Site and severity of pain (visual analogue scale).
- History of locking, pain and / or instability during throwing movements, joint swelling, or inability to extend the elbow (suggesting joint effusion).
- Paraesthesiae of the hand (ulnar nerve compromise at the level of the elbow).
- Any previous treatments of the elbow (synoviorthesis, intra-articular injections, surgery).

Clinical examination

Examine the patient standing, adequately exposed, and having both forearms in full extension on the sides. (Ensure you are familiar with the anatomy of the elbow – see Chapter 1: *Anatomy – The elbow joint*.)

Look from the front, side and back of the patient

- Observe, comparing both sides for the presence of swelling, effusion, deformity, scars, muscle wasting.
- Assess the carrying angle: with the forearms extended on the sides and the palms facing forward, the forearm and hands are normally slightly away from the body (physiological valgus 5° to 15°), permitting the forearms to clear the hips in swinging movements during walking.
- Look for frequently encountered pathological features in rheumatoid arthritis patients:
    - Bulging in the para-olecranon groove (effusion or synovial tissue proliferation)
    - Prominence of the olecranon (a sign of posterior subluxation of the elbow)

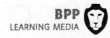

- Rheumatoid nodules on the posterior aspect of the elbow, and
- Bursitis
- Assess skin atrophy at steroid injection sites, or scars from previous surgery.

Feel

- Palpate (for tenderness):
  - The two epicondyles and the apex of the olecranon that form an equilateral triangle when the elbow is flexed 90° and a straight line when the elbow is in extension.
  - The radial head laterally.
  - Medially, for presence of supracondylar lymph nodes.

Move

- Flexion / extension 0–140°: Loss of extension provides a very sensitive clue to intra-articular elbow pathology.
- Pronation (70°) / supination (85°).

Special tests

- Evaluate mediolateral stability:
- Patient is examined lying supine; hold the patient's humerus with one hand, and with the other hand place the forearm in valgus (or in varus), while the elbow is flexed 20-30° (to remove the olecranon from the fossa). With the patient's abducted and externally rotated arm tucked under the examiner's shoulder, the medial collateral ligament may be palpated at the same time. The physiological laxity of the elbow between 10 and 20° of flexion, in varus and in valgus, does not exceed 5°.
- Assess anteroposterior stability (controlled exclusively by the collateral ligaments).
- Flex the forearm to 90° and hold it with one hand, while the other hand holds the humerus, and apply anteroposterior stress to the joint.
- Tests for epicondylitis
  - Tennis elbow (lateral epicondylitis): pain on resisted dorsiflexion of the wrist.
  - Golfer's elbow (medial epicondylitis): pain on resisted palmar flexion of the wrist.
- Offer to examine the joints above and below and perform neurological examination of the upper extremity.

Surgical pathology

Tennis elbow (lateral epicondylitis)

Tennis elbow manifests as pain over the lateral epicondyle of the elbow, radiating down the forearm, aggravated by active extension of the wrist. The presumed cause involves tendinosis of the insertion of extensor carpi radialis brevis. On examination, there is localised tenderness over the lateral epicondyle, exacerbated by gripping objects or resisted active extension of the wrist and fingers. The treatment is conservative with NSAIDs, physiotherapy and corticosteroid injections. Surgical release of the extensor origin at the elbow (with particular attention to that of extensor carpi radialis brevis) is indicated if conservative measures fail.

Student's elbow (olecranon bursitis)

Student's elbow refers to inflammation of the olecranon bursa (by excessive leaning on the elbow, infection, gout or rheumatoid arthritis). Treatment includes rest and NSAIDs and antibiotics for infected cases. Chronically enlarged or infected bursae may require surgical excision.

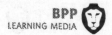

Golfer's elbow (medial epicondylitis)

Golfer's elbow presents with pain over the medial epicondyle, aggravated by resisted forearm pronation and wrist flexion. The treatment is the same with lateral epicondylitis (NSAIDs and physiotherapy). Surgery involves release of the common flexor origin for refractory cases.

Examination of the hand

Ask if the patient has any pain, ensure adequate exposure by asking them to roll their sleeves up above the elbow and place a pillow on their lap.

Look

- Inspect the elbow (joint above), looking for rheumatoid nodules, calcinosis, or plaques of psoriasis on the extensor surface.
- Ask the patient to place hands palm down, inspect the dorsal surface and comment on
  - Any obvious changes such as amputated digits.
  - Skin changes such as erythema, rash, sclerodactyly, Raynaud's phenomenon, digital gangrene, scars (previous corrective surgery).
  - Soft tissue: Thenar wasting, small muscle wasting (carpal tunnel syndrome, primary or secondary to RA), nodules around joints. Heberdens nodes are usually found at the distal interphalangeal joints (DIP) and Bouchard's nodes at the proximal interphalangeal (PIP) joints.
  - Nail abnormalities: Look for any pitting or onycholysis (psoriasis), sub-ungual calcinosis.
  - Joints: Look for any obvious swelling or deformity, and the pattern of involvement (symmetrical / asymmetrical); involvement of metacarpophalangeal (MCP) / PIP joints suggests rheumatoid arthritis; the DIP joints are usually involved in osteoarthritis.
  - Bones: Look for any asymmetry or deformity; ulnar deviation of the MCPs, often associated with radial deviation of the wrist, Boutoniere's, Swan neck (Figure 7.2), Z deformity of thumb etc.
- Inspect the palmar surface.
  - Skin changes: Palmar erythema, telangiectasiae, scars, pitting, contractures (Dupuytren's)
  - Soft tissue: Thenar wasting small muscle wasting (carpal tunnel, primary or secondary to RA).

Feel

- Assess the temperature of the joints with the dorsal surface of your hand, feeling over the wrist, MCP and IP joints; cold fingers distally could be suggestive of Raynauds.
- Palpate the wrist joint (tenderness) and over the anatomical snuff box (scaphoid fracture, De Quervains tenosynovitis).
- Characterise any joint swelling that is identified (hard – bony, boggy – soft tissue swelling, fluctuant – suggesting effusion of the joint). Palpate the MCP and IP joints (swelling, tenderness).

Move

- Assess joint mobility but also hand function:
  - With palms facing up, clench hands into a fist to bury the distal phalanges in the palm (reduced in arthritis).
  - Turn the fist so palms face down (pronation).

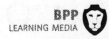

- Extend the little finger and then the remaining fingers (extensor tendons can be damaged especially in RA).
- Ask patient to place palm to palm (fixed flexion deformity) and then bring out elbows (wrist extension). Similarly place palms dorsum to dorsum (finger extension) and then bring out elbows in this position (wrist flexion).
- Assess hand function by asking the patient to:
  - Oppose the thumb to the tips of the remaining fingers on that hand.
  - Generate a pincer grip and try to pull it apart.
  - Generate a hook grip and try to undo.
  - Squeeze two fingers in a clenched fist.
  - Undo / do up a button.
  - Grip a piece of paper / your name card like a key, and attempt to pull it away (also a test of ulnar nerve function).
  - Write their name.

Central slip rupture - Boutonniere

Subluxed lateral band

Volar plate rupture - Swan neck

PIP in flexion
DIP in hyperextension

PIP in hyperextension
DIP in flexion

Figure 7.2 Boutonniere (left) and Swan neck (right) deformities of the hand

Vascular examination of the hand

- Feel for the radial and ulnar artery pulses.
- **Perform Allen's test**: Patient clenches fist and the radial and ulnar arteries are occluded with pressure; consequently the hand is unclenched and the return of erythema to the palm is observed on release of one of the arteries and repeated for the other.

Neurological examination

Motor

- Median nerve: Test the function of abductor pollicis brevis; with patient's palm facing up, stabilise the rest of patient's hand on the table and ask them to point with the thumb to the ceiling.
- Ulnar nerve: Test interossei of the hand with abduction and adduction.
- Radial nerve: Test wrist and finger extension.

Sensory (test grossly with soft touch)

- Volar aspect of index finger (median n. and C6).
- Volar tip of middle finger (C7).
- Volar tip of little finger (ulnar n. and C8).

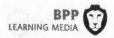

- First dorsal web space (radial n).
- With finger, run up dorsal surface of hand from tip of middle finger to the forearm (proximal neuropathy).

Surgical pathology

Carpal tunnel syndrome

Carpal tunnel syndrome (CTS) is a collection of symptoms and signs that occur following entrapment of the median nerve within the carpal tunnel.

Epidemiology

Carpal tunnel syndrome is a common condition with 37,745 carpal tunnel decompressions performed by the NHS in England in 2001. The prevalence of carpal tunnel syndrome in the general population ranges between 2.7 and 5.8%. Carpal tunnel syndrome is approximately three times more common in women than men.

Risk factors

The following have been associated with higher risk of CTS.

- Increasing age.
- Female sex.
- Increased body mass index (BMI).
- Square-shaped wrist, short stature, dominant hand.
- Race (white).
- Strong family susceptibility.
- Wrist fracture (Colles).
- Acute, severe flexion / extension injury of wrist.
- Space-occupying lesions within the carpal tunnel (eg, flexor tenosynovitis, ganglions, haemorrhage, aneurysms, anomalous muscles, various tumours, oedema).
- Diabetes.
- Thyroid disorders (usually myxoedema).
- Rheumatoid arthritis and other inflammatory arthritides of the wrist.
- Recent menopause (including post-oophorectomy).
- Renal dialysis.
- Acromegaly.
- Amyloidosis.
- Repeated activity involving severe force and extreme posture of the wrist / vibrating activity.

Clinical manifestations

- Intermittent pain, numbness and tingling, more common at night.
- Symptoms localised to the palmar aspect of the first to the fourth fingers and the distal palm (sensory distribution of the median nerve at the wrist).
- Patient relieves symptoms by shaking the hand / wrist.
- Autonomic symptoms: tight or swollen feeling in the hands and / or temperature changes (hands being cold or hot all the time) and rarely changes in sweating.
- Weakness / clumsiness.

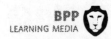

Examination findings

- Sensory deficit may be present on the palmar aspect of the first three digits and radial one half of the fourth digit.
- Motor examination: Wasting and weakness of the median-innervated hand muscles (LOAF muscles) may be detectable.
  L – First and second lumbricals
  O – Opponens pollicis
  A – Abductor pollicis brevis
  F – Flexor pollicis brevis

Special tests

- Tinel sign: Gentle tapping over the median nerve in the carpal tunnel region elicits tingling in the nerve's distribution (low sensitivity and specificity).
- Phalen sign: Tingling in the median nerve distribution is induced by full flexion (or full extension for reverse Phalen) of the wrists for up to 60 seconds (80% specificity but lower sensitivity).
- The carpal compression test: This test involves applying firm pressure directly over the carpal tunnel, usually with the thumbs, for up to 30 seconds to reproduce symptoms (sensitivity of up to 89% and a specificity of 96%).

Diagnostic work up

- Electrophysiologic studies including electromyography (EMG) and nerve conductions studies (NCS) are the first-line investigations in suggested CTS.
- MRI scan can exclude underlying causes in the carpal tunnel.

Management

- Treatment of underlying disease, if any.
- Conservative management of mild to moderate disease (EMG and NCS) includes:
  - Splinting the wrist at night time for a minimum of three weeks
  - Steroid injection into the carpal tunnel
  - Non-steroidal anti-inflammatory drugs (NSAIDs) and / or diuretics
- Surgical treatment is indicated for severe disease, or when conservative management fails and includes carpal tunnel release.

Anatomy of the Carpal tunnel

It is formed by the bony elements of the wrist forming a concave arch on the palmar side of the wrist (the sulcus carpi) and by the flexor retinaculum, a sheath of tough connective tissue.

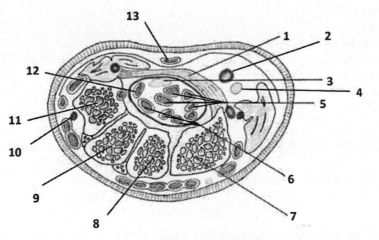

1. Flexor retinaculum
2. Ulnar artery
3. Median nerve
4. Ulnar nerve
5. Flexor digitorum superficialis (4 tendons)
6. Flexor digitorum profundus (4 tendons)
7. Hamate
8. Capitate
9. Trapezoid (Lesser multangular)
10. Radial artery
11. Trapezium (Greater multangular)
12. Flexor carpi radialis tendon
13. Palmaris longus tendon

Figure 7.3. Axial view of the wrist and carpal tunnel
Based on Gray H (1918), Anatomy of the Human Body, 20th edition, Lea & Febiger, Philadelphia.
(*This image is in the public domain because its copyright has expired. This applies worldwide.*)

It contains
- A total of *9 flexor tendons*
  - Flexor digitorum profundus (4)
  - Flexor digitorum superficialis (4)
  - Flexor pollicis longus (1)
- The *median nerve*

Examination of the spine

Expose the patient down to their underwear. Start with the patient standing, then lying prone and finally lying supine.

Patient standing
Look

- Inspect for scars (previous surgery), lumps (abscess, tumours) or sinuses (deep infections).
  - 'Cafe au lait' spots indicate neurofibromatosis and hairy patches are associated with congenital spinal abnormalities (dysraphism, myelomeningocele).
  - Look for features of specific syndromes, such as the low hairline of and short neck of Klippel-Feil (fusion or absence of cervical vertebrae), Sprengel shoulder (undescended scapula).
- Evaluate for any asymmetry in the shoulder height, loin creases (scoliosis) or iliac crest levels (leg length discrepancy) between two sides. If the patient consistently stands with one knee bent despite equal leg lengths (antalgic position), this may indicate nerve root tension or osteoarthritis. Lateral tilt may be a sign of a prolapsed intervertebral disc.
- Look from the side for kyphosis and lordosis or the presence of gibbus (acute angular deformity with bony prominence).
- Inspect for any associated anomalies of the hands or feet, eg syndactyly, pes cavus, which may be part of a syndrome.
- Observe the patients' gait.

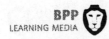

Feel

- With the back of the hand assess for temperature (inflammation, abscess).
- Examine for tenderness over the bony, intervertebral or paravertebral areas and feel for any bony prominence or steps.

Move

- Flexion: Flexion of the cervical spine should bring the patient's chin to their suprasternal notch.

  No flexion happens in the thoracic spine, because it is splinted by the ribcage.

  To evaluate the flexion of the lumbar spine, mark two spots about 10cm apart; these should separate by a further 5cm.
  - **Forward bend test**: Flexion accentuates any scoliosis by causing a rib prominence (rib hump) on the convexity of the curve and a loin crease on its concavity. Postural scoliosis disappears on forward bending; if the scoliosis disappears on sitting, it may be due to leg shortening.
- Extension: Ask the patient to arch backwards, keeping the knees straight. For the cervical spine alone, extension should result in the patient's nose or forehead being parallel to the ceiling.
  - **Wall test**: Ask the patient to stand with his/her back against a wall. Observe if heels, buttocks, shoulders and occiput all touch the wall; if impossible, think of fixed flexion deformity.
- Lateral flexion: Ask the patient to run a hand down the ipsilateral thigh on one side, and then the other and look for asymmetry in the range of movement between sides.
- Rotation: Stabilise the patient's pelvis with both hands, and ask the patient to twist / turn to either side, looking for asymmetry of range of movement. No rotation is noted in the lumbar spine, because the facet joints are vertical. Rotation of the cervical spine should place the cheek parallel to shoulder.

Patient lying prone

Look

Watch the patient climb onto the examination couch.

Move

Femoral nerve stretch: acutely flex the knee with the thigh resting on the couch, or extend the hip with the knee in moderate flexion. If pain is elicited, the test is positive.

Patient lying supine

Look

Watch the patient turn over onto his / her back.

Move

- **Straight leg raise (SLR)**: Keep the knee extended and passively flex the hip by lifting the heel off the examination couch (normal angle of elevation 80–90°). If restricted by pain radiating from the back to below the knee there is evidence of sciatic nerve root irritation. Tension on the sciatic nerve by dorsiflexion of the ankle can increase pain. If the pain on SLR is felt in the contralateral limb (cross-leg pain or cross-sciatic tension), there may be a central disc prolapse with a risk of cauda equina syndrome.

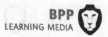

- **Lasegue's test:** Allow the hip to be fully flexed to reduce tension. If when the knee is extended from this flexed hip / knee position, the pain is reproduced, Lasegue's test is positive.
- Offer to assess the patient's hip ('joint below').

Following a standard full neurological examination of both lower limbs, any deficit secondary to nerve root compression should follow an anatomical distribution, (dermatome or myotome). Signs such as superficial tenderness, non-anatomical motor or sensory deficits, painful SLR but with the patient comfortably sitting forward with legs extended on the examination couch etc, indicate non-organic cause of symptoms.

Examination of foot and ankle

Look

- Expose the whole lower leg and foot and examine the patient's shoes if available.
- Ask the patient to walk and observe the walking gait, looking for:
  - A high stepping gait (foot drop or equinovarus).
  - An antalgic gait (ankle or posterior foot pain), which in case of forefoot pain has a short propulsive phase.
- Inspect the foot shape and particularly:
  - The medial arch (obliterated in pes planus, exaggerated in pes cavus).
  - The hindfoot (looking from behind) and look for varus (pes cavus) or valgus deformity (pes planus); in the latter more toes are seen on the lateral side of the leg when looking from behind ('too many toes' sign).
- Ask the patient to sit on the examination couch with both lower legs hanging over the side, if possible, and examine the foot from a lower level than the couch, if available.
  - Evaluate the overall foot shape and comment on any deformity. Look for a flat foot or a cavus foot (Figure 7.4).
  - Evaluate the condition of the skin, nails, muscle wasting, and bony prominences.

Feel

Ask the patient about any pain and request permission to feel the foot and tender areas, if any.

- Evaluate the skin temperature and indirectly in this way assess its perfusion. The temperature will be increased in inflammation or infection of the soft tissue or joints.
- Feel the ankle, systematically checking in succession the anterior joint line, the lateral gutter and lateral ligaments, the syndesmosis, the posterior joint line, the medial ligament complex and the medial gutter.
- Also palpate from laterally towards the dorsum of the foot and then towards medially.
  - Laterally, from distal to proximal, palpate the styloid process of the fifth metatarsal, posterior to it the groove in the cuboids for the peroneus longus tendon, the peroneal tubercle, the sinus tarsi (soft tissue depression just anterior to the lateral malleolus) and the dome of talus (made prominent by plantar flexing ankle).
  - Medially, from proximal to distal, palpate the first metatarso-cuneiform joint, the navicular tubercle (most obvious bony prominence in front of medial malleolus where the tibialis posterior tendon inserts), the head of talus (felt just behind the navicular, by everting and inverting the midfoot), the sustentaculum tali (one fingerbreadth below medial malleolus, serves as an attachment for the spring ligament and supports the talus), and the medial malleolus.
- Palpate the first metatarsal head and MTPJ, the metatarsal heads and web spaces.

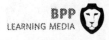

Move

- Ankle movements
  - Active: ask the patient to lift foot up (dorsiflex) and down (plantarflex).
  - Passive: For dorsiflexion, place one hand on the heel with the same forearm supporting the foot, while the other hand supports the tibia. Dorsiflex the ankle by lifting the forearm under the foot (normal ROM 55°). The ROM of plantarflexion is 15°.
- Subtalar: With one examining hand placed on the calcaneus and the thumb and index finger of the other hand on the talar head / neck, apply varus and valgus stress; the hand on the calcaneus feels for movement of the talus (normal = 5° in each direction).
- Midtarsal (talo-navicular and calcaneo-cuboid joints): Hold the calcaneus with one hand and move the forefoot medially and laterally with the other hand (adduction 20° and abduction 10°).
- Tarsometatarsal: There is no active motion, but test the joints for stability (by pushing each joint up and down).
- First MTPJ: The normal ROM is 70–90° dorsiflexion and 45° plantar flexion.

Perform neurovascular examination of the foot

Special tests

Muscle tests

Evaluate the good function of the muscles by performing the following tests:

- Tibialis posterior muscle and tendon: From behind, ask the patient to do a single foot tiptoe test on both sides; if abnormal, the affected heel cannot get off the ground.
- Tibialis anterior muscle and tendon: Ask the patient to walk on his heels with his feet inverted; the tibialis tendon can be seen prominent.
- Peroneals: Ask the patient to walk on the medial border of his feet.

Stability tests

- For the ankle perform **the anterior drawer test** (stability of anterior talofibular ligament): Stabilise the distal part of leg with one hand and apply anterior force to the heel with the other hand, in attempt to subluxate the talus anteriorly from beneath the tibia.
- **Talar tilt** (anterior talofibular and the calcaneofibular ligaments): The patient is seated and with the ankle and foot unsupported in 10 to 20° of plantar flexion; stabilise the medial aspect of the distal part of leg, just proximal to medial malleolus, with one hand and apply inversion force slowly to the hindfoot with the other hand; the lateral aspect of the talus should be palpated during inversion of hindfoot to determine if tilting is occurring at ankle.

Achilles tendon test (Simmonds / Thompson)

With the patient prone squeeze the calf; if movement is noted at the ankle the Achilles tendon is intact.

Pes planus (flat foot)

A variation in the normal contour of the foot in which its longitudinal arch is reduced so that, on standing, the medical (inner) border of the foot is close to or touching the ground. It is normal up to the age of three years (physiological flat foot). The pathological forms are classified according to aetiology into:

- Congenital: The condition presents at or around birth, due to structural anomalies arising in utero.
- Acquired
  - Static: commonest type, developmental in origin.
  - Posterior Tibial Tendon (PTT) dysfunction: secondary to degenerative changes in the tendon or excess physical activity.
  - Traumatic.
  - Paralytic.
  - Inflammatory (infiltration of the ligaments and plantar fascia of the foot following gonorrhoea, acute rheumatism or rheumatoid arthritis).

Pes cavus

A deformity of the foot in which clawing of the toes is combined with a raising of the long arch of the foot. Classified according to aetiology:

- Idiopathic: Family history is present with a hereditary developmental weakness of the muscles of the forefoot.
- Secondary to
  - Spina bifida (overt or occult).
  - Poliomyelitis.
  - Friedreich's Ataxia.
  - Pyramidal or Extrapyramidal syndromes (e.g. cerebral palsy).
  - Progressive peroneal palsy.
  - Direct trauma to the foot.
  - Myopathies (eg muscular dystrophy).
  - Plantar fibromatosis.
  - Congenital talipes equinovarus.

Further reading

- Dormandy, J ed (1989) *European consensus document on critical limb ischaemia.* Berlin: Springer Verlag.
- Dumontier C. Examen Clinique du Coude *Maitrise Orthopédique* No. 77, Octobre 1998 www.maitrise-orthop.com/corpusmaitri.orthopaedic/no. 77 dumontier/index us. shtml.
- Ederle J, Featherstone R and Brown MM. Percutaneous transluminal angioplasty and stenting for carotid artery stenosis. *Cochrane Database of Systematic Reviews 2007,* Issue 4. Art. No.: CD000515. DOI: 10.1002/14651858.CD000515.pub3.
- EVAR trial participants: Endovascular aneurysm repair and outcome in patients unfit for open repair of abdominal aortic aneurysm (EVAR Trial 2): randomised controlled trial. *Lancet* 2005; 365 (9478): 2187–92.
- Garden, RS, Stability and union in subcapital fractures of the femur *J Bone Joint Surg Br*; 1961; 46: 630–647.
- Greenhalgh, RM, Brown, LC, Kwong, GP, *et al.* Comparison of endovascular aneurysm repair with open repair in patients with abdominal aortic aneurysm (EVAR trial 1), 30-day operative mortality results: randomised controlled trial. *Lancet* 2004; 364: 843.
- International Carotid Stenting Study investigators. Carotid artery stenting compared with endarterectomy in patients with symptomatic carotid stenosis (International Carotid Stenting Study): an interim analysis of a randomised controlled trial. *The Lancet* 2010; 375 (9719): 985-997.
- Martin, RM, Fish, DE. Scapular winging: anatomical review, diagnosis, and treatments. *Curr Rev Musculoskelet Med* 2008; 1(1): 1–11.
- MRC Asymptomatic Carotid Surgery Trial (ASCT) Collaborative Group. Prevention of disabling and fatal strokes by successful carotid endarterectomy in patients without recent neurological symptoms: randomised controlled trial. *The Lancet* 2004; 363 (9420): 1491-1502.
- NHS (2011). *NHS Abdominal Aortic Aneurysm Screening Programme.* Available at: aaa.screening.nhs.uk.
- Rothwell, PM *et al.* Analysis of pooled data from the randomised controlled trials of endarterectomy for symptomatic carotid stenosis. *The Lancet* 2003; 361 (9352): 107-116.
- Schmedt, CG, Sauerland, S, Bittner, R, Comparison of endoscopic procedures v Lichtenstein and other open mesh techniques for inguinal hernia repair: a meta-analysis of randomised controlled trials *Surg Endosc* 2005; 19(2): 188–99.
- Sutton, G *et al. Developing Measurable Indicators for the Quality of Care of Hip Fracture Patients.* Institute of Public Health, University of Cambridge.
- The UK Small Aneurysm Trial Participants. Mortality results for randomised controlled trial of early elective surgery or ultrasonographic surveillance for small abdominal aortic aneurysms. *Lancet* 1998; 352: 1649–1655.
- Walker MD *et al.* Endarterectomy for asymptomatic carotid artery stenosis. JAMA. 1995; 273 (10): 1421-1428.
- Wheeless' Textbook of Orthopaedics (2011). Available at: www.wheelessonline.com/

Chapter 8
Procedural skills

Overview

This chapter focuses on the procedures that core surgical trainees are expected to master and practise safely on the wards, in an emergency setting and in the operating theatre. They can be examined either in the form of theoretic questions or in the context of a procedural skills simulating station. Such examination stations occur not only during the MRCS Part B exam, but have also been used during interviews in the selection process for appointments to surgical training grades. The objectives for the examiners (or interviewers) are to be reassured that candidates practicse along the guidelines of safety and have sound psychomotor skills. These procedures are part of the daily routine of junior doctors and are performed in large numbers; however, in exam (or interview) conditions, with the superimposed stress pressures, it is important that you perform the requested tasks according to 'textbook' guidelines – do *not* 'cut corners' and ensure you emphasise patient and operator safety. The technical aspects for these procedures are inseparable from the underlying basic medical science. Therefore, as well as providing a step-by-step guide for performing the commonest practical tasks, we also discuss relevant anatomical, physiological and clinical implications or topics for exam questions.

Intravenous access and fluid management

Peripheral intravenous cannulation

This is a commonly performed procedure with associated risks of infection (local and systemic), thrombophlebitis and embolism. Intravenous cannulae may be contaminated by the patient's skin flora at the insertion site or by the introduction of other organisms via the cannula hub or injection port; the associated bacteraemia rate is about 1 per 3,000 cannulae or 0.2 per 1,000 intravenous cannula-days. The most commonly isolated organisms are Coagulase-negative Staphylococci (35%). Staphylococcus aureus is the second most common (25%) organism.

Procedure (variations in practice conform to local microbiology policies)

- Introduce yourself and confirm the patient's identity.
- Explain the procedure, obtaining verbal consent.
- The ideal position would have the patient lying or sitting with their arm resting on a pillow.
- Apply the tourniquet above proposed site and identify a suitable vein (superficial with a few centimetres' length). Warn the patient about discomfort from the tourniquet.
- Decontaminate your hands before and after each patient contact and before applying examination gloves. Use correct hand hygiene procedure.
- Put on the gloves and clean the overlying skin with 2% chlorhexidine gluconate in 70% isopropyl alcohol and allow drying. If the patient has a sensitivity use a single use povidone-iodine solution.
- Remove the cannula from the package and check it is functioning correctly. Fold down the wings and open and close the port.
- Warn the patient of a 'sharp scratch' and to remain still.
- Insert the cannula at an angle of 20–40° through the skin with the bevel facing upwards.
- Observe for 'flashback' of blood into the hub of the cannula.
- Carefully thread the cannula into the vein with one hand while holding the needle still. This should bring the needle to the entrance of the cannula.
- Release the tourniquet and press over the vein at the tip of the cannula while removing the needle.
- Dispose of the needle in the sharps bin immediately.
- If appropriate obtain blood samples for laboratory tests.
- Place cap on the cannula and fix in place with a semi-permeable transparent dressing to allow observation of the insertion site.
- Flush the cannula through top port using syringe of normal saline. Watch the vein for any swelling in the subcutaneous tissue due to misplacement of the cannula.
- Date of insertion should be recorded in the notes.
- The cannula site should be inspected every 24 hours. In cases of discomfort or increasing inflammatory signs, the cannula should be resited immediately.

Gauge	External diameter (mm)	Length (mm)	Maximum flow (ml/min)	Colour
14G	2.1	45	290	Orange
16G	1.7	45	172	Grey
18G	1.3	45	76	Green
20G	1.0	33	54	Pink
22G	0.8	25	25	Blue

Table 8.1. Sizing of peripheral cannulae

External jugular vein cannulation

The external jugular vein (1) lies superficially in the neck extending from the angle of the jaw across sternocleidomastoid (2, 3) passing deep to drain into the subclavian vein. It can be used in emergency situations to provide essential venous access.

Procedure

- Introduction, patient ID check, description of the procedure and consent as above.
- Decontaminate hands and put on a pair of gloves.
- With the patient supine, tilt their head down by 10° if possible and identify the external jugular vein.
- Clean as above and using a small needle inject 1–2ml of 1% lignocaine subcutaneously around the insertion site (if time allowing).
- Take care not to inject local anaesthetic directly into the vein.
- Turn the patient's head to the side (if appropriate).
- Attach a 5ml syringe to the cannula and insert the cannula in the direction of the ipsilateral nipple.
- Aspirate while advancing checking for venous blood.
- Dispose of sharps and fix the cannula using dressing.
- Flush with normal saline, return the patient to a comfortable position and document the procedure.

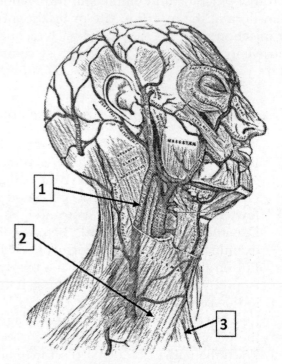

Figure 8.1 Anatomy of the veins of the neck
Based on Gray H (1918) Anatomy of the Human Body, 20th edition, Lea & Febiger, Philadelphia.
(*This image is in the public domain because its copyright has expired. This applies worldwide.*)

Central venous access

Central lines usually contain 1–3 individual lumens, each providing a separate port of access for administration of drugs or fluids. Longer term devices consist of subcutaneous cuffs and are tunnelled under the skin. This reduces infection and improves comfort. Absolute contraindications for insertion include superior vena cava syndrome and infection at the insertion site. Relative contraindications are: coagulopathy; newly inserted pacemaker wire; recent cannulation of internal jugular vein (check contralateral side); and prior neck surgery.

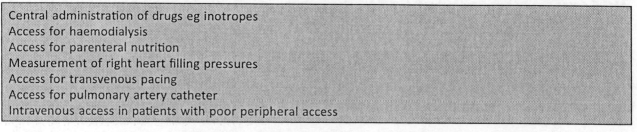

Central administration of drugs eg inotropes
Access for haemodialysis
Access for parenteral nutrition
Measurement of right heart filling pressures
Access for transvenous pacing
Access for pulmonary artery catheter
Intravenous access in patients with poor peripheral access

Table 8.2. Indications for insertion of central line

NICE Guidelines 2002 Central Venous catheters – ultrasound locating devices (Adapted from NICE, 2002)

Two-dimensional (2-D) imaging ultrasound guidance is recommended as the preferred method for insertion of central venous catheters (CVCs) into the internal jugular vein (IJV) in adults and children in elective situations and should be considered in most clinical circumstances where CVC insertion is necessary either electively or in an emergency situation. It is recommended that all those involved in placing CVCs using two dimensional (2-D) imaging ultrasound guidance should undertake appropriate training to achieve competence. Audio-guided Doppler ultrasound guidance is not recommended for CVC insertion.

Equipment for insertion of CVC

- Trolley
- Sterile gown / gloves
- Local anaesthetic
- Heparinised saline flush
- Ultrasound probe
- Cardiac monitor
- Dressing pack
- Antiseptic solution
- 2 small needles (19G, 25G)
- Dressing
- Central line kit (Seldinger)

Femoral vein access / cannulation

This is suitable for patients with severe coagulopathies as it is the most easily compressible site, but carries a higher risk of infection. It is also a useful site in patients with superior vena cava obstruction.

Anatomy (Figure 8.2)

The femoral vein passes medially and parallel to the femoral artery in the upper thigh, which runs at the mid-inguinal point (between the ipsilateral anterior superior iliac spine and the pubic symphysis). Remember the NAVEL of the femoral triangle: laterally to medially, Nerve, Artery, Vein, Empty space and lymphatics.

Procedure

Palpate the femoral artery at the level of the inguinal ligament and insert the needle 1–1.5cm medial and 2cm caudal to the artery. Insertion above the level of the inguinal ligament may cause bowel injury or retroperitoneal haematoma.

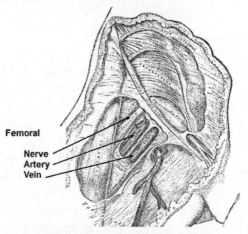

Femoral
Nerve
Artery
Vein

Figure 8.2. Femoral vein access
Based on Gray H (1918) Anatomy of the Human Body, 20th edition, Lea & Febiger, Philadelphia.
(*This image is in the public domain because its copyright has expired. This applies worldwide.*)

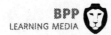

335

Internal jugular and subclavian vein access – insertion sites

Internal jugular vein (1, Figure 8.3)

Runs vertically in the neck under the anterior border of sterocleidomastoid muscle in a sheath with the carotid artery and vagus nerve. The anatomical landmarks include the mastoid process, carotid pulse and the depression between the two heads of sternocleidomastoid immediately above the clavicle.

- Palpate the carotid artery identifying its course.
- Insert the needle into the apex of the triangle made by intersection of heads of sternocleidomastoid at an angle of 30–40°.
- Direct the needle towards the ipsilateral nipple.

Subclavian vein (2, Figure 8.3.)

Runs over the first rib anterior to the scalene muscles. The vein joins the internal jugular vein to become brachiocephalic vein at the medial border of the anterior scalene muscle. The subclavian artery lies posterior and superior to the vein. The pleura extends to the proximal portion of the first rib near the origin of the brachiocephalic vein. Thoracic and right lymphatic ducts cross the anterior scalene muscle to enter the superior portion of the subclavian vein lateral to the origin of the brachiocephalic vein. Insertion sites are either the intersection of the middle and lateral thirds of the clavicle or the midpoint of the clavicle. The needle should be inserted 0.5–1cm below the clavicle aiming towards the sternal notch.

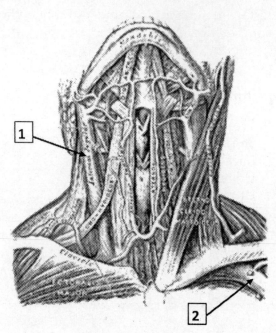

Figure 8.3 Anatomy of internal jugular and subclavian veins.
Based on Gray H (1918) Anatomy of the Human Body, 20th edition, Lea & Febiger, Philadelphia.
(*This image is in the public domain because its copyright has expired. This applies worldwide.*)

Procedure

- Introduction, patient ID check, description of the procedure and consent as before.
- Carefully position the patient (remove pillow, rotate head away, Trendelenburg position) and set up monitoring equipment (ECG for monitoring dysrythmias).
- Wash your hands, use sterile gloves and gown, prepare the skin and apply fenestrated drape.
- Choose the skin entry point as above.
- Using a small 25G needle inject 1% lignocaine to create a skin wheal, followed by a 19G needle to infiltrate the deeper tissues.
- Pass the needle slowly, gently aspirating on the syringe.
- Upon entry into the vessel occlude the needle to prevent air entrapment and carefully insert the Seldinger wire (J tipped).
- Withdraw the wire if any atrial or ventricular arrhythmias develop.
- Use the blade to make a small skin incision at the entry site of the wire.
- Insert dilator and advance to shoulder.
- Insert catheter, remove wire and suture into place.
- Dress the site and document procedure in patient's notes.

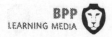

Early	Late
Bleeding	Venous thrombus formation
Haematoma	Thrombophlebitis
Arterial injury	Sepsis
Air embolism	Endocarditis
Subcutaneous / mediastinal emphysema	Chylothorax
Arrhythmias	Nerve injury
Pneumothorax / haemothorax	Development of arteriovenous fistula

Table 8.3. Complications of central venous cannulation

Central venous pressure

The central venous pressure (CVP) describes the pressure of blood in the superior vena cava near the right atrium of the heart. It is measured with the patient lying flat and expressed in cm H_2O above a point level with the right atrium. The normal value in a spontaneously breathing patient is between 0–8cm H_2O. The CVP equals the right atrial pressure. This pressure correlates with the amount of blood returning to the heart (right ventricular preload) and the ability of the heart to pump it further. CVP is affected by changes in venous blood volume or venous tone.

Increased CVP	Decreased CVP
Hypervolaemia	Hypovolaemia
PEEP (Positive end expiratory pressure)	Septic shock (vasodilation)
Tension pneumothorax	Increased venous compliance
Pleural effusion	Deep inhalation
Cardiac failure	

Table 8.4. Causes of altered CVP

Central venous waveform

The central venous waveform (Figure 8.4) reflects the events of cardiac contraction. Variations in pressure occurring during the cardiac cycle create a characteristic waveform. The central venous pressure and waveforms are also influenced by changes in intrathoracic pressure with respiration; the CVP decreases slightly with inspiration and increases slightly with forced exhalation and positive pressure (PEEP).

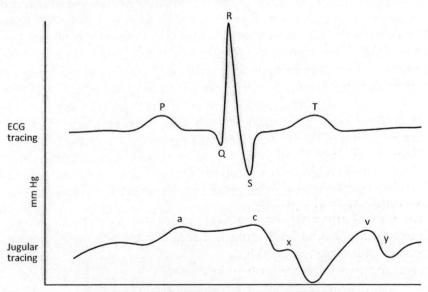

Figure 8.4. Central venous pressure waveform

- a wave: Due to increased atrial pressure during contraction. It occurs just after the P wave on ECG.
- c wave: Caused by elevation of tricuspid valve into right atrium during isovolumetric contraction. It corresponds with the end of the QRS complex on the ECG.
- x descent: Caused by right ventricular contraction pulling the tricuspid valve away from the atrium. It occurs just before the T wave of the ECG.
- v wave: Caused by the pressure produced when the blood filling the right atrium comes up against a closed tricuspid valve. It occurs at the end of the T wave on the ECG.
- y descent: Caused by the tricuspid valve opening in diastole with blood flowing into the right ventricle. It occurs before just before the P wave on the ECG.

Pathological waveforms

- Atrial fibrillation: Absent a waves.
- In atrioventricular dissociation: a waves are dramatically increased ('cannon waves') as the atrium contracts against a closed tricuspid valve.
- Tricuspid regurgitation: The c wave and x descent will be replaced by a positive wave of regurgitation as blood flows back into the right atrium during ventricular contraction. This can cause an elevated CVP measurement.
- Cardiac tamponade: All pressures will be elevated, and the y descent will be nearly absent.
- Tricuspid stenosis: Enlarged a wave with a muted y descent.

Fluid resuscitation

Methods of assessment and monitoring of fluid balance

- History: Alerts to likelihood of fluid deficit (eg vomiting / diarrhoea / haemorrhage) or excess (eg from intraoperative fluids).
- Weighing: 24-hour change in weight (performed under similar conditions) is the best measure of change in fluid balance and is simple to carry out by bedside.
- Fluid balance charts: They can have inherent inaccuracies in measurement and recording and do not measure insensible loss. There can be a large cumulative error over several days. Good measure of changes in urine output, fistula loss, gastric aspirate, etc.
- Urine output < 0.5 ml/kg of body weight per hour in adults is commonly used as indication for fluid infusion, but in the absence of other features of intravascular hypovolaemia it can be due to the normal oliguric response to surgery. Urine quality (eg urine / plasma urea or osmolality ratio) is just as important, particularly in the complicated patient.
- Blood pressure: Cuff measurements may not always correlate with intra-arterial monitoring. It does not necessarily correlate with flow and can be affected by drugs, etc. Nonetheless, a fall is compatible with intravascular hypovolaemia, particularly when it correlates with other parameters such as tachycardia, decreased urine output, etc.
- Capillary refill: Slow refill is compatible with, but not diagnostic of, volume deficit. It can be influenced by changes in temperature and peripheral vascular disease.
- Autonomic responses: Pallor and sweating, particularly when combined with tachycardia, hypotension and oliguria are suggestive of intravascular volume deficit, but can also be caused by other complications, eg pulmonary embolus or myocardial infarction.
- Skin turgor: Diminished in salt and water depletion, but also caused by ageing, cold and wasting.
- Dry mouth: Usually due to mouth breathing, but compatible with salt and water depletion.
- Sunken facies: May be due to starvation or wasting from disease, but compatible with salt and water depletion.
- Serum biochemistry: Indicates ratio of electrolytes to water in the extracellular fluid and is a poor indicator of whole body sodium status. Hyponatraemia is most commonly caused by

water excess. Hypokalaemia nearly always indicates the need for potassium supplementation. With high outputs the magnesium levels shoudl also be monitored closely. Blood bicarbonate and chloride concentrations measured on point of care blood gas machines are useful in patients with acid-base imbalance including iatrogenic hyperchloraemia.

- Urine biochemistry: Urine sodium concentration reflects renal perfusion and a low value (< 20mmol/L) indicates renal hypoperfusion. Urine potassium measurement is helpful in assessing the cause of refractory hypokalaemia. Urine urea excretion increases several fold in catabolic states (eg sepsis) and is an indication for provision of additional free water to avoid hypernatraemia and uraemia.

Treatment of hypovolaemia

The fluid challenge is a method by which the circulating volume can be safely restored to physiological need. Small boluses of fluid can be administered to create a known incremental rise in circulating volume, which can be assessed by the haemodynamic changes. Trends rather than fixed points are assessed to determine the fluid status of the patient. Intravenous boluses of colloid or crystalloid fluid (200–250ml) are recommended. (There is no evidence that resuscitation with colloids reduces the risk of death, compared to resuscitation with crystalloids, in patients with trauma, burns or following surgery as shown by a Cochrane Collaborative Study performed by Perel and Roberts in 2011 – a systematic review of 65 randomised controlled trials).

Following bolus administration, the effects can be monitored by measuring changes in the stroke volume, central venous pressure (or pulmonary artery wedge pressure PAWP), blood pressure, pulse, urine output and capillary refill. Such changes in the CVP / PAWP will depend on the initial circulating volume. Stroke volume is measured during fluid challenges rather than cardiac output as a decrease in the heart rate with a fluid challenge may result in a reduction in cardiac output despite an increase in the stroke volume. If there is a rise in the CVP / PAWP reassess after five to ten minutes to see if the rise persists. If the pressure returns to a lower level implying underfilling, further fluid boluses may be administered until the parameter normalises. However if the pressure remains high above normal range, this implies possible overfilling and caution should be taken. A 3mmHg increase in CVP / PAWP indicates an adequate circulating volume (Figure 8.5).

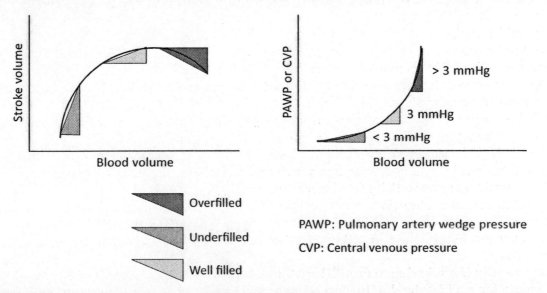

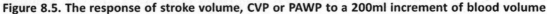

Figure 8.5. The response of stroke volume, CVP or PAWP to a 200ml increment of blood volume

All responses should also be assessed together with clinical responses. In cases of suspected or known congestive cardiac failure smaller fluid boluses of 50–100 ml can be administered and the response monitored. In situations where the central venous pressure remains in the normal range or higher but no similar improvements are seen in the blood pressure and urine output, inotropic / vasopressor support needs to be considered to maintain organ perfusion. Various studies have shown promising results with intraoperative oesophageal Doppler monitoring for fluid status optimisation, leading to a significant reduction in hospital stay.

Fluid	Na+	K+	Ca^{2+}	Mg^{2+}	Cl−	$HCO3^-$	pH	Osmolality	Plasma volume T½ (min)
Body compartment									
Plasma	142	4	2.5	1	100	25	7.4	280	
Interstitial fluid	145	4	2.4	0.9	118	27	7.4	280	
Intracellular fluid	12	155	0	15	8	10	7.2	280	
Secretions									
Saliva	50–70	15–20	–	–	10–15	30–50	6–7		
Gastric juice	150	5–10	–	–	100–160	10–20	1–3.5		
Bile	180–220	6–8	–	–	60–70	60–70	7–8		
Pancreatic juice	160	4	–	–	30–60	80–120	8–8.3		
Small bowel	140	4	–	–	100	25	7.8–8		
Crystalloids									
N. saline (0.9% NaCl)	154	–	–	–	154	–	5	300	80
Hartmann`s	131	5	2	–	111		6.5	275	68
Dextrose 4% Saline 0.19%	31	–	–	–	31	–	4.5	286	
Dextrose 5%	–	–	–	–	–	–	4.2	278	19
Bicarbonate 8.4%	1000	–	–	–	–	1000	8	2000	–
Colloids									
Gelofusine	154	0.4	0.4	0.4	120–125	–	7.4	274	180
Dextran 40	154	–	–	–	154	–	3.5–7.0	280–324	180
Dextran 70	154	–	–	–	154	–	5.0	280–324	1500
HAS 4.5%	100–160	<2.25	–	–	100–160	–	5.5	200–310	1000

Table 8.5. Electrolyte composition (mmol/L), pH and osmolality (mOsm/kg) of body compartments, secretions and commonly used intravenous fluids

Blood cultures

Blood culture sampling is an important investigation with significant implications for the diagnosis of patients with infection and administration of appropriate treatment. Caution must be taken to assure the quality and clinical value of blood cultures by avoiding sample contamination and 'false positive' readings. For this reason it is important that blood cultures are taken for the correct clinical indication, at the correct time and using the correct method. Reports from NHS Trusts and equipment suppliers suggest that the contamination rate could be as high as 10%. Common sources of contamination include the patient's skin, the equipment used to take the sample and transfer it to the culture bottle, the health professional's hands and the general environment.

* Abnormal core temperature
* Focal signs of infection
* Tachycardia, altered blood pressure (low or raised) or respiratory rate (raised)
* Chills or rigors
* Altered white blood cell count (raised or extremely low) and inflammatory markers (C-reactive protein, erythrocyte sedimendation rate)
* Confusion (new / worsening)

Table 8.6. Signs and symptoms of bacteraemia

Signs of sepsis may be minimal or absent in the very young and the elderly. After assessing the patient and identifying possible bacteraemia or sepsis, blood cultures should be taken **before** the administration of antibiotics. If a patient is on antibiotics, blood cultures should ideally be taken immediately before the next dose, with the exception of paediatric patients. Ideally blood cultures should be documented in the patient's notes including date, time, indications and site. With suspected bacteraemia, it is generally recommended that two sets of cultures are taken at separate times (5–60 minutes later) from separate sites. If suspecting bacterial endocarditis three separate sets of cultures should be taken. Do not use existing peripheral lines / cannulae. (If a central line is present, blood may be taken from a separate peripheral site, particularly if a central line infection is suspected; the peripheral vein sample should be collected first.)

Procedure

* Ensure hand hygiene, check patient's ID, provide brief explanation, obtain verbal consent.
* Label bottles with appropriate patient information.
* Check blood culture bottles are not out of date and clean any visibly soiled skin.
* Use a pair of gloves, apply a disposable tourniquet and palpate to identify the vein.
* Using 2% chlorhexidine in 70% isopropyl alcohol impregnated swabs, clean the tops of culture bottles (allow drying for 1 minute) and also the skin (allow drying for 30 seconds). If culture is being collected from a central venous catheter, disinfect the access port.
* Connect winged blood collection set to adaptor and insert the needle into cleaned site.
* Place adaptor cap over blood collection bottle and pierce septum.
* Collect sample using graduation lines to gauge quantity.
* Inoculate aerobic bottle first. Aim for 10ml blood per bottle.
* If collecting blood for other tests, take cultures first.
* Apply dressing to puncture site and dispose of sharps appropriately.
* Gently mix bottles by inversion, wash hands and document the procedure in the patient's notes.
* (Alternatively use syringe to collect sample but do not change needles between bottles.)

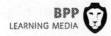

Urinary catheterisation

Urethral catheterisation

This is a routine medical procedure facilitating direct drainage of the urinary bladder. Catheters may be inserted as an in / out procedure for immediate drainage, left in for short-term drainage (eg during surgery), or left indwelling for long-term drainage for patients with chronic urinary retention. They are widely used in the diagnosis and treatment of urological problems, and in the resuscitation and monitoring of critically ill patients. Urethral catheterisation is contraindicated in the presence of traumatic injury to the lower urinary tract. In such cases a retrograde urethrogram is recommended to exclude any urethral injury before catheter insertion.

Diagnostic evaluation
   Obtaining urine sample for analysis
   Measure residual urine volume
   Accurate measurement of urine output in critically ill patients
   Cystogram, cystourethrogram, assessing vesicoureteric reflux
Therapeutic (short term)
   Acute urinary retention
   Epidural anaesthesia
   Instillation of drugs into bladder (chemotherapy in bladder cancer)
   Abdominal / pelvic surgery
   Management of patients with spinal injuries, neuromuscular degeneration
   Urinary diversion for decubitus ulcers or perineal infections
   Prevention of urethral obstruction by blood or clots (irrigation)
Therapeutic (long term)
   Refractory bladder outlet obstruction
   Neurogenic bladder
   Palliative care in terminally ill or severely impaired patients
   Prolonged and chronic urinary retention

Table 8.7. Indications for urethral catheterisation

Choice of catheter

- Choice of catheter depends on the size of the patient's urethral canal, the expected duration of catheterisation (e.g. intermittent or indwelling), any allergies (to latex or plastic) and the indications for catheterisation.
- Sizes of catheters
   - Diameters: 5fr, 6fr, 8fr 10fr, 12fr, 14fr, 16fr, 18fr, 20fr, 22fr, 24fr, 26fr.
   - The higher the number the larger the diameter of the catheter.
   - 1Fr = 0.3mm (i.e. a 24fr catheter is 8mm in diameter)
- Types (Figure 8.6):

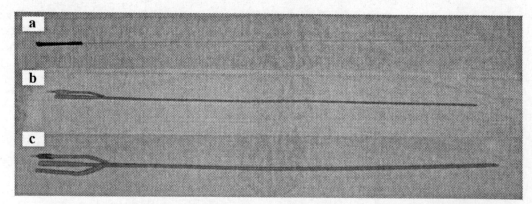

Figure 8.6. Types of urinary catheters: one-way (a), two-way (b), three-way (c)

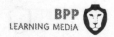

- Straight-single use catheters (a): They have a single lumen with a small 1¼ cm opening.
- Two-way Foley catheters (b): An inflatable balloon encircles the tip near the lumen or opening of the catheter.
- Three-way Foley catheter (retention catheters) (c): They have three lumens that encircle the body of the catheter. One lumen drains the urine through the catheter into a collection bag. The second lumen holds the sterile water when the catheter balloon is inflated and is also used to deflate the balloon. The third lumen maybe used to instil medications into the bladder or provide a route for continuous bladder irrigation.

Procedure: male catheterisation

- Wash your hands, confirm the patient's identity, explain procedure and obtain verbal consent.
- Place the patient in supine position with legs extended and flat on the bed.
- Set up trolley and unpack equipment including a catheter pack, a collecting bag (simple bag or urometer) and the catheter to be used (check correct catheter and intact balloon).
- Don a pair of gloves (you can wear two pairs and remove the first after cleaning).
- Use gauze to hold the penis and then clean it with saline working away from the meatus.
- Tear a hole in the centre of the drape and place over the penis.
- Retract the foreskin, clean properly and instil 10ml of lubricant into the meatus.
- Position a kidney dish between patient's thighs to catch spillage.
- Tear away small plastic portion over tip of catheter, taking care not to touch the catheter.
- Insert the tip of catheter into urethral meatus and advance slowly by feeding from the bag.
- Lift the penis to an angle of 60°–90° and continue advancing.
- When passing the prostate, resistance may be felt which can be countered by adjusting the angle of the penis to a horizontal position between the patient's legs.
- On entering the bladder, urine should flow freely.
- Advance the catheter to the bifurcation to ensure the balloon is beyond the urethra.
- Warn the patient as you inflate the balloon with 10ml of water (30ml in certain catheters) checking for pain. Ensure you have seen urine draining before inflating.
- Gently pull back on the catheter until the balloon engages with the bladder neck.
- Attach catheter bag, replace foreskin, clean and redress the patient.
- Remove gloves, wash hands, document the procedure and residual volume in the patient's notes.
- If resistance is noted at the prostate gland, examine the prostate for enlargement or nodules and arrange a urology referral.

Procedure: female catheterisation

- Wash your hands, confirm the patient's identity, explain procedure and obtain verbal consent.
- Place the patient in supine position with knees flexed and hips abducted with heels together.
- Set up trolley, unpack equipment (check correct catheter), and don a pair of gloves.
- Hold labia apart with non dominant hand.
- Clean genitalia properly (pubis-anus direction), drape appropriately and instil 5ml of lubricant gel into the urethral meatus.
- Position a kidney dish between patient's thighs to catch spillage.
- Tear away small plastic portion over the tip of catheter.
- Taking care not to touch the catheter, insert its tip into urethral meatus and advance slowly by feeding from bag. On entering the bladder, urine should flow freely.
- Advance the catheter to the bifurcation to ensure the balloon is beyond the urethra.

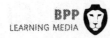

- Warn patient as you inflate the balloon with 10ml of water checking for pain. Ensure you have seen urine draining before inflating.
- Gently pull back on the catheter until the balloon engages with the bladder neck.
- Attach catheter bag, remove gloves, wash hands and document the procedure in the notes.

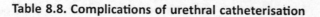

Infection: urethritis, cystitis, pyelonephritis
Bleeding
Pain
Urethral perforation or stricture
Creation of false passage
Paraphimosis (if foreskin left retracted)

Table 8.8. Complications of urethral catheterisation

Suprapubic catheterisation (Bonanno)

Indications

This can be a safer alternative in cases where the urethral route is contraindicated or not possible, such as urethral trauma, urethral or bladder neck obstruction, benign prostatic hypertrophy, and prostatic carcinoma.

Contraindications

- The absence of an easily palpable distended bladder.
- Previous lower abdominal pelvic surgery.
- Pelvic cancer with or without radiation therapy.
- Previous arterial surgery – femoral – femoral crossover

If a suprapubic catheter is necessary in these cases, insertion can be guided by flexible cystoscopy.

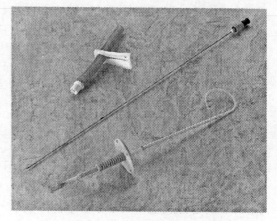

Figure 8.7. A Bonanno catheter

Procedure

- Wash your hands, confirm the patient's identity, explain procedure and obtain verbal consent.
- Place the patient in supine position with legs extended and flat on the bed. Ensure the pelvis is squared off.
- Set up trolley, unpack equipment and confirm full bladder (bladder scan / percussion).
- Don a pair of gloves, clean suprapubic area with antiseptic solution and drape appropriately.
- The insertion point is 2cm above the pubic symphysis.
- Infiltrate the insertion site with Lignocaine 1% and insert the 18G needle into the catheter.
- Push catheter needle through the anterior abdominal wall.
- Check position of the catheter in bladder by removing plug and aspirating urine.
- Disconnect the needle from the catheter and advance until disc flat against skin.
- Withdraw the needle completely.
- Attach catheter to a drainage bag.
- Suture catheter to the abdominal wall.
- Remove gloves, wash your hands and document the procedure in the patient notes.

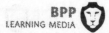

- Recommendations for safe practice in the insertion of suprapubic catheters (SPLs) have recently been published by the British Association of Urological Surgeons (Harrison *et al* 2011).

Low urine output

The normal urine output in adults ranges between 0.5 and 1 ml/kg of body weight per hour.

- Oliguria is defined as a urine output of less than 0.5ml/kg/hr for at least two consecutive hours or a daily urine output of less than 400 ml/day (about 15ml/hr).
- Anuria is the production of < 100ml of urine/day (absolute anuria equals no urine output).

Adequate urine output depends on satisfactory renal perfusion pressure, which is determined by the cardiac output, normal renal tubular function and the absence of any distal obstruction. Poor urine output may be an indicator of renal ischaemia, which if ignored, could lead to acute tubular necrosis and acute renal failure.

Clinical examination findings may include a dry mouth, cool peripheries, hypotension and tachycardia. Examination should also focus on excluding any obstruction (distended bladder) and excessive losses through drains etc. Investigations should help establish the cause of oliguria and assess the renal function: serum urea and creatinine, urine sodium and osmolality, renal ultrasound, and cardiac investigations.

Management of these patients must start with initially excluding any obstruction, then assessing the impact of a fluid bolus on both central venous pressure and urine output. All nephrotoxic drugs should be stopped. If measures fail, critical care input should be considered. In cases of established acute renal failure, renal replacement therapy may be required. This can be in the form of haemodialysis or haemofiltration. Indications for commencing such therapy are: uncontrollable hyperkalaemia; severe fluid overload with pulmonary oedema; uraemia (to prevent encephalopathy); and persistent / severe acidosis. (Also see Chapter 4 – *Renal physiology and critical care*.)

Pre-renal causes	Renal causes
Hypovolaemia (most common cause) • Dehydration, typically because of inadequate perioperative fluid management • Fluid depletion (vomiting, losses from nasogastric tube, diarrhoea, high output stoma, diuretic therapy, heat, fever, burns) • Sepsis • Haemorrhage	• Intrinsic renal disease • Following prolonged period of hypovolaemia • Nephrotoxic drugs (eg gentamicin) • Acute exacerbation of pre-existing renal disease
Renal hypoperfusion	**Post-renal causes**
• Drugs (non-steroidal anti-inflammatory drugs, angiotensin converting enzyme inhibitors, angiotensin II receptor antagonists, cyclo-oxygenase 2 inhibitors) • Hepatorenal syndrome • Acute heart failure • Myocardial infarction, arrhythmia, iatrogenic fluid overload • Abdominal compartment syndrome	• Urinary tract outflow obstruction • Obstructed catheter • Benign prostatic hypertrophy • Tumour compression of urinary outflow • Expanding hematoma or fluid collection
Oedema states	
• Acute heart failure (see above) • Nephrotic syndrome • Decompensated liver disease	

Table 8.9. Causes of postoperative oliguria

Insertion of nasogastric tube

This involves the passage of a plastic tube through the nose down the oesophagus into the stomach. This is a commonly performed procedure on surgical patients, and good understanding of its indications, contraindications, complications and technique is essential (Tables 8.10, 8.11). Enteral tubes are made of various materials, including latex, silicone, polyurethane and polypropylene, which is the most common material used. The simplest nasogastric tube is the Levin tube, which has a single lumen and multiple distal holes used for diagnostic aspiration of stomach contents or simple instillation of therapeutic agents. The tubes come in various bores: small – 10, medium – 12, large – 16. A fine bore tube can be used for short term nutritional support, whereas larger tubes are reserved for decompressing obstruction.

Indications
- Emptying stomach contents (prolonged ileus, in intubated patients to prevent aspiration)
- Decompression of gastric outlet or small bowel obstruction
- Delivery of oral agents – contrast medium, activated charcoal
- Nutrition
- Diagnostic aspiration of gastric contents – suspected upper gastrointestinal haemorrhage (poor sensitivity)

Contraindications
- Maxillofacial trauma with cribriform plate injury
- Oesophageal disorders – strictures, diverticulae – risk of perforation
- Unstable cervical spine injuries
- Nasal CPAP
- Relative contraindication – severe coagulopathy, variceal bleeding.

Table 8.10. Indications and contraindications for insertion of nasogastric tube

Equipment

- Gloves and gown
- Lubricant
- Appropriate sized nasogastric tube
- Anaesthetic spray
- Glass of water with straw
- Bowl for vomiting
- Bladder syringe
- Stethoscope
- Tape to secure tube

Procedure (Figure 8.8)

- Wash your hands, confirm the patient's identity, explain procedure and obtain verbal consent.
- Don a pair of gloves.
- Position the patient upright or in the high Fowler position (placement of the patient in a semi-sitting position by raising the head and trunk 90°, the knees may or may not be flexed).
- Examine to decide which nostril to insert the tube in.
- Measure the distance from xiphisternum to earlobe and then to the tip of nose (Figure 8.8).
- Can anaesthetise nasal cavity and posterior oropharynx with local anaesthetic spray.
- Lubricate the last few centimetres of the tube, insert tube into nostril and advance posteriorly.
- The tube will pass a corner at the nasopharynx.

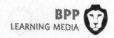

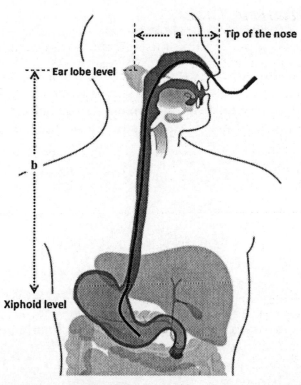

Figure 8.8 Insertion of nasogastric tube. The minimum length required to advance the tube is equal to a+b.

- Once the tube is at the level of the larynx, stop and have the patient sip water through a straw, co-ordinating the advancement of the tube with their swallow. This technique helps to ensure the tube enters the oesophagus and not the trachea.
- Advance the tube to the pre-measured distance and secure it to the patient's nose with tape.
- Confirmation of tube position:
  - Inject 30cc of air into the tube while auscultating over the epigastrium (borborygmus).
  - Aspirate gastric contents and check pH (<6). Note patients receiving H_2 antagonists or PPIs may have an unusually high pH.
  - Use a CXR to confirm position (below diaphragm) before feeding.

Minor	Major
Epistaxis Sinusitis Sore throat	Oesophageal perforation Pneumothorax Aspiration Intracranial placement

Table 8.11. Complications of nasogastric tubes

Nasogastric feeding

This is one of the simplest methods of enteral feeding. It is reliant on adequate gastric emptying. In cases of gastric atony the tube can be sited beyond the pylorus, as high gastric residuals and distention can cause vomiting and potentially lead to aspiration. Gastric residual volumes can be judged by spigotting the tube and aspirating intermittently (four-hourly). Feed can be administered from a large reservoir system of up to two litres. It is preferable to administer the feed continuously rather than intermittently to minimise bloating. Complications of feeding include: diarrhoea (approximately 10% patients); vitamin / mineral / trace element deficiencies; and blockage of the feeding tube. Note also that enteral feeding can react with certain orally administered drugs such as warfarin and digoxin.

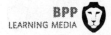

Scrubbing and gowning

Hand washing

Preoperative hand washing aims to reduce the number of normal and transient flora on the hands and to minimise the growth of bacteria under the gloves while operating. Prior to entering the theatre all jewellery should be removed and fingernails should be kept short. A single use sterile nail brush should be used but continual use is not advised as damage to the skin may occur.

Properties of the ideal scrub solution

- Significant reduction of transient and resident flora
- Effective against a wide spectrum of microorganisms
- Persistent effect after application (in case of glove puncture)
- Not damaging to skin

Povidone-iodine (PVP-I) is a stable chemical complex of polyvinylpyrrolidone (povidone, PVP) and elemental iodine (9.0% to 12.0%). It serves as an iodophor, slowly liberating free iodine that kills eukaryotic or prokaryotic cells through iodination of lipids and oxidation of cytoplasmic and membrane compounds. PVP-I exhibits a broad range of microbicidal activity against bacteria, fungi, protozoa, and viruses. The slow release of iodine minimises toxicity towards mammalian cells.

Chlorhexidine is a chemical antiseptic, effective on both Gram-positive and Gram-negative bacteria (although it is less effective with some Gram-negative bacteria). It has both bactericidal and bacteriostatic mechanisms of action, by causing membrane disruption.

Chlorhexidine gluconate 4% with soap is an ideal agent with a prolonged effect, whereas povidone-iodine soap solutions have a shorter duration of action, but both have a wide spectrum of activity. Alcohol antiseptics are as effective as the more conventional antiseptic detergent solutions with a wide spectrum of antimicrobial activity without any more damage to skin.

The recommendations by the World Health Organisation (WHO) are that if alcohol based antiseptics are to be used, a prior wash with non-medicated soap should be performed on entering the operating theatre, followed by at least three applications of hand rub for a period of three to five minutes. These alcohol based antiseptics have been shown to reduce resident skin flora levels rapidly, taking up to six hours to return to baseline.

A Cochrane review (Tanner *et al*, 2008) of ten randomised controlled trials analysed the effects of surgical hand antisepsis on surgical site infections. The authors concluded that alcohol rubs used by the surgical team in preparation for surgery are just as effective, if not more, in preventing surgical site infections. The evidence from four studies suggested that chlorhexidine gluconate based scrubs are more effective than povidone-iodine solutions in terms of the number of colony forming units on the hands.

Hand washing technique (from fingers to elbows, four minutes)

- Adjust water temperature and flow to avoid splashing.
- During washing, raise hands to above elbows so water runs down away from the hands.
- Use elbows to dispense antiseptic solution.
- Rub palm to palm with fingers interlaced.
- Rub right palm over left dorsum of hand and left palm over right dorsum of hand.
- Rub backs of fingers with the opposing palms with the fingers interlocked.
- Grasp the thumb of the opposing hand and rub by rotating the hand.
- Repeat with the other thumb and hand.
- Rub the palm of each hand with the clasped fingers of the opposing hand.
- Rub the left wrist and arm to within a few centimetres of the elbow using the right hand.
- Repeat for the other arm.
- If this is the first scrub of the session, brush under the nails, avoiding the skin.
- Wash the forearms again but stop one-third of the way from the elbow.
- Rinse hands and arms thoroughly, keeping hands up so water runs to the elbows.
- At arm's length use the first towel to dry one hand and arm.
- Pat, not rub, the skin dry working towards the elbow.
- Drop the towel on reaching the elbow.
- Repeat using the second towel for the other arm.

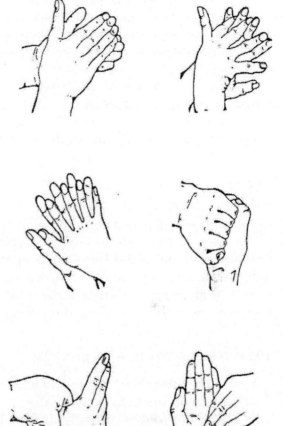

Figure 8.9. Hand washing technique
Reproduced with permission from H. Ali

Gloves

Gloves must be of high quality, low in extractable latex proteins and powder-free. There is evidence that adhesions and postoperative wound complications can be attributed to glove powder transferring latex proteins from the surface of the glove. An increased use of latex gloves has led to an increase in the incidence of latex allergy (between 28%–67% in high risk healthcare workers in the US). The allergy may take some time to develop. Gloves should also be pyrogen-free to prevent misdiagnosed pyrexia. Glove puncture is common place in surgery, particularly in procedures lasting longer than two hours. Between 50% and 92% of perforations pass undetected. It is possible for approximately 40,000 organisms to pass through a pin hole in a glove in a 20-minute period. Double gloving is recommended for certain procedures using an underglove. The inner glove should be a half size larger than the outer to optimise sensitivity, dexterity and comfort.

Masks

Traditionally masks were thought to reduce the bacterial contamination of wounds. However today they are more used to protect the surgeon. It is believed that approximately 36 bacteria are released per 100 spoken words. Masks are usually only effective for short periods as the increasing moisture reduces the filtering quality. Evidence now suggests that there is no increase in surgical site infections after operations carried out by surgeons without masks, except in the presence of a respiratory tract infection due to increased bacterial numbers in the oropharynx. Masks are also part of the universal precautions to prevent the possible spread of blood-borne viruses. A Cochrane review (Lipp *et al*, 2002) set out to determine whether disposable surgical face masks worn by the team during clean surgery prevents postoperative surgical wound infection. A total of four trials were included involving 2,113 participants. No statistically significant difference in infection rates between the masked and unmasked groups was found in any of the trials.

Gowns

Wearing theatre scrubs decreases possible bacterial contamination and decreases the number of desquamated skin flakes. The ability of the gown to be impermeable to moisture is paramount as this decreases the transmission of bacteria from the skin surface. For short durations (less than two hours) and minimal blood loss (less than 100ml) a 1 ply gown is recommended. However with longer durations of two to four hours or with 100–500ml of blood loss or procedures involving the chest or abdominal cavity a 2 ply reinforced gown is recommended. Gowns are considered to be sterile from the shoulders to the level of the sterile field and from just below the elbows.

Procedure: gowning and gloving

- Grasp the pre-folded sterile gown by the neckline with both hands and step back from the table into an unobstructed area.
- Holding the folded gown with the inside towards you, locate the neckline of the gown and holding the gown with both hands allow the gown to unfold in front of you. Do not touch the outside of the gown.
- Holding the unfolded gown at shoulder level, push both hands and arms into the sleeves simultaneously keeping your hands inside the cuffs.
- Using the cuff of the gown as a mitten, open the inside wrappers of the glove packaging and with the left hand lift the right glove from the wrapper by the cuff.
- Extend the right forearm with the palm upwards. Place the palm of the glove against the palm of the protected hand, thumb to thumb with the fingers pointing towards the elbow.
- Hold securely the cuff of the glove, and with the other protected hand, stretch the glove cuff over the end of the right sleeve and hand. The cuff of the glove is now over the stockinette cuff of the gown with the hand still inside the sleeve.
- Pull the glove over the extended fingers until it completely covers the stockinette cuff.
- Using the gloved hand, pick up the other glove from the package and repeat the above steps.

Surgical Site Infections (SSI)

Surgical site infections refer to infections that develop in wounds created by an invasive surgical procedure. Surgical site infections make up 14% of healthcare associated infections in UK hospitals. Significant morbidity is associated with SSIs with over a third of postoperative deaths associated in part with them. They are responsible for increased hospital stay and significant additional healthcare costs.

The Centres for Disease Control and Prevention recognise three levels of SSI.

- Superficial incisional: Affecting skin and subcutaneous tissue. These can be recognised by local signs such as swelling, redness, pain or the drainage of pus.
- Deep incisional: Affecting the fascial and muscle layers. These can be recognised by the presence of pus or an abscess, fever, tenderness over the wound or separation of the wound edges exposing the deeper tissues.
- Organ or space infection: Involves any part of the anatomy other than the incision that is opened or manipulated e.g. joint or peritoneum. These infections may be indicated by the drainage of pus or the formation of an abscess detected by histopathological or radiological examination or during re-operation.

Risk factors for SSIs include older age, smoking, obesity, alcoholism, diabetes mellitus, poor nutritional state, immunosuppressive medication and underlying illness (eg anaemia, jaundice, renal disease). These contribute to the risk of SSIs in three ways: by increasing the risk of endogenous contamination; increasing the risk of exogenous contamination; or reducing the efficacy of the general immune response.

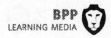

Preoperative phase	
Preoperative showering	Advise patients to shower / bathe either the day before or on the day of surgery.
Hair removal	Hair should not be routinely removed to reduce risk of infection. If necessary electric clippers with single use heads should be used on the day of surgery.
Patient clothing	Patients should be given appropriate specific theatre wear. Ensure patient's comfort and dignity. All jewellery and artificial nails should be removed preoperatively.
Staff clothing	Staff should wear specific theatre clothing in appropriate areas.
Bowel contamination	Mechanical bowel preparation should not be routinely used to decrease the risk of surgical site infection.
Antibiotic prophylaxis (Use local antibiotic policies)	Antibiotic prophylaxis should be given for: • clean surgery involving prosthesis/implant • clean-contaminated surgery • contaminated surgery Antibiotic treatment should be administered for dirty / infected wounds
Intraoperative phase	
Hand decontamination	Prior to the first surgery the team should use an aqueous antiseptic surgical solution with single use brush. Washing before further surgeries should be using either an alcohol based hand rub or antiseptic solution.
Gowns / Gloves	Sterile gowns should be worn during the operation. In cases of high risk for perforation of glove or contamination, wearing two pairs is advisable.
Antiseptic skin preparation	Immediately prior to commencing surgery prepare the site with an antiseptic solution-povidone-iodine or chlorhexidine. Ensure the area has dried by evaporation before using diathermy. Ideally diathermy should not be used for the incision.
Maintaining patient homeostasis	Patient temperature and oxygenation should be monitored throughout the surgery. An oxygen saturation of > 95% should be maintained. In non-diabetic patients insulin should not be routinely used to control glucose levels.
Antiseptic / antimicrobial cleaning of wound	Re-disinfection of the wound or administration of topical antimicrobial agents should not be performed to reduce the risk of surgical site infection.
Postoperative phase	
Dressing change / postoperative cleaning	All dressings should be changed using an aseptic non-touch technique. For the first 48 hours following surgery saline should be used for cleaning. Patients should be advised they may shower safely 48 hours after surgery. Topical antimicrobial agents should not be used for wounds healing by primary intention.
Wounds healing by secondary intention	Appropriate interactive dressings should be used under guidance of the local tissue viability team. Eusol and gauze or other moist gauze dressings should not be used.
Antibiotics for surgical site infection	In cases of surgical site infection antibiotics covering all most likely organisms should be administered in accordance with local policies. Input from the local microbiology department should be sought.

Table 8.12. Recommendations for reducing SSI (Adapted from NICE, 2008)

Basic suturing skills

Basic suturing is an essential psychomotor skill used in everyday surgical practice. Together with adopting a good technique, it is important to develop a thorough understanding of all aspects of wound management. Wounds encountered must be assessed independently. Factors such as location, size of wound, time since injury, contamination, tissue loss and patient factors (age, nutritional status and comorbidities) must be addressed. Wound locations such as face, hands and perineum can be more complex for cosmetic reasons. Other common locations such as scalp and trunk are often simpler. Lacerations and wounds suffered from blunt force trauma may often require debridement and revision of the wound edges before closure can be contemplated. A thorough irrigation of the wound before closure is paramount to minimise the risk of infection. Heavily contaminated wounds or those inflicted more than eight hours prior to treatment should be considered for being left open to heal by secondary intention.

Wound healing

The following phases are noted during the process of wound healing.

1. Haemostasis

The first stage of healing is to establish haemostasis as vessels may have been severed by the trauma. Blood vessel injury leads initially to contraction of the arterioles. Platelets and plasma proteins adhere to the site releasing cytokines. Both the intrinsic and extrinsic clotting pathways are activated. The platelet plug becomes converted into a clot consisting of fibrin and stabilised by fibronectin.

2. Inflammation

This next phase commences within the first six to eight hours. This involves dilation of the capillaries and the formation of an exudate. Polymorphonuclear leucocytes engorge the wound, removing bacteria and scavenging any tissue debris. Macrophages exude from the blood vessels aiding the cleansing process. The macrophages also initiate the multiplication of endothelial cells, duplication of smooth muscle cells and angiogenesis by secreting growth factors.

3. Granulation

Within five to seven days fibroblasts migrate to the wound laying down collagen (initially type III, then replaced by type I). Fibroblasts produce glycosaminoglycans and fibronectin which contribute to matrix deposition. The growth factors stimulate and modulate angiogenesis. Within 24 hours cells begin to migrate from the periphery and adnexal structures. Their division over the next two to three days leads to the formation of a thin layer of epithelial cells bridging the wound.

4. Remodelling

After the third week the wound begins constant remodelling which may continue for years. Collagen is constantly degraded and deposited within the wound. Myofibroblasts cause contraction of the wound, seen more in healing by secondary intention (see below). The maximum tensile strength of the wound is achieved by the 12th week and the resultant scar has only 80% of the strength of the initial skin in that location.

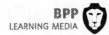

Primary, secondary and tertiary intention

Three types of wound repair are described according to the type and timing of surgical intervention:

- Primary intention (most surgical wounds, well repaired lacerations): The wound edges are brought together by adhesive strips, sutures or staples. The wound edges are easily apposed; there is little tissue loss and minimal scarring.
- Secondary intention: The wound is left open due to tissue loss, infection or excessive trauma. The wound edges come together by granulation and contraction, resulting in a broader scar. The healing process can be slow due to the presence of infection. Regular wound care is essential.
- Tertiary intention (delayed primary closure): The wound is initially cleaned, debrided and left open for four to five days. This method allows for a decreased infection rate after surgical closure a few days later. It provides superior cosmetic appearance to the closure of a contaminated wound.

Factors affecting wound healing

- Nutrition: Malnutrition leads to a depressed immune system, increasing the risk of wound infection and therefore delayed healing.
- Steroid treatment: Glucocorticoids inhibit the healing process by acting on fibroblasts and altering the collagen deposition.
- Foreign bodies / infection: They prolong the inflammatory response.
- Excess mobility: Impairs healing and time to full recovery.
- Vascular supply: Perhaps one of the most important factors affecting healing. This includes both arterial supply and venous drainage.

Suture materials

Certain procedures place specific requirements upon suture material. The time requirement for wound support varies in different tissues from days to weeks, months and long term for certain prostheses.

• Sterile, pulls through tissue easily • Does not promote tissue response on absorption • Easy to handle • Non-allergenic	• Does not stimulate bacterial growth • Predictable tensile strength • Inexpensive • Should not shrink in the tissues

Table 8.13. Properties of an ideal suture material

An absorbable suture loses most of its strength within 60 days. These can be either monofilament or multifilament. The process of absorption occurs by enzymatic proteolysis and hydrolysis. Synthetic sutures are preferred because hydrolysis is a more stable mechanism than proteolysis allowing a more stable absorption. Monofilament sutures are smooth and pass easily through tissues. Knotting must be performed carefully together with delicate handling of the suture by instruments to prevent fracturing. Multifilament sutures have a much larger surface area than monofilament material, making them easier to handle and knot. They can however drag on passing through tissue, stimulating a reaction.

Suture	Type	Tensile strength retention	Mass absorption rate	Contraindications	Frequent use
Glycolide and lactide	Absorbable, braided, coated	28 days	56–70 days	As absorbable should not be used where prolonged approximation of tissues under stress required	Ophthalmology
Glycolide and lactide (rapid absorption)	Absorbable, braided and coated	10–14 days	42 days	Should not be used in tissues that heal slowly	Closure of skin and mucosa
Polydioxanone	Absorbable, monofilament	56 days	180 days	As absorbable should not be used where prolonged approximation of tissues under stress required	Abdominal and thoracic closure, colorectal surgery
Polyglactin 910	Absorbable, braided and coated	50% at 21 days	60–90 days	As absorbable should not be used where prolonged approximation of tissues under stress required	General surgery, suturing and ligation
Polyglecaprone	Absorbable, monofilament	21 days	90–120 days	Not for use in neural tissue, cardiovascular, microsurgery	Subcuticular skin suturing
Silk	Non absorbable, braided	Loses most or all in 1 year	Cannot be found after about 2 years	Not for use for placement of vascular prostheses or heart valves	General surgery, suturing and ligation
Braided polyamide	Non absorbable, braided	Loses 15–20% per year	Degrades at 15–20% per year	None	Ligating and suturing – general closure
Monofilament polyamide	Non absorbable, monofilament	Loses 15–20% per year	Degrades at 15–20% per year	None	Skin closure
Polypropylene	Nonabsorbable monofilament	Indefinite	Non absorbable	None	General, plastic, skin closure

Table 8.14. Suture materials

Suturing a simple skin laceration

Equipment

- Dressing pack
- Small needle
- 10ml syringe
- Local anaesthetic
- Gauze
- Cleaning solution
- Dressing

- Sterile gloves
- Sutures
- Needle holder
- Forceps (toothed)
- Suture scissors
- Sharps bin

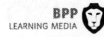

Procedure

- Wash hands, introduce yourself, confirm patient's ID, explain procedure and obtain consent.
- Assess the wound to decide on suture material and check history regarding trauma.
- Check and inject local anaesthetic.
- Clean hands again, don a pair of gloves, clean and drape the wound appropriately.
- Make sure the wound is clean (if not irrigate) and all foreign bodies removed.
- Use needle holder and toothed forceps and hold the needle two-thirds of the way from the tip.
- Lift the skin edge carefully without damaging it and pierce skin at 90°.
- Rotate wrist to bring needle into middle of wound.
- Grasp needle with instrument rotating it out of the wound.
- Evert other skin edge and pass needle through at 90°.
- Perform a knot (hand tie or instrument tie).
- Leave a few millimetres of the end to allow easy removal of suture.
- Once completed, dispose of sharps safely and wash hands.
- Administer antibiotics and / or tetanus prophylaxis if necessary.
- Give instructions to patient regarding signs of infection (increased pain, swelling, redness, fever).
- Give instructions to patient regarding suture removal: four to five days then replace with strips for face wounds, seven to ten days for scalp and trunk, 10 to 14 days for limbs and 14 days for joints.
- Document the procedure in the patient's notes.

Types of tissue repair with sutures

- Interrupted sutures: The needle should be inserted and exited at right angles to the tissue. Avoid dragging the needle through tissue, follow the curve. The distance from the entry point to the edge of the wound should be similar to the thickness of the tissue sutured. The distance between each suture should be double the thickness of the tissue.
- Continuous sutures: Insertion similar to above, after tying first suture; the remaining sutures are placed in a continuous manner until the far end of the wound where the knot is tied. It is useful to have an assistant present to follow the suture maintaining tension.
- Mattress sutures: These may be vertical or horizontal and are useful for ensuring eversion or inversion of the wound edges. The initial suture is placed as above following which the

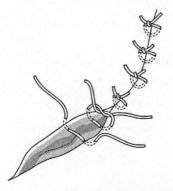

**Figure 8.10. Interrupted suture
(Reproduced with permission from
Olek Remesz/cc-BY-2.5)**

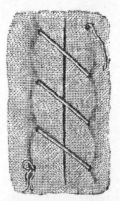

**Figure 8.11. Continuous suture
Based on Dechambre A (1884) Dictionnaire
Encyclopédique des Sciences Médicales. 13th edition,
Masson, Paris.** *(The image is in the public domain
because its copyright has expired.
This applies worldwide)*

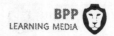

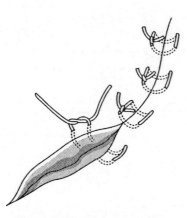

Figure 8.12. Mattress suture

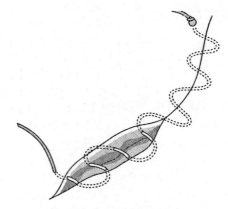

Figure 8.13. Subcuticular sutures

needle is reversed and taken back either vertically or horizontally to the previous traverse. This allows good apposition of the edges.

- Subcuticular sutures: This technique results in a neat scar if the wound edges can be approximated without tension. The suture material used can be either absorbable or non-absorbable. The suture is initially fixed at one end of the wound with a buried knot. This is then followed by small bites of subcuticular tissues on alternate sides of the wound into the intradermal layer. Cross the gap in the wound at right angles to avoid distorting the skin.

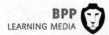

Tissue biopsy

In this section the techniques of excision biopsy, core biopsy and fine needle aspiration cytology are described with step-by-step instructions and relevant clinical tips.

Excision of skin lesion / excision biopsy

Procedure

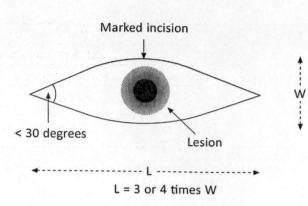

Figure 8.14 Excision of skin lesion

- Wash hands, introduce yourself, confirm patient's details, explain procedure and obtain consent.
- Assess the wound to decide on suture material.
- Check local anaesthetic (type, strength, expiry date).
- Choose combination with adrenaline to minimise oozing, except from organs with terminal perfusion (ie digits, penis).
- Inject local anaesthetic, wash hands again and don a pair of gloves.
- Clean and drape the wound appropriately.
- Plan an elliptical incision, lying along the tension lines (Langer's lines).
- If the lesion is benign, leave a 1mm margin. In malignant cases a larger lateral and deep margin is required; warn patient that re-excision to larger margins may be required.
- Estimate the planned width of the ellipse; the length (L) should be three times the width (W).
- A skin marker can be used to mark the incision.
- Keep the scalpel perpendicular to the skin while making the incision.
- Excise ellipse of skin and part of subcutaneous tissue.
- Close the wound after undermining the skin on each side,if necessary, to minimise tension.
- Close the wound with interrupted or subcuticular sutures.
- Dispose of sharps safely and wash hands.
- Place lesion in an appropriately labelled container, usually in formalin solution, unless fresh biopsy is planned when no formaline should be used.
- Give instructions to patient regarding signs of infection.
- Document the procedure in the patient's notes.

Fine needle aspiration cytology (FNAC) and biopsy

Biopsy is defined as the removal of a sample of tissue for laboratory examination in order to establish the presence or extent of a particular disease. The common biopsy techniques practised today include open, core, endoscopic and fine needle aspiration cytology (FNAC). Developments in imaging techniques have led to an expansion in the anatomical sites amenable to FNAC. One of the most successful applications to date remains in the diagnosis of breast cancer.

FNAC aims to collect an adequate representative sample of a particular lesion in order to make a cytological diagnosis (based on appearances of cells and cell groups) as opposed to a histological diagnosis (that is based on appearances of cells within a tissue). FNAC is an inexpensive technique requiring less laboratory time and fewer reagents. It can be used in a variety of settings by radiologists (image guided), physicians or surgeons and is relatively painless. It is important to be aware of the limitations of such a cytological diagnostic technique; FNAC cannot distinguish between invasive and in situ carcinoma of the breast, and follicular adenoma and carcinoma of the thyroid gland.

Feature	FNAC	Tissue core biopsy
Results available	Usually same day	Commonly following day
Anaesthesia	Not required	Needed occasionally
Complications	Minor	Can be serious
Inadequate specimens	Common	Rare
Cost	Low	Higher
Cellular sampling	Smaller numbers of cells	Large numbers of cells
Tissue architecture	Not preserved	Preserved in sample

Table 8.15. Comparison between FNAC and core biopsy

Procedure for FNAC

- Equipment needed: 20ml syringe, 21 G (green) needle, two glass slides.
- Wash hands, confirm patient's identity, explain the procedure and obtain verbal consent.
- Set up equipment and don a pair of gloves.
- Clean skin area with alcohol swab.
- Hold the lesion between thumb and index finger with non-dominant hand.
- Insert needle to skin and once the lesion is reached apply 6–10ml of suction, advancing the tip of needle into lesion. If thyroid nodule is sampled do not apply suction.
- Pass needle through lesion several times at various planes.
- Release suction and withdraw needle when either blood or fluid in the needle hub.
- Material is drawn into needle by capillary action.
- Can use needle without syringe in highly vascular sites (thyroid gland).
- On removing the needle put firm pressure on the area to control any bleeding.
- Gently express material onto a glass slide using the residual 5ml of dead space in the syringe.
- Usually prepared by direct smears; material is expressed onto slide and spread out to form a single layer either by using the needle or sandwiching between two slides.
- Slides can be air dried or fixed with alcohol.
- Remove gloves, wash hands and document procedure in patient's notes.
- Causes of non-diagnostic samples include needle missing lesion, no lesion present, inexperienced operator, aspiration of cystic / necrotic lesion, and low yield of cells.
- Complications include bleeding, damage to neighbouring structures, pneumothorax (breast FNAC), and seeding of tumour (extremely rare).

Image-guided FNA

Deep seated lesions are often sampled by radiologists via various imaging techniques. Ultrasound is the simplest method allowing real time guidance of the needle in any plane. CT scanning allows sampling of lesions almost anywhere in the body. Common sites include the lungs, liver and retroperitoneum. Lung lesions are also amenable to sampling via fluoroscopy which allows real time guidance in two planes. A relatively newer method, the endoscopic ultrasound, allows diagnosis and staging of pancreatic, gastric and oesophageal lesions.

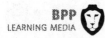

Specific sites for FNAC

- Breast: FNAC together with core biopsy have become central to the diagnosis of breast cancer. Lesions can be sampled via stereotactic FNAC with the use of mammograms. FNAC of the breast is reported on a scale of C1 to C5 (see Chapter 7 – *Breast examination*). In cases of insufficient information, a tissue core biopsy can be performed, which can distinguish between in situ and invasive carcinoma.
- Thyroid: This is one of the first line investigations for thyroid nodules. The procedure can be performed in the outpatient setting using a small needle. Care should be taken to minimise suction in vascular organs. FNAC is unable to distinguish between follicular adenoma and follicular carcinoma.
- Lymph nodes: FNAC may be used to differentiate between reactive lymphadenopathy and specific conditions. Where FNAC does not reveal a diagnosis, excision biopsy can be performed. FNAC can be used in the diagnosis of lymphoma followed by biopsy for staging purposes.

Core biopsy

This involves obtaining a core of tissue to confirm a diagnosis or undertake further analysis. It is useful to discuss the sample with a pathologist beforehand to confirm how it should be preserved. In cases of impalpable lesions radiological imaging may be required. The most commonly used method is the Trucut needle. This needle contains a trough for collecting the sample.

Procedure

- Wash hands, confirm patient's identity, explain the procedure and obtain verbal consent.
- Set up equipment, don a pair of gloves and clean skin area with alcohol swab.
- Inject a small amount of local anaesthetic over the subcutaneous lesion raising a bleb.
- Make a small cut (2mm) in the overlying skin with a fine scalpel to allow smooth passage of the needle.
- Steady the lesion between the fingers of one hand.
- Pass the closed needle through the incision into the lesion.
- Push the central needle into the lesion.
- Holding the central needle still, advance the outer sheath which cuts and encloses the tissue in the trough.
- Remove the whole closed needle system and inspect the sample.
- Maintain pressure on biopsy site for at least five minutes and watch out for bleeding.
- Insert sample in appropriately labelled container.
- Remove gloves, wash hands and document the procedure in the patient's notes.

Open biopsy

- Incision biopsy: This refers to removal of a section of a large structure. The aim is to provide enough sample for analysis but not excise the diseased tissue. It is useful to try to include junctional tissue between pathological and normal tissue. The sample can either be taken as a wedge from the edge of the lesion, closed with sutures, or as an ellipse in the centre.
- Excision biopsy: This refers to the complete removal of a lesion with a margin of normal tissue around the lesion, particularly if malignancy is suspected. A good example is in the diagnosis of small melanomas.

Further reading

- Al-Khafaji, AH and Webb, AR. Fluid resuscitation. *BJA, Contin Educ Anaesth Crit Care Pain* 2004; 4: 127–131.
- Department of Health (2011) *Reducing healthcare associated infections.* Available at: www.clean-safe-care.nhs.uk.
- Harrison, SC, Lawrence, WT, Morley, R, Pearce, I, Taylor, J. British Association of Urological Surgeons' suprapubic catheter practice guidelines. *BJU Int* 2011, 107(1): 77–85.
- *Intercollegiate Basic Surgical Skills Participant Handbook.* Edited by Roy McCloy 4th Revised edition. The Royal College of Surgeons of England. September 2010.
- Lipp, A, Edwards, P. Disposable surgical face masks for preventing surgical wound infection in clean surgery. *Cochrane Database Syst Rev* 2002; (1): CD002929.
- Mitchard, JR, Romaine, KE, Shepherd, NA. Principles and techniques of biopsy with special reference to fine needle aspiration cytology. *Surgery (Medicine Publishing)* (28): (2): 38–42.
- Needle biopsy (2011). Available at: www.youtube.com/watch?v=Kl-NoRjoeMI
- NICE (2002) *TA49 Central Venous Catheters – Ultrasound locating devices.* Available at: www.nice.org.uk/nicemedia/live/11474/32461/32461.pdf.
- NICE (2008) *CG74 Surgical site of infection.* Available at: www.nice.org.uk/CG74fullguideline.
- Perel, P, Roberts, I. Colloids vs crystalloids for fluid resuscitation in critically ill patients. *Cochrane Database Syst Rev* 2011; (3): CD000567.
- Recommendations for safe practice in the insertion of supra public catheters (SPLs) have recently been published by the British Association of Urological surgeons (Harrison *et. al.* 2011).
- Stroud, M, Duncan, H, Nightingale, J. BSG Guidelines for enteral feeding in adult hospital patients. *Gut* 2003; 52 (Suppl VII): vii1–vii12.
- Tanner, J, Swarbrook, S, Stuart, J. Surgical hand antisepsis to reduce surgical site infection. *Cochrane Database Syst Rev* 2008; (1): CD004288.

References

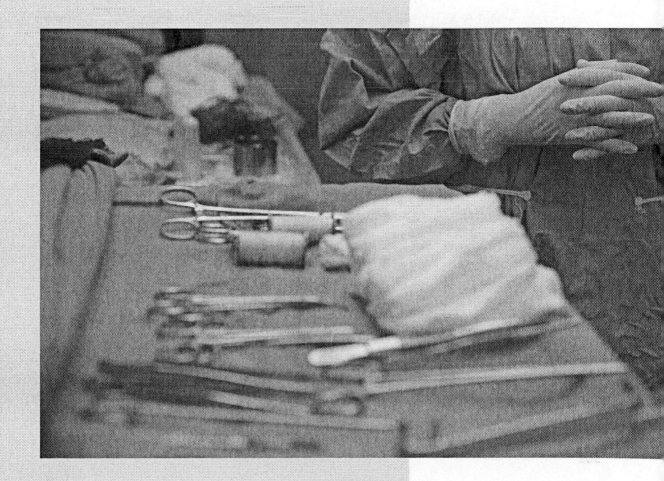

References

Anderson, I. (2003) Care of the Critically Ill Surgical Patient. 2nd edition. London: Hodder Arnold Publication.

Ayub, K, Imada, R, Slavin, J. Endoscopic retrograde cholangiopancreatography in gallstone-associated acute pancreatitis. Cochrane Database Syst Rev 2004 18; (4): CD003630.

Bodger, K, Trudgill, N. (2006) Guidelines for oesophageal manometry and pH monitoring (British Society of Gastroenterology). [Online] Available at: www.gastroscan.ru/literature/pdf/bodger01.pdf [Accessed 14 February 2013].

British Association of Day Surgery (2004) Day Case Laparoscopic Cholecystectomy. [Online] Available at: http://www.daysurgery.net/bads/joomla/files/Handbooks/LaparoscopicCholecystectomy.pdf [Accessed 14 February 2013].

British Medical Association, Board of Medical Education (2004). Communication Skills Education for Doctors: An Update, November 2004. London: British Medical Association.

Couinaud, C (1957) Le foie: études anatomiques et chirurgicales. Paris: Masson.

Dechambre, A (1884) Dictionnaire Encyclopédique des Sciences Médicales. 13th edition. Paris: Masson.

Dormandy, J ed (1989) European consensus document on critical limb ischaemia. Berlin: Springer Verlag.

Ederle J, Featherstone R and Brown MM. Percutaneous transluminal angioplasty and stenting for carotid artery stenosis. Cochrane Database of Systematic Reviews 2007, Issue 4. Art. No.: CD000515. DOI: 10.1002/14651858.CD000515.pub3.

Ewing, JA. Detecting alcoholism. The Cage questionnaire. JAMA/1984 12; 252 (14) 1905–7.

Garden, RS, Stability and union in subcapital fractures of the femur J Bone Joint Surg Br; 1961; 46: 630–647.

Gurusamy, KS, Samraj, K, Fusai, G and Davidson, BR. Early versus delayed laparoscopic cholecystectomy for biliary colic. Cochrane Database Syst Rev 2008; (4): CD007196.

Harrison, SC, Lawrence, WT, Morley, R, Pearce, I, Taylor, J. British Association of Urological Surgeons' suprapubic catheter practice guidelines. BJU Int 2011, 107(1): 77–85.

International Carotid Stenting Study investigators. Carotid artery stenting compared with endarterectomy in patients with symptomatic carotid stenosis (International Carotid Stenting Study): an interim analysis of a randomised controlled trial. The Lancet 2010; 375 (9719): 985-997.

Lau, H, Lo, CY, Patil, NG, Yuen, WK. Early versus delayed-interval laparoscopic cholecystectomy for acute cholecystitis: a meta-analysis. Surg Endosc 2006; 20(1): 82-7.

Lipp, A, Edwards, P. Disposable surgical face masks for preventing surgical wound infection in clean surgery. Cochrane Database Syst Rev 2002; (1): CD002929.

Martin, DJ, Vernon, DR, Toouli, J. Surgical versus endoscopic treatment of bile duct stones. Cochrane Database Syst Rev 2006; (2): CD003327.

MRC Asymptomatic Carotid Surgery Trial (ASCT) Collaborative Group. Prevention of disabling and fatal strokes by successful carotid endarterectomy in patients without recent neurological symptoms: randomised controlled trial. The Lancet 2004; 363 (9420): 1491-1502.

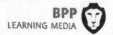

NCEPOD (2005) An Acute problem? [Online] Available at: www.ncepod.org.uk/2005report/introduction.html [Accessed on 15 March 2013].

NHS (2000) High Quality Care For All: NHS Next Stage Review Final Report. [Online] Available at: http://www.dh.gov.uk/prod_consum_dh/groups/dh_digitalassets/@dh/@en/documents/digitalasset/dh_085828.pdf [Accessed on 15 March 2013].

NHS (2000) The NHS Plan: A plan for investment, a plan for reform. [Online] Available at: http://www.dh.gov.uk/prod_consum_dh/groups/dh_digitalassets/@dh/@en/@ps/documents/digitalasset/dh_118522.pdf [Accessed on 15 March 2013].

NICE (2002) TA49 Central Venous Catheters – Ultrasound locating devices. [Online] Available at: www.nice.org.uk/nicemedia/live/11474/32461/32461.pdf [Accessed 14 February 2013].

NICE (2004) TA83 Hernia-laparoscopic surgery (review) guidance. [Online] Available at http://publications.nice.org.uk/laparoscopic-surgery-for-inguinal-hernia-repair-ta83. [Accessed 15 March 2013].

NICE (2005, updated 2011) CG27 Referral guidelines for suspected cancer.[Online] Available at: www.nice.org.uk/nicemedia/live/10968/29814/29814.pdf [Accessed 14 February 2013].

NICE (2008) CG65 Perioperative hypothemia (inadvertent): full guideline. [Online] Available at: guidance.nice.org.uk/CG65/Guidance/pdf/English [Accessed 14 February 2013].

NICE (2008) CG74 Surgical site of infection. [Online] Available at: www.nice.org.uk/nicemedia/line/11743/42379/42379.pdf [Accessed 14 February 2013].

NICE (2009) Early and locally advanced breast cancer: Diagnosis and treatment. [Online] Available at: http://www.nice.org.uk/nicemedia/pdf/CG80NICEGuideline.pdf [Accessed 15 March 2013].

NICE (2010) CG92 (Venous thromboembolism reducing the risk. [Online] Available at: www.nice.org.uk/nicemedia/live/12695/47195.pdf [Accessed 14 February 2013].

NICE (2011) CG88 Low back pain. [Online] Available at: www.nice.org.uk/cg88fullguidelines [Accessed 14 February 2013].

Nienhuijs, S, de Hingh, I. Conventional versus LigaSure hemorrhoidectomy for patients with symptomatic Hemorrhoids. Cochrane Database Syst Rev 2009; 2009; Jan 21; (1): CD006761.

Perel, P, Roberts, I. Colloids vs crystalloids for fluid resuscitation in critically ill patients. Cochrane Database Syst Rev 2011; (3): CD000567.

Purkayastha S et al. Laparoscopic v open surgery for diverticular disease: a meta-analysis of nonrandomized studies. Dis Colon Rectum 2006; 49(4): 446–63.

Rothwell, PM et al. Analysis of pooled data from the randomised controlled trials of endarterectomy for symptomatic carotid stenosis. The Lancet 2003; 361 (9352): 107-116.

Sanabria, AE, Morales, CH, Villegas, MI. Laparoscopic repair for perforated peptic ulcer disease. Cochrane Database Syst Rev 2005; (4): CD004778.

Scott ish Intercollegiate Guidelines Network (2008) Management of Acute Upper and Lower Gastrointestinal Bleeding. A National Clinical Guideline. [Online] Available at: www.sign.ac.uk/pdf/sign105.pdf [Accessed 14 February 2013].

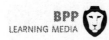

References

Tanner, J, Swarbrook, S, Stuart, J. Surgical hand antisepsis to reduce surgical site infection. Cochrane Database Syst Rev 2008; (1): CD004288.

Thomas, PD, Forbes, A, Green, J, Howdle, P, Long, R, Playford, R, Sheridan, M, Stevens, R, Valori, R, Walters, J, Addison, GM, Hill, P, Brydon, G (2003) Guidelines for the investigation of chronic diarrhoea. 2nd edition. Gut 2003; 52: v1–v15

Toorenvliet, BR, Swank, H, Schoones, JW, Hamming, JF, Bemelman, WA. Laparoscopic peritoneal lavage for perforated colonic diverticulitis: a systematic review. Colorectal Dis 2010; 12(9): 862–7.

UK Working Party on Acute Pancreatitis. UK guidelines for the management of acute pancreatitis. Gut 2005; 54: 1 – 9.

Walker MD et al. Endarterectomy for asymptomatic carotid artery stenosis. JAMA. 1995; 273 (10): 1421-1428.

Watson A et al (2005) Guidelines for the Diagnosis and Management of Barrett 's Columnarlined oesophagus. [Online] British Society of Gastroenterology. [Online] Available at: www.bsg. org.uk/images/stories/docs/clinical/guidelines/oesophageal/Barretts _Oes.pdf [Accessed 14 February 2013].

Wilson, JMG and Jungner, G (1968) Principles and Practice of Screening for Disease. Geneva: World Health Organisation.

Index

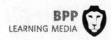

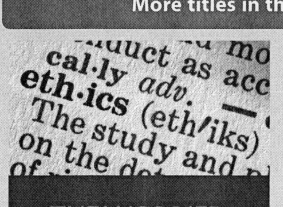
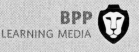

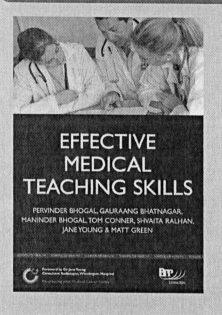
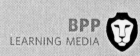

More titles in the Progressing your Medical Career Series

EFFECTIVE
COMMUNICATION
SKILLS FOR
DOCTORS

TERESA PARROTT & GRAHAM CROOK

£19.99
September 2011
Paperback
978-1-445379-56-2

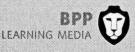
BPP
LEARNING MEDIA

Would you like to know how to improve your communication skills? Are you looking for a clearly written book which explores all aspects of effective medical communication?

There is an urgent need to improve doctors' communication skills. Research has shown that poor communication can contribute to patient dissatisfaction, lack of compliance and increased medico-legal problems. Improved communication skills will impact positively on all of these areas.

The last fifteen years have seen unprecedented changes in medicine and the role of doctors. Effective communication skills are vital to these new roles. But communication is not just related to personality. Skills can be learned which can make your communication more effective, and help you to improve your relationships with patients, their families and fellow doctors.

This book shows how to learn those skills and outlines why we all need to communicate more effectively. Healthcare is increasingly a partnership. Change is happening at all levels, from government directives to patient expectations. Communication is a bridge between the wisdom of the past and the vision of the future.

Readers of this book can also gain free access to an online module which upon successful completion can download a certificate for their portfolio of learning/Revalidation/CPD records.

This easy-to-read guide will help medical students and doctors at all stages of their careers improve their communication within a hospital environment.

More titles in the Progressing your Medical Career Series

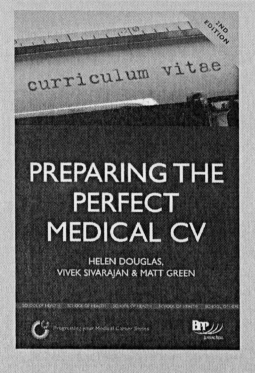

PREPARING THE PERFECT MEDICAL CV

HELEN DOUGLAS,
VIVEK SIVARAJAN & MATT GREEN

£19.99
October 2011
Paperback
978-1-445381-62-6

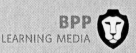
Are you unsure of how to structure your Medical CV? Would you like to know how to ensure you stand out from the crowd?

With competition for medical posts at an all time high it is vital that your Medical CV stands out over your fellow applicants. This comprehensive, unique and easy-to-read guide has been written with this in mind to help prospective medical students, current medical students and doctors of all grades prepare a Medical CV of the highest quality. Whether you are applying to medical school, currently completing your medical degree or a doctor progressing through your career (foundation doctor, specialty trainee in general practice, surgery or medicine, GP career grade or Consultant) this guide includes specific guidance for applicants at every level.

This time-saving and detailed guide:

- Explains what selection panels are looking for when reviewing applications at all levels.

- Discusses how to structure your Medical CV to ensure you stand out for the right reasons.

- Explores what information to include (and not to include) in your CV.

- Covers what to consider when maintaining a portfolio at every step of your career, including, for revalidation and relicensing purposes.

- Provides examples of high quality CVs to illustrate the above.

This unique guide will show you how to prepare your CV for every step of your medical career from pre-Medical School right through to Consultant level and should be a constant companion to ensure you secure your first choice post every time.